Paramedic Research

Principles, Designs and Methods

Julia Williams

and

Graham McClelland

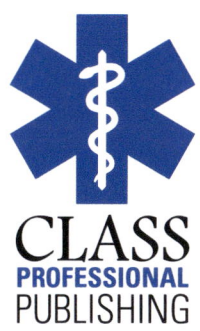

Class Professional Publishing have made every effort to ensure that the information, tables, drawings and diagrams contained in this book are accurate at the time of publication. The book cannot always contain all the information necessary for determining appropriate care and cannot address all individual situations; therefore, individuals using the book must ensure they have the appropriate knowledge and skills to enable suitable interpretation. Class Professional Publishing do not guarantee, and accept no legal liability of whatever nature arising from, or connected to, the accuracy, reliability, currency or completeness of the content of *Paramedic Research: Principles, Designs and Methods*. Users must always be aware that such innovations or alterations after the date of publication may not be incorporated in the content. Please note, however, that Class Professional Publishing assume no responsibility whatsoever for the content of external resources in the text or accompanying online materials.

Text © Julia Williams and Graham McClelland 2025

All rights reserved. Without limiting the rights under copyright reserved above, no part of this publication may be reproduced, stored in or introduced into a retrieval system, or transmitted, in any form or by any means (electronic, mechanical, photocopying, recording or otherwise) without the prior written permission of the publisher of this book.

The information presented in this book is accurate and current to the best of the authors' knowledge.

The authors and publisher, however, make no guarantee as to, and assume no responsibility for, the correctness, sufficiency or completeness of such information or recommendation.

Printing history
This first edition printed in 2025.

The authors and publisher welcome feedback from the users of this book.

Please contact the publisher:
Class Professional Publishing,
The Exchange, Express Park, Bristol Road, Bridgwater TA6 4RR
Telephone: 01278 472 800
Email: info@class.co.uk
Website: www.classprofessional.co.uk

Class Professional Publishing is an imprint of Class Publishing Ltd
A CIP catalogue record for this book is available from the British Library

Paperback ISBN: 9781801611350
ePDF: 9781801611374
ePUB: 9781801611367
Cover design by Nicky Borowiec
Designed and typeset by PHi Business Solutions Ltd
Printed in the UK by Hobbs

This book is printed on paper from responsible sources. Refer to local recycling guidance on disposal of this book.

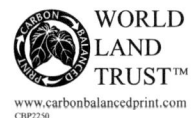

Product safety information can be found at https://www.classprofessional.co.uk/terms-of-use/gpsr-statement/

This book is dedicated to the memory of Professor Malcolm Woollard, a true pioneer and leading light in the field of paramedic research. His unwavering dedication to advancing the science and practice of paramedicine has left an indelible mark on the profession. Professor Woollard's pioneering spirit, pursuit of excellence and profound commitment to research serve as an enduring inspiration to us all. May his legacy continue to guide and inspire future generations of paramedic researchers.

Contents

Foreword	vii
Preface	ix
About the authors	xi
List of tables	xvii
List of figures	xix
List of boxes	xxi

SECTION 1

1 Introduction: paramedic research: what is it all about? — 3
Julia Williams and Graham McClelland

2 Why do we need evidence-based practice? — 9
Jamie Scott and Karl Bloomer

3 Making sense of the research process — 19
Kristy Sanderson and Larissa Prothero

4 Clinical audit, quality improvement, service evaluation and innovation: what are they? — 29
Duncan Robertson and Mary Peters

5 Research paradigms — 41
Cheryl Cameron, Adam Greene and Alan M. Batt

6 The role of existing literature in research: searching, retrieving and evaluation — 55
William Broughton and Ian Maconochie

7 Developing research questions: avoiding the 'so what' factor — 69
Scott Devenish and Julia Williams

SECTION 2

8 Quantitative research design — 83
Helen Snooks and Christopher Stein

9 Data collection in observational studies — 101
Tim Edwards and Jack Barrett

Contents

10 Data collection in experimental studies   115
Ruth Fisher and Elicia Austin

11 Making sense of quantitative data   123
John Talbot, Hayley Stagg and Anthony Herbland

12 Qualitative research design   141
Georgina Murphy-Jones and Joel Symonds

13 Qualitative data collection   157
Mike Brady and Enrico Dippenaar

14 Making sense of qualitative data   173
Ursula Rolfe and Alison Porter

15 Mixed methods research design   189
Gregory A. Whitley and Scott Munro

SECTION 3

16 Ethics and governance in research   203
Georgette Eaton and Helen Pocock

17 Involving service users in research   213
Sarah Black and Karl Charlton

18 Health economics: its role in health research   221
Jamie Miles and Peter McMeekin

19 Sharing research findings   233
James Yates and Pete Gregory

20 Developing a successful research proposal   245
Janette Turner and Andy Newton

21 Obtaining research funding: hints and tips   255
Graham McClelland and Fiona Bell

22 Research careers for paramedics   265
Kim Kirby and Graham McClelland

23 Conclusion: next steps   273
Graham McClelland and Julia Williams

References   275
Index   295

Foreword

It is my pleasure to introduce *Paramedic Research: Principles, Designs and Methods*, a vital resource that sheds light on the critical nexus of research and practice in paramedicine. As someone deeply entrenched in the world of evidence-based care, I understand firsthand the profound impact that well-conducted research can have on shaping the future of paramedic practice and patient outcomes.

Although focusing on paramedicine, this book offers valuable insights and practical guidance which will be useful to a wide range of health and care professionals. In an age where evidence-based practice is paramount, this text provides readers with the tools they need to engage in meaningful research that drives innovation and improves care delivery.

From foundational research principles to ethical considerations and practical methodologies, each chapter contributes to advancing the science and practice of paramedicine through rigorous research.

I am confident that *Paramedic Research: Principles, Designs and Methods* will inspire and empower paramedics and other health professionals to embrace research as a powerful tool for improving patient care and driving positive change in their respective fields.

Professor Richard Lyon, PhD, MBE
Consultant in Emergency Medicine at the Royal Infirmary of Edinburgh
Director of Research and Innovation, Kent, Surrey and Sussex Air Ambulance
Professor of Prehospital Emergency Care at the University of Surrey

Preface

As the field of paramedicine continues to evolve, so too does the importance of evidence-based practice and research. In this exciting and timely textbook, we embark on a journey through the fundamental principles and practical applications of paramedic research.

Paramedic Research: Principles, Designs and Methods offers a comprehensive exploration of the paramedic research landscape, from its historical roots to its future trajectories. Through the collaborative efforts of esteemed authors, each chapter delves into key aspects of paramedic research, providing invaluable insights and practical guidance for both novice and seasoned researchers alike.

In Section 1, we set the stage with an examination of the evolution of paramedic research and the various methodologies that drive it forward. From understanding the importance of evidence in informing practice, to navigating the intricacies of research paradigms, this section lays the groundwork for the chapters to come.

Section 2 explores the nuts and bolts of research design and data collection, whether quantitative, qualitative or mixed methods. Readers will gain a fundamental understanding of how to design studies and analyse data effectively to generate meaningful insights that can inform paramedic practice.

Ethical considerations and the role of governance in research are explored in Section 3, alongside practical guidance on engaging with service users, understanding health economics and disseminating research findings. Additionally, invaluable advice on developing research proposals, securing funding and exploring career pathways in research equips readers with the tools they need to embark on their own research journeys.

This text would not have been possible without the support of our research communities, as well as Class Professional Publishing. We have been writing through times of great change in healthcare, in part due to the COVID-19 pandemic. We thank all our authors for continuing to support this publication while at the same time managing to navigate the challenges brought to the forefront by the pandemic, with many of us maintaining patient-facing roles during those years. Equally, we thank everyone at Class Professional Publishing for believing that we would complete this textbook in spite of these unique and additional pressures.

Preface

As editors, we are delighted to present this practical resource to the research communities. We extend our deepest gratitude to the contributing authors for their expertise and dedication in shaping this textbook. They have written with passion, expert knowledge and a desire to make the content meaningful and accessible to all. It is our sincere hope that *Paramedic Research: Principles, Designs and Methods* will inspire and empower paramedics and other health and care professionals to engage in research endeavours that drive innovation and advance the field for years to come.

Julia Williams and Graham McClelland

About the authors

Editors

Julia Williams, PhD, PGCert ED, PG Cert, Dip HE, FCPara. Professor of Paramedic Science and Director of the Paramedic Clinical Research Unit (ParaCRU) at the University of Hertfordshire, UK. Head of Research at the College of Paramedics, UK. Head of Research, South East Coast Ambulance Service NHS Foundation Trust, UK. ORCID: https://orcid.org/0000-0003-0796-5465.

Julia, a registered paramedic and Professor of Paramedic Science at the University of Hertfordshire, has been involved in paramedic education and development since 1996. As Head of Research for the College of Paramedics, she actively promotes paramedics' contributions to clinical research and advocates for their involvement in health and care research studies. Julia has extensive experience with qualitative, quantitative and mixed methods research in paramedic practice, emergency and urgent care, paramedic education and workforce wellbeing, both in the UK and overseas. She has led research in the South East Coast Ambulance Service NHS Foundation Trust since 2005 and is a member of the National Ambulance Research Steering Group (NARSG). Julia has served on multiple trial steering groups, funding panels, and committees. She is also the Editor-in-Chief of the British Paramedic Journal and has mentored several paramedic PhD students. She firmly believes that a career in paramedic research is full of opportunities and exciting challenges, and hopes this book will be a valuable resource for everyone interested in research at all different levels.

Graham McClelland, PhD, MClinRes, BSc (Hons), FCPara. Vice-Chancellor's Fellow and Assistant Professor in Health, Northumbria University, UK. Visiting Professor, University of Hertfordshire, UK. Honorary Research Fellow, North East Ambulance Service NHS Foundation Trust, UK. Visiting Clinical Researcher, Stroke Research Group, Newcastle University, UK. ORCID: https://orcid.org/0000-0002-4502-5821.

Graham is a registered paramedic and Vice-Chancellor's Fellow at Northumbria University. Graham joined the North East Ambulance Service in 2003 and worked in a variety of clinical roles until he started getting involved in research which took him down a different career path. Graham is a pragmatic, applied healthcare researcher who has been involved in studies across the breadth of conditions encountered by paramedics, but his main focus has been on stroke. In addition to this, Graham has

About the authors

served on the editorial board of the British Paramedic Journal since it was set up, is a reviewer for multiple journals and funding bodies and has been a member of both NHS and university ethics committees. Graham is privileged to be able to support, mentor and supervise paramedics from internships through to PhD students. He thinks this is an exciting time to be involved in prehospital and emergency care research, and hopes that paramedic researchers will continue to seek ways to improve the care delivered to patients.

Contributors

Elicia Austin, BSc (Hons), AFHEA, MCPara. School of Health and Social Work, University of Hertfordshire, UK. South Central Ambulance Service NHS Foundation Trust, UK. ORCID: https://orcid.org/0009-0003-6306-3287.

Jack Barrett, PhD, BSc (Hons), BSc (Hons), MCPara. Senior Paramedic Research Fellow, South East Coast Ambulance Service NHS Foundation Trust, UK. ORCID: https://orcid.org/0000-0002-0040-537X.

Alan M. Batt, PhD, PGCME. Assistant Professor, Queen's University, Canada and Associate Professor, Monash University, Australia. ORCID: https://orcid.org/0000-0001-6473-5397.

Fiona Bell, PhD, BSc (Hons). Head of Research and Development, Yorkshire Ambulance Service NHS Trust, UK. ORCID: https://orcid.org/0000-0003-4503-1903.

Sarah Black, DClinRes, PGDip, BSc (Hons). Head of Research, Audit and Quality Improvement, South Western Ambulance Service NHS Foundation Trust, UK. ORCID: https://orcid.org/0000-0001-6678-7502.

Karl Bloomer, MSc, BA (Hons), MCPara. Consultant Paramedic, Northern Ireland Ambulance Service Health and Social Care Trust, UK. ORCID: https://orcid.org/0000-0002-7822-4528.

Mike Brady, PhD, PGDip, ACP, BSc (Hons), Dip HE. Cyfarwyddwr Clinigol Cynorthwyol/Parafeddyg Ymgynghorol ar gyfer Gofal Clinigol o Bell, Ymddiriedolaeth Brifysgol GIG Gwasanaethau Ambiwlans Cymru, which translates to Assistant Clinical Director/Consultant Paramedic for Remote Clinical Care, Welsh Ambulance Services NHS Trust, UK. ORCID: https://orcid.org/0000-0001-6675-9149.

William Broughton, MSc, PGCert, BSc (Hons), FCPara. Professor of Paramedicine, Buckinghamshire New University, UK. ORCID: https://orcid.org/0000-0002-9764-9433.

Cheryl Cameron, M Ed. Advanced Care Paramedic, Director of Operations, Canadian Virtual Hospice, Canada. ORCID: https://orcid.org/0000-0002-4085-7995.

Karl Charlton, MRes. Research Paramedic, North East Ambulance Service NHS Foundation Trust, UK. ORCID: https://orcid.org/0000-0002-9601-1083.

Scott Devenish, PhD, MVocED, FACPara. Professor of Paramedicine, Australian Catholic University, Australia. ORCID: https://orcid.org/0000-0001-9118-0163.

About the authors

Enrico Dippenaar, PhD, MSc, PGCert. Honorary Research Associate, University of Cape Town, South Africa. ORCID: https://orcid.org/0000-0001-8406-7373

Georgette Eaton, DPhil (Oxon), MSc, PGCert, BSc (Hons), FHEA, MCPara. Consultant Paramedic, Urgent Care, London Ambulance Service NHS Trust, UK. ORCID: https://orcid.org/0000-0001-9421-2845.

Tim Edwards, PhD, MSc, MSc, BSc (Hons), BA (Hons), MCPara. London Ambulance Service NHS Trust, UK ORCID: https://orcid.org/0000-0001-6084-932X.

Ruth M. Fisher, MSc, Dipl, DipHE, PGCert, BSc (Hons), MCPara, MRCSEd, FHEA. Senior Lecturer, Queen Margaret University, UK. Yorkshire Ambulance Service NHS Trust, UK. ORCID: https://orcid.org/0000-0003-3959-4021.

Adam Greene, MSc. Critical Care Paramedic Unit, BC Emergency Health Services, Canada. ORCID: https://orcid.org/0000-0002-4366-9455.

Pete Gregory, MEd, BSc (Hons), FCPara. ORCID: https://orcid.org/0000-0001-9845-0920.

Anthony Herbland, PhD, MA, PGCert, FHEA. Programme Lead for MRES in Health and Social Care, University of Hertfordshire, UK. ORCID: https://orcid.org/0000-0001-6182-4191.

Kim Kirby, PhD, MClinRes, MCPara. Senior Research Fellow, University of the West of England, UK. South Western Ambulance Service NHS Foundation Trust. ORCID: https://orcid.org/0000-0002-8092-7978.

Ian Maconochie, FRCPCH, FRCPI, FRCEM, PhD. Professor of Practice in Paediatric Emergency Medicine, Imperial College London, UK. Consultant in Paediatric Emergency Medicine, Imperial College Healthcare Trust NHS, UK. ORCID: https//orcid.org/0000-0001-6319-8550.

Peter McMeekin, PhD, MSc, BA (Hons). Professor at Northumbria University, UK. ORCID: https://orcid.org/0000-0003-0946-7224.

Jamie Miles, PhD, MSc, ClinRes, PGDip, DipHE, MCPara. Advanced Clinical Practitioner, Barnsley Hospital NHS Foundation Trust, UK. Visiting Research Fellow, Oxford University, UK. ORCID: https://orcid.org/0000-0002-1080-768X.

Scott Munro, PhD, PGDip, PGCert, BSc (Hons), MCPara. Lecturer, School of Health Sciences, University of Surrey, UK. Critical Care Paramedic, South East Coast Ambulance Service NHS Foundation Trust, UK. ORCID: https://orcid.org/0000-0002-0228-4102.

Georgina Murphy-Jones, MA, PGDip, PGCert, BSc (Hons), MCPara. Deputy Director of Clinical Assessment and Pathways, London Ambulance Service NHS Trust, UK. ORCID: https://orcid.org/0000-0002-6681-1506.

Andy Newton, PhD, MSc, PGCE, IMCDip, FCPara. Chief Executive Officer, Newton, London, UK. Chair of HPAC. ORCID: https://orcid.org/0000-0002-6708-8524.

About the authors

Mary Peters, MSc. Head of Patient Safety, North West Ambulance Service NHS Trust, UK. ORCID: https://orcid.org/0000-0003-0628-7084.

Helen Pocock, PhD, MSc, PGCHPE, BSc (Hons), MCPara. Senior Research Paramedic, South Central Ambulance NHS Foundation Trust, UK, Warwick Medical School, University of Warwick, UK. ORCID: https://orcid.org/0000-0001-7648-5313.

Alison Porter, PhD. Associate Professor of Health Services Research, Faculty of Medicine, Health and Life Science, Swansea University, UK. ORCID: https://orcid.org/0000-0002-3408-7007.

Larissa Prothero, BSc (Hons), PhD, BSc (Hons). Research Paramedic, East of England Ambulance Service NHS Trust, UK. ORCID: https://orcid.org/0000-0002-5440-8429.

Duncan Robertson, MClinRes, MSc. Chief Paramedic Officer, South Central Ambulance Service NHS Foundation Trust, UK. ORCID: https://orcid.org/0000-0002-6205-6558.

Ursula Rolfe, PhD, MPhil, BSc (Hons), BA (Hons), PG Cert Ed. Associate Professor Paramedic Science Faculty of Health and Social Sciences, Bournemouth University, UK. ORCID: https://orcid.org/0000-0003-3914-2607.

Kristy Sanderson, PhD, BSc (Psych) (Hons), FRSPH. Professor in Applied Health Research, School of Health Sciences, University of East Anglia, UK. ORCID: https://orcid.org/0000-0002-3132-2745.

Jamie Scott, MSc, PgCert, MCPara. Lecturer in Paramedic Science, Ulster University, UK. Advanced Paramedic Practitioner: ORCID: https://orcid.org/ 0000-0003-2402-021X.

Helen Snooks, PhD, BSc (Hons). Professor of Health Services Research, Swansea University, UK. ORCID: https://orcid.org/0000-0003-0173-8843.

Hayley Stagg, PhD, MMath. Senior Information Analyst, North East Ambulance Service NHS Trust, UK. ORCID: https://orcid.org/0009-0005-4693-1921.

Christopher Stein, PhD, MSc Med. Professor of Emergency Medical Care, University of Johannesburg, South Africa. ORCID: https://orcid.org/0000-0003-3874-6847.

Joel Symonds, PGDip, BSc, MCPara. Advanced Practitioner (Critical Care), Scottish Ambulance Service NHS Trust, UK. ORCID: https://orcid.org/0000-0003-4841-3499.

John Talbot, MSc, PGCert, BSc (Hons). Primary Care Paramedic, Visiting Lecturer University of Hertfordshire. ORCID: https://orcid.org/0009-0003-6070-0834.

Janette Turner, MSc. (Retired) Reader in Emergency and Urgent Care Research, SCHARR, University of Sheffield, UK. ORCID: https://orcid.org/0000-0003-3884-7875.

About the authors

Gregory Adam Whitley, PhD, MSc, PGCert, BSc (Hons), MCPara. Paramedic Research Fellow, East Midlands Ambulance Service NHS Trust, UK. Associate Professor in Paramedic Science, School of Health and Care Sciences, University of Lincoln, UK. ORCID: https://orcid.org/0000-0003-2586-6815.

James Yates, MSc, DipIMC, MCPara. Specialist Paramedic, Critical Care, Great Western Air Ambulance Charity, UK. Advanced Paramedic, South West Neonatal Advice and Retrieval, UK. ORCID: https://orcid.org/0000-0002-2520-0602.

List of tables

Table 4.1	Summary of characteristics of the different activities	39
Table 5.1	Paramedic researcher engagement with paradigms	51
Table 6.1	Different types of literature review	57
Table 6.2	Guides to development of review or evidence synthesis	58
Table 6.3	Structures for development of research questions	59
Table 6.4	Example of developing search terms to answer a PICO question	61
Table 6.5	Illustration of results from PubMed search	62
Table 6.6	Example of combining searches in PubMed	62
Table 6.7	Example of widening a search strategy	63
Table 6.8	Examples of critical appraisal frameworks	66
Table 7.1	Example of using the funnel model	73
Table 7.2	Example of a research question structured using O'Leary's framework	78
Table 11.1	Reporting the descriptive analysis of nominal variable (i.e. gender)	125
Table 11.2	Reporting the descriptive analysis of ordinal data with frequencies and percentages	126
Table 11.3	Reporting the descriptive analysis of normally distributed data	127
Table 11.4	Reporting of the descriptive analysis of skewed continuous data	127
Table 11.5	Data on mortality outcomes from the CRASH-2 trial comparing tranexamic acid (TXA) to placebo in bleeding trauma patients	128
Table 11.6	Eight-year mortality hazard rate estimates for each year	130
Table 11.7	Guide for selecting the appropriate statistical tests for discerning statistical differences	133
Table 11.8	Guide for selecting the appropriate statistical tests for statistical correlation or association analysis	134
Table 11.9	Assessing accuracy of diagnostic tests	136
Table 13.1	Developing questions for a qualitative questionnaire	164
Table 15.1	Methods of integration	191
Table 20.1	Plan of investigation	249

List of figures

Figure 2.1	The Ottawa model of research use	15
Figure 5.1	The elements of a research paradigm	42
Figure 5.2	The research paradigm spectrum	45
Figure 6.1	Example of PubMed MeSH tree structure	61
Figure 6.2	Example of a PRISMA flow diagram	64
Figure 7.1	Example of narrowing down a research problem into a specific focus area	71
Figure 7.2	Refining the research problem into a question	71
Figure 9.1	The Recognition Of Stroke In the Emergency Room (ROSIER) data collection tool	113
Figure 11.1	Example of a normal distribution for systolic blood pressure with mean of 120 and standard deviation of 10	124
Figure 11.2	Non-normal distribution of survival probability relative to time to defibrillation	125
Figure 11.3	Kaplan–Meier survival curves	130
Figure 11.4	CCR probability distribution graph	138
Figure 15.1	Procedures for mixed methods sequential designs	192
Figure 15.2	Procedures for the Prehospital Pain Management in Children study	193
Figure 15.3	Procedures for the mixed methods convergent design	195
Figure 15.4	Procedures for the prehospital stroke care study	196
Figure 15.5	Philosophical branches and divisions	199
Figure 18.1	QALY gain example	227
Figure 18.2	Decision tree model for epilepsy patients in the ambulance service	230
Figure 18.3	Markov model example	230
Figure 18.4	Discrete event simulation	231

List of boxes

Box 2.1	Relevance of research to HCPC standards of proficiency for paramedics	11
Box 4.1	Brief history of clinical audit in the NHS	31
Box 4.2	Clinical guidelines for management of chest pain of suspected cardiac origin	32
Box 6.1	Quick search task	56
Box 7.1	Hypothetical example of a research problem	70
Box 10.1	An example of a quasi-experimental design	118
Box 12.1	An example of a generic qualitative study	144
Box 13.1	An example of a survey collecting qualitative and quantitative data	162
Box 13.2	An example of an observational study	164
Box 13.3	An example of a study using photo-elicitation	170
Box 14.1	An example of an ethnographic study using mid-range theory	175
Box 14.2	An example of a study using an abductive approach to analysing feedback to paramedics	176
Box 14.3	An example of a study using content analysis	178
Box 14.4	An example of a study using framework analysis	179
Box 14.5	An example of a study using thematic analysis	180
Box 14.6	An example of a study using grounded theory	181
Box 14.7	An example of a study using conversation analysis	182
Box 14.8	An example of a study using discourse analysis	183
Box 14.9	An example of a team approach to qualitative analysis	185
Box 14.10	An example of verifying qualitative data	186
Box 16.1	Seven requirements of ethical research	207
Box 17.1	Top tips for involving service users in research	220
Box 19.1	Key points in presentations	239
Box 20.1	Characteristics of a good research proposal	253
Box 21.1	Examples of funding bodies	257

SECTION 1

Chapter 1

Introduction: paramedic research: what is it all about?

Julia Williams and Graham McClelland

> **Purpose of this chapter**
>
> Completion of this chapter will help you to:
> - identify how this book can contribute to learning about research in paramedicine
> - outline what is meant by the term 'paramedic research'
> - understand the importance of research for the paramedic profession.

Introduction

Over the past few decades, from the mid-1990s to the present day, the landscape of paramedic research has undergone a remarkable transformation, ushering in a new era of evidence-based practice and innovation. The end of the 1990s was a pivotal period in the history of prehospital care, with a growing interest in research among paramedics and healthcare professionals alike. This era witnessed the emergence of pioneering figures like Malcolm Woollard, a distinguished paramedic professor and trailblazer in the field of research in the UK. Woollard's contributions not only laid the groundwork for paramedic research, but also served as a catalyst for its integration into mainstream healthcare practices.

Since then, paramedic research has evolved from its nascent stages into a multidisciplinary domain utilising diverse methodologies, from clinical trials to qualitative studies. The significance of research in this context cannot be overstated, as it provides the foundation for advancing the quality, safety and effectiveness of paramedic practice, whether paramedics are working in prehospital care or any other setting.

By fostering a culture of inquiry and critical thinking, paramedics are empowered to consider evidence-based interventions that are grounded in robust scientific evidence, bridging the gap between theory and practice. By systematically evaluating interventions and protocols through rigorous inquiry, or exploring experiences and other phenomena, paramedic research contributes to the ever-expanding body

Chapter 1 — Introduction: paramedic research: what is it all about?

of evidence that informs clinical decision making and policy formulation. To fully harness the transformative power of research, it is imperative for paramedics to not only understand its relevance, but also actively engage in its pursuit. By providing accessible opportunities for education, training and mentorship, we can enable paramedics to embrace research as an integral component of their practice.

In expanding research capability and capacity among our own professional workforce, the importance of interprofessional and interdisciplinary collaboration must not be overlooked. We are working at a time when health and social care challenges are complex and multifaceted, and collaboration across disciplines is essential for generating comprehensive solutions. By fostering partnerships between paramedics, academic discipline experts, researchers, clinicians and other healthcare stakeholders, we can bring together diverse perspectives and expertise to tackle pressing healthcare issues in practice, management, education, policy and service delivery.

Equally vital is the involvement of patients and the public in research processes. By actively engaging stakeholders from the outset, researchers can ensure that studies are designed to address the needs and preferences of those directly impacted by paramedic practice. Through meaningful involvement in all stages of the research process, from study design to dissemination of findings, patients and the public become true partners in advancing the science of health and social care, no matter what the discipline.

What do we mean by 'paramedic research'?

Terminology has its uses, but it can also lead to confusion if there is no shared understanding of the term. Paramedicine is still defining its parameters and meanings, and this is also true when it comes to paramedic research. We have been asked before whether it means research undertaken by paramedics, research about the paramedic profession, or both? Or something else completely? There may not be consensus on this, but when we refer to paramedic research, we are broadly talking about studies, investigations or inquiries undertaken to enhance the understanding, effectiveness and quality of care provided by paramedics. This could be in any setting where paramedics are working, whether that is ambulance services, primary care, tertiary care, industry, education, prisons, acute hospitals – the list is growing.

Sometimes this involves prehospital care, which may include emergency medical care delivery. By implication, prehospital indicates the patient is likely to go to hospital and in the 21st century this is not necessarily the case for all our patients, and certainly does not reflect the work of the whole of our workforce. However, on many occasions it is totally appropriate to refer to prehospital care, and in this book, we want to be inclusive of all roles and settings related to our profession. So sometimes we will refer to prehospital care and other times we might refer to unplanned or unscheduled, urgent and/or emergency care. The phrase 'paramedic research' just appears to be a more encompassing term than 'prehospital' or 'out of hospital' as it relates to all situations, settings and roles which affect paramedics and their working practices.

The paramedic profession is in a state of flux and we are still defining our scopes of practice – and there are many. Hopefully, research will add to our understanding of these areas as we continue to grow as a profession. We need to acknowledge that there is no simple phrase that encompasses everything that paramedics do and, therefore, most of the time in this book we are likely to refer to research relating to paramedic practice or the paramedic profession.

At the same time as wanting to include all paramedics and our associated workforce, we also want to embrace opportunities for interprofessional research and multidisciplinary working. Paramedic research, while focused on improving care provided by paramedics, is not exclusive or undertaken in isolation. On the contrary, it encourages collaboration and interdisciplinary approaches to problem-solving within the broader healthcare landscape. Rather than promoting siloed working, paramedic research actively seeks to engage with other healthcare professionals, researchers, academics and stakeholders to foster a comprehensive understanding of unscheduled and/or unplanned, urgent and/or emergency care and its integration into the larger health and social care systems as well as other organisations. You can see the dilemma here as we cannot write this out in full all the time, which is why authors frequently shorten it to prehospital or paramedic research, more for convenience than necessarily as an accurate delimiter of the settings.

Paramedic research examines various aspects of paramedic practice, including, but not limited to, the following:

- Clinical interventions, such as evaluating the effectiveness of specific medical treatments or procedures administered by paramedics.
- Patient experiences and outcomes, focusing on the perspectives, needs and experiences of patients receiving paramedic treatment and management, as well as the factors influencing their outcomes and satisfaction.
- Workforce well-being, examining the health and well-being of paramedics and other emergency care staff working in different settings.
- Education and training, investigating the efficacy of different education/training programmes, simulation exercises or educational strategies in preparing paramedics to manage their expanding practices whether they are related to emergency medical services, health promotion or primary care, to name a few.
- Evolving technology and equipment, exploring the use of new technologies, devices or equipment in improving the delivery of paramedic treatment/ management and patient outcomes.
- Paramedic career development, investigating the impact of different elements whether related to clinical, management, education, research or entrepreneurship.
- Development of protocols and guidelines, assessing the impact of different protocols and guidelines on patient outcomes and resource utilisation.
- Workflow and systems, exploring organisations and integration of the paramedic workforce within the broader health and care systems to optimise patient outcomes and experiences, promoting integrated care and collaboration across the health and social care professions.

Chapter 1 — Introduction: paramedic research: what is it all about?

Overall, paramedic research aims to generate evidence that informs best practice, enhances patient care and contributes to the ongoing advancement of the profession. The areas presented here are not exhaustive, and throughout this textbook we will look at different elements of paramedic research, but even then, we will only have space to scratch the surface of the many research studies that have been undertaken in recent years related to the paramedic profession. It is notable how far the profession has come since the turn of of the century, when there were fewer research studies related to the paramedic profession and very few being initiated and led by paramedics.

Does paramedic research have to be led by paramedics?

The simple reply is 'No, but ...' – there is always a 'but', isn't there?

While we might not agree on everything, many people recognise that paramedicine is diverse in nature. How many times have you heard people say that paramedics need to be prepared to provide services 24/7 to manage patients spanning the age continuum from birth to death, presenting as low acuity through to high acuity (and everything in between), including physical and mental health presentations? Our work exposes us to interactions with different health and care providers, including emergency physicians, GPs, nurses, midwives, specialists, social workers, fire service staff, police, prison officers and other hospital and community healthcare staff. Paramedics often work alongside these professionals, and their research efforts reflect this collaborative spirit.

Furthermore, paramedic research recognises the interconnectedness of different facets of healthcare delivery. It acknowledges that, for example, improvements in prehospital care can have effects on patient outcomes, resource utilisation, and health and care system efficiency. Therefore, paramedic research often intersects with areas such as emergency medicine, trauma care, mental health, public health, end-of-life care and healthcare policy, contributing to a more holistic understanding of health and care service delivery.

In promoting collaboration and interdisciplinary approaches, paramedic research helps break down silos between different healthcare specialties and fosters a culture of shared learning and innovation. Ultimately, paramedic research can serve as a bridge, connecting various stakeholders and disciplines in pursuit of improved patient outcomes and a more efficient healthcare system.

So, paramedic research does not exclusively have to be led by paramedics and we should work collaboratively, of course, to build as strong a team as possible to support the project. We have the expectation, however, that as more paramedics become expert researchers, we will see growth in the numbers of paramedics taking the lead in research teams as chief investigators on studies pertaining to our profession. We are seeing that trend emerge, and we must enable more paramedics to develop the prerequisite skills and knowledge for them to be effective in these roles. Through a comprehensive exploration of research principles, methodological approaches and real-world applications, this book endeavours to support paramedics with the knowledge and skills necessary to embrace the complexities of researching contemporary paramedicine and ultimately to become research leaders in the future.

Welcome to *Paramedic Research: Principles, Designs and Methods*

Here, we introduce you to the structure of this book which we hope will serve as a roadmap for paramedics, researchers and other health and care professionals, offering invaluable insights into the principles, methodologies and applications of paramedic research.

In this introductory section, we explore the foundation for understanding the significance of paramedic research, highlighting challenges in the use of specific terminology.

The chapters in Section 1 provide a comprehensive overview of key concepts and frameworks essential for conducting paramedic research. We delve into the distinctions between research, clinical audit, quality improvement, service evaluation and innovation, highlighting their respective roles in driving improvement and innovation in paramedic and prehospital care. Furthermore, we emphasise the paramount importance of evidence in informing practice, guiding readers as to how to make sense of research processes and develop rigorous research questions. Navigating the research process can be daunting, but do not be put off. Section 1 equips readers with the knowledge and tools necessary to begin to address the complexities of research design and methodology. From understanding different research paradigms to critically evaluating existing literature and developing research proposals, we invite readers to engage with paramedic research effectively and meaningfully.

In Section 2, we go deeper into quantitative and qualitative research design and data collection methods. Whether exploring observational data, conducting experiments or engaging in, for example, ethnography or phenomenology, readers gain insights into making sense of both quantitative and qualitative data. Additionally, we explore mixed methods research design, offering a holistic approach to understanding complex phenomena in paramedicine.

Section 3 addresses critical issues such as ethics and governance in research, the involvement of service users and an introduction to health economics. We explore strategies for sharing research results and findings, developing research proposals, securing funding and navigating career pathways in research.

Summary

As we wrap up our introduction, we hope we have effectively outlined the scope of this book. Our team of international authors brings a wealth of experience, expertise and knowledge in research, all of which they are eager to share with you. Whether you are starting your first research project, advancing in your research career or

Chapter 1 — Introduction: paramedic research: what is it all about?

are simply curious about the importance of research and evidence in paramedicine, *Paramedic Research: Principles, Designs and Methods* will be a valuable resource and guide, contributing to the development of excellence in paramedic research.

Useful resources

- Griffiths P and Mooney G (eds) (2011). *The Paramedic's Guide to Research: An Introduction.* Maidenhead: McGraw-Hill Education.
- Olaussen A, Bowles KA, Lord B and Williams B (eds) (2022). *Introducing, Designing and Conducting Research for Paramedics*. Chatswood: Elsevier Health Sciences.
- Siriwardena AN and Whitley GA (eds) (2022). *Prehospital Research Methods and Practice*. Bridgwater: Class Professional Publishing.

Chapter 2

Why do we need evidence-based practice?

Jamie Scott and Karl Bloomer

> **Purpose of this chapter**
>
> Completion of this chapter will help you to:
> - discuss the origins of evidence-based medicine
> - explore the relevance of evidence-based practice to paramedicine
> - identify the role of knowledge translation
> - examine the challenges of getting evidence into practice in unscheduled urgent and emergency care settings.

Introduction

The landscape of healthcare has witnessed a transformative shift over the past 30 years, with the emergence of evidence-based approaches contributing to improved patient outcomes and well-informed decision making. There are different definitions of 'research' and various understandings of the term 'evidence' but generally, research refers to systematic investigation aimed at generating new knowledge or validating existing knowledge, while evidence refers to the reliable and valid data derived from such research that support or refute clinical practices and decision making.

This chapter embarks on a journey to trace the origins of evidence-based medicine, (sometimes called evidence-based practice (EBP), evidence-informed practice or evidence-based healthcare), contextualise its applicability within the paramedicine domain, shed light on the role of knowledge translation and explore some of the intricate challenges associated with implementing EBP in the dynamic context of unscheduled urgent and emergency care settings.

What is evidence-based practice?

An evidence-based approach to medicine was first proposed by the medical doctor and researcher Professor Archie Cochrane in 1972. Concerned that most treatment decisions were not based on clinical evidence, he proposed that researchers should

Chapter 2 — Why do we need evidence-based practice?

collaborate to systematically review all the best available clinical trials in each speciality area (Cochrane et al., 1989). This would produce the best-quality evidence on which to base treatment decisions, and would ultimately lead to the formation of the Cochrane Library of systematic reviews.

However, the term 'evidence-based practice' was not commonly used until 1991, when Professor Gordon Guyatt, of McMaster University in Ontario, highlighted that most clinical decision making relied on clinical intuition, clinical experience, pathophysiological rationale and the opinion of senior clinicians (Guyatt, 1991). He proposed a move away from this model to one based on high-quality, clinically-relevant research, and set about designing educational programmes and textbooks on the subject.

Then, in 1996, Dr David Sackett and his colleagues elaborated on this, explaining that EBP is a combination of research evidence and clinical expertise, as well as the values and preferences of the individual patient (Sackett et al., 1996). They formally defined EBP as:

> ... the conscientious, explicit and judicious use of current best evidence in making decisions about the care of the individual patient. The practice of evidence-based medicine means integrating individual clinical expertise with the best available external clinical evidence from systematic research.
>
> (Sackett et al., 1996, p. 71)

At an organisational level, EBP is the use of the latest knowledge and evidence derived from research activities, clinical audit, quality improvement and service evaluation, to evaluate the risks, benefits and costs of an intervention in a particular setting. These findings are then used to inform the production of clinical guidelines, standard operating procedures and protocols that assist individual clinicians in making clinical decisions. Evidence-based practice aims to ensure that patients receive the most effective care possible, based on the best available evidence while recognising the importance of incorporating patients' values and beliefs wherever possible.

Individual clinicians engage in EBP by developing the skills and knowledge to critically evaluate the evidence, and the clinical guidelines based upon it, and using it to inform clinical decision making. This is achieved through appropriate education (for example, undergraduate degree) and ongoing continuing professional development (CPD) activities such as:

- reflective practice
- critical appraisal of peer-reviewed journals
- peer review
- conferences
- engaging with research activities
- clinical placements
- mentorship.

Why is evidence-based practice still important in the 21st century?

The role of the paramedic has evolved significantly since the introduction of professional registration in the UK in 2000. This began a process of professionalisation that has progressed at a pace unmatched by other health and care professions.

Trait theory identifies three key pillars of a profession; registration, self-regulation and possessing an exclusive body of knowledge (First et al., 2012). Professional registration and self-regulation for paramedics were achieved through the Health Professions Council (HPC), which is now the Health and Care Professions Council (HCPC), and by the formation of what is now known as the College of Paramedics, the central professional body representing UK paramedics.

Registration with the HCPC has the additional benefit of protecting the paramedic title and providing standards of proficiency for the profession. Of particular relevance to research are standards 12 and 13 (Box 2.1).

Box 2.1

Relevance of research to HCPC standards of proficiency for paramedics

- 12.2 demonstrate awareness of the principles and applications of scientific enquiry, including the evaluation of treatment efficacy and the research process
- 12.10 understand the principles of evaluation and research methodologies which enable the integration of theoretical perspectives and research evidence into the design and implementation of effective paramedic practice
- 13.8 recognise a range of research methodologies relevant to their role
- 13.9 recognise the value of research to the critical evaluation of practice
- 13.10 critically evaluate research and other evidence to inform their own practice
- 13.11 engage service users in research as appropriate

Source: HCPC (2023).

The development of an exclusive body of knowledge is ongoing as there were significant gaps in the prehospital evidence base (Wood, 2012) and historically many prehospital clinical guidelines and protocols were based on evidence gathered in other settings. Generation of evidence specific to the prehospital environment and other settings in which paramedics work is required in order to ensure patients receive the best possible care based on up-to-date evidence.

Evidence-based practice is a dynamic process, with our understanding of best practice evolving over time in response to a constant stream of new evidence. As such, engaging with research and the evolving evidence base will always be a key foundation of modern paramedic practice.

Chapter 2 — Why do we need evidence-based practice?

How are paramedics contributing to evidence-based practice?

The profession has more recently been contributing to its own specific evidence base, generated by an ever-increasing and diverging range of sources. UK paramedics, as part of their professional development, and more recently as part of the HCPC registration requirements, have been completing undergraduate and postgraduate programmes, with the first of these starting in 1998 (University of Hertfordshire, 2021). These not only incorporated introductions to research methodology and theory, but often required students to produce their own empirical research projects. The move to higher education has contributed to an increasing number of research projects including paramedics undertaking substantial doctoral and postdoctoral research projects (Paramedic PhD, 2021).

The demand for EBP has influenced UK NHS ambulance trusts to expand their research capacity by forming research and development departments, staffed by emerging in-house staff with expertise in the area. Within these departments, we have seen the growing development of specific 'research paramedic' roles, allowing much larger studies to be undertaken by ambulance services with paramedic research leads or those who are heavily involved in research (McClelland, 2013). These formal research posts allow paramedics to undertake a range of research duties, from designing research through to increasing participant recruitment, data collection and analysis, and publishing an increasing number and range of studies.

As ambulance trusts successfully demonstrate an ability to deliver high-quality research on time and to budget, there is an increasing commercial interest in partnering with them and their paramedic workforce to undertake pharmaceutical and non-pharmaceutical trials. Large multicentre trials, such as the AIRWAYS-2 (Benger et al., 2018) and PARAMEDIC2 and 3 studies (Perkins et al., 2018; Couper et al., 2024), have allowed a much larger number of paramedics to experience essential trial aspects, such as patient recruitment, while providing valuable contributions to the profession's evidence base.

Outside dedicated research roles and academic settings, it is important to acknowledge that paramedics across all settings are contributing to EBP. Local journal clubs and professional development events offer paramedics opportunities to reflect on emerging evidence, as well as contributing through informal presentations and peer reviews. Indeed, many paramedics, especially those in UK ambulance trusts, act in mentorship roles, as practice educators, facilitating the translation of clinical theory from universities into practical experiences for students, and ultimately reflection upon this experience – the very essence of EBP.

Along with the more traditional roles in ambulance services, paramedics are working in a range of primary, urgent care and hospital settings. These relatively new roles are enabling increased collaboration in research projects and trials, and facilitating access for paramedics to established research networks, a key strategic objective of the Council for Allied Health Professions Research (CAHPR) (Eaton et al., 2018). It is from within these settings that paramedics are able to develop an evidence base to support and validate these new and emerging roles, generating evidence that is transferrable into the clinical practice of the modern paramedic.

Opportunities for dissemination of the profession's own evidence base, both within the UK and internationally, have increased and become commonplace in recent years. The UK now has a number of annual national research conferences relevant to the paramedic profession, such as those from the College of Paramedics and the 999 EMS Research Forum (Health Services Research Team, 2021). These organisations, and others such as the McNally Project in Canada and the Australasian College of Paramedicine, are building research capacity within the profession and working to ensure that a stronger evidence base is created. The success of research expansion in the paramedic profession has led to an increase in the number of dedicated peer-reviewed journals, with the *British Paramedic Journal*, *Paramedicine* and the *Journal of Paramedic Practice* emerging within recent years.

How should we be expanding the evidence base underpinning paramedic practices?

Within the UK, it is still the case that a majority of paramedics practise within NHS ambulance trusts (although that majority has decreased over the years), where practice is largely directed by guidelines such as those published by the Joint Royal Colleges Ambulance Liaison Committee (JRCALC). These guidelines have at times relied heavily on established evidence bases, particularly those from in-hospital and other acute settings, creating an evidence base that may not always have been appropriate for the prehospital setting (Ball, 2005). This was highlighted as an area of concern in 2010 in the Department of Health report 'Building the evidence base in prehospital urgent and emergency care: a review of research evidence and priorities for future research' (Department of Health, 2010).

Over the years, this situation has been changing with the growth of conducting and validating clinical research in clinical environments where paramedics practise. One example demonstrating this was the push for early intravenous antibiotics for the treatment of suspected sepsis in the prehospital setting by ambulance paramedics. It was well established from hospital data that earlier antibiotic administration in sepsis improved outcomes, and for some time the suggestion of paramedics administering these appeared to be an obvious next step. However, studies conducted in prehospital settings have questioned the effectiveness of simply shoehorning this into paramedic practice, with research showing no improvement in patient outcomes with prehospital antibiotic use (Alam et al., 2018). The end result was more research being needed before this is implemented more widely.

It is not only essential to validate external research, but equally important to establish the evidence base for new practice as it is developing and becoming part of the changing roles for paramedics. There is an ever-increasing emphasis placed on paramedics within ambulance trusts to move away, where appropriate, from assessment, stabilisation and transport of patients to autonomously diagnosing, treating and referring an increasing share of patients where it is safe to do so. This is

Chapter 2 — Why do we need evidence-based practice?

an area that has attracted several research studies, and one identified as a priority by the National Ambulance Service Medical Directors (NASMeD, 2014; Bell and Fitzpatrick, 2016).

As the role of paramedics continues to evolve, the profession itself must play a key part in the establishment of its evidence base. Encouragingly, as changing scopes of practice take paramedics into specialist and advanced roles, there are more opportunities to engage with research and develop the paramedic evidence base. However, Harris et al. (2020) caution that research is often the most overlooked pillar of advanced practice, and advocate use of frameworks to help embed continual development and evaluation of the evidence into practice-based settings, and not relying on colleagues based solely in academia.

These views are shared by many experts in the field of EBP and to establish this culture and ensure its continued expansion, we need to do more than identify the priorities. Undergraduate programmes need to not only introduce students to EBP, but to embody and incorporate it into every feasible aspect of pre- and post-registration education. Likewise, it must be part of everyday clinical practice, ideally with clinicians afforded dedicated research/CPD time and access to EBP tools and clinical mentorship, in order to identify evidence gaps and actively expand the profession's evidence base.

Knowledge translation – what is this and how do we do it?

Knowledge translation is the assimilation of new evidence into current clinical practice. In other words, it is how we translate the evidence gathered from research into better clinical practice that improves patient outcomes.

Knowledge translation is defined by the World Health Organization (WHO) as:

> *… the synthesis, exchange, and application of knowledge by relevant stakeholders to accelerate the benefits of global and local innovation in strengthening health systems and improving people's health.*
>
> (WHO, 2021b)

The WHO (2012) has published detailed descriptions and discussions on the strengths and weaknesses of several well-known models of knowledge translation. The Ottawa Model of Research Use (Figure 2.1), for example, is an easy-to-use model that defines key elements of knowledge translation and has a heavy focus on knowledge translation in clinical practice (WHO, 2012).

In the prehospital setting, the most well-known example of how knowledge is translated from research evidence to clinical practice is the JRCALC guidelines. These guidelines are intended to synthesise relevant evidence and inform good clinical practice amongst paramedics working on frontline emergency ambulances.

An example of how evidence derived from research is translated into JRCALC guidelines was the update of the head injury algorithm following the results of the CRASH-3 trial (CRASH-3 Trial Collaborators, 2019). The aim of this international,

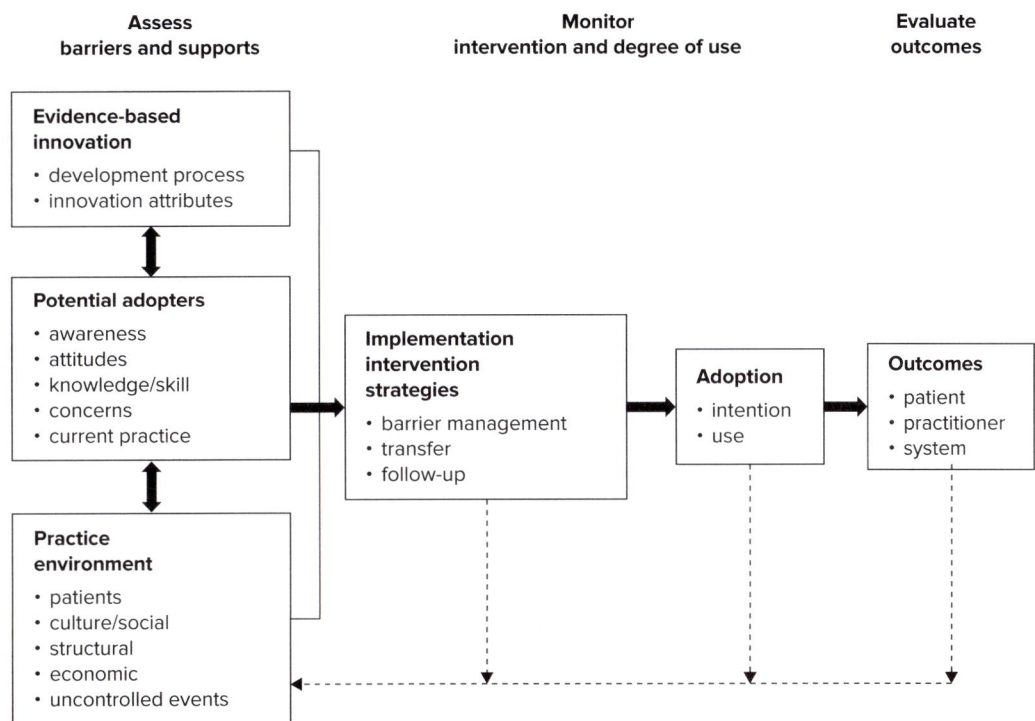

Figure 2.1 The Ottawa model of research use.

Source: Logan J and Graham ID (1998). Toward a comprehensive interdisciplinary model of health care research use. *Science Communication*, 20(2): 227–246.

Reproduced with permission from the author, Ian Graham.

double-blind, placebo-controlled trial was to provide evidence about the effect of the antifibrinolytic drug tranexamic acid (TXA) on mortality and disability in patients who had sustained a traumatic brain injury. The authors concluded that TXA was a safe, cost-effective drug intervention that could reduce death from traumatic brain injury by up to 20% (CRASH-3 Trial Collaborators, 2019). Following publication of the results of CRASH-3, the JRCALC updated its head injury algorithm to recommend that paramedics administer TXA to patients aged over 18 who have a known or expected head injury, with a Glasgow Coma Scale score of less than 12, where the injury has occurred in the last three hours.

Interestingly, after the results of CRASH-3 were released, members of the National Ambulance Research Steering Group (NARSG) contacted Professor Ian Roberts, the chief investigator of the CRASH studies, to ask to bring the trial into the prehospital setting. These early discussions resulted in some ambulance services being involved in the development and implementation of CRASH-4, which is an example of co-construction and collaboration in developing the evidence base.

Although JRCALC guidelines are used to inform paramedic clinical practice, the modern paramedic is also required to be an autonomous practitioner, who can critically analyse and assimilate varying forms of evidence to inform/improve their own practice. This can be achieved through reading, engaging with or producing research, reflecting on their practice, seeking feedback on their practice, and improving their background knowledge through CPD activities.

However, several of the ambulance services' guidelines are based on evidence from other settings or on the expert opinion of contributors. This raises questions around the validity of applying findings outside the context of the research, and highlights the importance of prehospital knowledge generation by the paramedic profession, who are the experts in their own clinical setting.

An autonomous clinical practitioner must be able to critically analyse these guidelines and the evidence they are based on, weighing this against other clinical guidelines (such as National Institute for Health and Care Excellence, Scottish Intercollegiate Guidelines Network) and evidence from other sources of peer-reviewed research.

Challenges to getting the evidence into practice in unscheduled urgent and emergency care

'But we've always done it this way...'

Despite the wealth of clinical knowledge and the increasing numbers of publications, paramedics are not alone in their encounters with fellow clinicians who, for whatever reason, are unaware of or resistant to certain evidence bases (Boswell and Cannon, 2020).

Paramedics must not only be aware of available evidence but understand how to critically evaluate it, and ultimately how to use this to inform their practice where appropriate. Introductions to research-informed practice and evidence hierarchies have been part of paramedic and university programmes in the UK for some time, but many currently-practising clinicians have received no formal education on research and EBP.

Challenges and barriers encountered at an individual level can include a lack of awareness about research and its benefits, and the clinician not feeling capable or confident enough to accurately evaluate research or transition it into their practice (Rosser, 2012; Samarkandi et al., 2018). There is also evidence to demonstrate that higher-education qualifications above pre-registration degrees (MSc and PhD) lead to a greater likelihood that clinicians will adopt and use research in their practice (Omery and Williams, 1999). As the paramedic profession continues to develop specialist and advanced roles, an increasing number of paramedics are expected to undertake these higher education courses and develop greater confidence in translating research into their practice. This will have the combined effect of combatting barriers at the level of the individual clinician, and at an organisational and institutional level by building the clinical workforce knowledge in EBP (Carroll et al., 1997; Meats et al., 2009).

A range of organisational challenges, often outside the ability of individual clinicians to immediately rectify, also exist at local, Trust and even national levels. For example, local journal clubs, the benefits of which are well established, can struggle to function in certain areas where clinicians are isolated from others equally interested in research and EBP, or the time and facilities may neither exist nor be supported by local organisations. Protected study and CPD time for most paramedics is still not a common phenomenon, a complaint noted among many clinical professionals as a barrier to keeping up with the latest EBP even before facing other challenges implementing it into practice (Rosser, 2012; Houser, 2015).

Support at organisational level for EBP is vital, and clinicians experiencing even passive resistance, such as managerial apathy, can quickly find themselves and any collective efforts to implement the science up against a very real barrier. In order for a culture of enquiry and EBP to thrive, there needs to be an environment with deliberate support and practical infrastructure to facilitate it (Slade et al., 2018). We can see this in those NHS Trusts and hospitals where dedicated research staff exist; these Trusts are early adopters of new EBP, and ultimately have better patient-centred outcomes (Ozdemir et al., 2015). These dedicated research staff can also act as catalysts, encouraging an evidence-based change in practice where needed, and aiding those staff less familiar with appraising findings (Carroll et al., 1997).

Summary

In conclusion, this chapter seeks to provide an enriched understanding of evidence-based healthcare, tracing its historical origins and assessing its relevance in paramedicine. By exploring the role of knowledge translation and addressing challenges in the implementation of evidence-based approaches in unscheduled urgent and emergency care settings, this chapter aims to contribute to the advancement of evidence-driven patient-centred care.

Useful resources

- The JBI provides the latest research and evidence-based guidelines regarding patient care, treatment options and interventions. JBI EBP Database: https://jbi.global/jbi-ebp-database

Chapter 3

Making sense of the research process

Kristy Sanderson and Larissa Prothero

> **Purpose of this chapter**
>
> Completion of this chapter will help you to:
> - outline the key steps in a research process
> - identify various methodological approaches and methods
> - highlight the importance of involving different stakeholders and groups in paramedic research.

Introduction

This chapter provides an overview of the research process from research question formalisation to project wrap-up. You can read these steps as a sequential list or dip into each step as you need, as not all steps will be relevant to all types of studies or research questions, and some steps can occur concurrently. Further detail on many of these steps is provided in subsequent chapters.

1. Choose a topic that is relevant to practice and policy.
2. Review the literature to identify gaps in knowledge.
3. Identify stakeholders and key research partners (including patient and public involvement).
4. Formulate the research aims, questions, hypotheses and objectives.
5. Choose appropriate study design and methodologies.
6. Write the protocol and estimate financial and/or in-kind resources needed.
7. Apply for funding (if applicable).
8. Obtain ethics, governance and other approvals as appropriate.
9. Data collection.
10. Analysis.

Chapter 3 — Making sense of the research process

11. Write-up.
12. Dissemination and impact activities.

Where needed, repeat steps 8–11 for multiphase or multicomponent studies.

Key stages of the research process

Step 1: Choose a topic that is relevant to practice and policy

Clinicians, student clinicians and those working for and with health and care services are often drawn to their first research project by curiosity about something they have experienced or learned about in practice: Why did that clinical scenario not go as planned? Why do we do things in that order? What caused that near-miss incident? Why do some people but not others improve with this treatment? Why can't we use that medical device too?

Research projects are also selected from lists of research priorities periodically published by major research funders (such as government and third sector), government departments, professional bodies, charities and patient advocacy groups.

Some funding bodies will also commission research on a topic, where the research questions are provided to the research community and researchers bid or tender to deliver the prescribed research. Recently in the UK, the James Lind Alliance Emergency Medicine Research Priority Setting Partnership provided direction for National Institute for Health and Care Research Commissioned Funding Calls (National Institute for Health and Care Research, 2021b).

Step 2: Review the literature to identify gaps in knowledge

Replication is important in science, but you don't want to repeat research that has already been done without also contributing something new. An important step in the research process is having a solid understanding of the research that has already been produced for your topic (Lund et al., 2016). This could be research published in journal articles, book chapters, government reports or student dissertations.

Research can be the first study of its kind (for example, first-in-human clinical trials) or can explore whether known interventions work the same in different populations from the ones for which they were developed (for example, medicines developed for in-hospital use being used in the ambulance setting). To decide whether you need to do a formal review of the existing evidence, known as a systematic review, check that a relevant review doesn't already exist for your question by searching bibliographic healthcare databases and dedicated review libraries (for example, Cochrane Library www.cochranelibrary.com/; BestBets https://bestbets.org/; PROSPERO www.crd.york.ac.uk/prospero/). University-based library services often offer support with literature searching, and with the growth in paramedic research, an increasing array of systematic reviews are being published. Literature searching is covered in Chapter 6.

Key stages of the research process

Step 3: Identify stakeholders and key research partners, including patient and public involvement

A critical ingredient to successful research that makes a real-world difference is answering questions that matter to end-users. By 'end-users', we mean people who will use and/or benefit from your research. This includes patients and their families, the general public, clinicians, healthcare providers, healthcare funders and policy makers.

Consulting with these groups will give you confidence that you are addressing questions that are important to people, and you will be more likely to produce research that will be put into practice and therefore increase the chances of having impact.

If you are seeking external project funding for your research, to be competitive you will almost certainly need to demonstrate that these consultations have taken place. Involving individuals as 'experts with lived experience' from the outset will increase the quality of the research being undertaken and prevent poor research questions (Pratt, 2021). Involvement of these important stakeholders should continue throughout the delivery of a research project, with them having the opportunity to have roles such as co-investigator or advisory group member and facilitate project data analysis or findings dissemination.

Tips for involving patients and services users are covered in Chapter 17.

Step 4: Formulate the research aims, questions, hypotheses and objectives

Time spent formulating compelling and answerable research questions is always time well spent. A good research question should be focused, researchable, feasible, specific and relevant (McCombes, 2023). Most studies will have an over-arching aim or question, which will anchor the research and be reflected in the titles of journal articles.

For some studies it may be appropriate to have one or more hypotheses, or formal statements, which predict what the research will find. The planned research activities will support or refute a hypothesis. Furthermore, all studies will have objectives, which are the steps to be taken to address their aim(s).

Writing a good question is explored further in Chapter 7.

Step 5: Choose study design and methodologies

The choice of study design and associated methodologies is heavily influenced by the research question.

- *Descriptive studies* that seek to understand how often people get certain health conditions or access suitable healthcare are often addressed by large epidemiological studies known as prevalence or incidence studies (descriptive epidemiology).

Chapter 3 — Making sense of the research process

- *Causal questions*, including intervention studies, will require a study that allows inference of causality, such as a randomised controlled trial.
- *Exploratory studies*, such as those seeking to understand a phenomenon or how people experience a health event or care episode, may best be addressed through qualitative or experiential designs and methods.

Quantitative, qualitative and mixed methods approaches are covered in more detail in Section 2 of this book.

It may be possible to answer your research question using existing data, or what is known as secondary data sources. This could be existing original data from previous research studies, from healthcare databases or registries, or government administrative data. These data may be quantitative, qualitative or a mix of both. Studies adopting meta-analytical approaches, for example Bauer et al. (2020), analyse the findings of previously performed scientific studies, answering the same research question. Meta-analysis can offer researchers a powerful approach to draw robust conclusions, and use of existing data is cost-effective, as the high front-end cost of data collection has already been undertaken.

Step 6: Write the protocol and estimate financial and/or in-kind resources needed

Once you have determined the aims and design of your study, you need to prepare a document that summarises how you will conduct the study. This is called a research protocol (or research proposal). A protocol is a key research document that details the rationale for a study and all the methods and process steps that will be undertaken to deliver the study. Protocols are formal documents that should have version numbers, an audit trail of changes and are 'locked' once finalised and approved. Any subsequent protocol amendments are then saved as a new version of the document, may need approval from funders and ethics/governance bodies, and then are 'locked' again. Most health or health funding authorities will have guidance on what a protocol should include. Example templates for research conducted in the NHS (UK) can be found on the Health Research Authority website.

A protocol will often be developed iteratively – an initial protocol will be written to support an application for funding which, if successful, will be finalised as part of ethical and governance approval processes. As the protocol includes detailed information on how the research will be conducted, it is essential in helping estimate the financial or other resources needed to deliver the study. Questions which may need to be answered in your protocol include the following.

- How many people will you be recruiting to your study?
- How long do you think this will take?
- Do you need research staff to do the recruiting or will potential participants be responding to publicly distributed invitations and self-enrolling, such as with online surveys?

- If it is an interventional study, what are the intervention delivery costs?
- Who will be doing the analysis, and how long will they be involved with the study?
- Do you need to purchase specialist software or equipment?
- How will you disseminate your study findings and do you need to budget for publication costs, workshops, social media, etc.?

All these considerations inform the budget and resource estimates. This will all inform the timeline for your activities, often represented in the form of a Gantt chart which is a visual representation of a schedule of activities.

Protocol development is explored further in Chapter 20.

Step 7: Apply for funding

Securing financial support is necessary for the delivery of most research studies. Experimental studies that require significant personnel time and specific expertise, such as a randomised controlled trial to test a new practice or treatment, and studies that have substantial recruitment costs, such as those that involve hundreds or thousands of participants, require funding.

However, not all research seeks or needs dedicated funding. Studies conducted as part of a clinician's or academic's usual work may be done within existing resources. Studies undertaken by students may have minimal financial support requirements or needs that are met by their university. Some research studies use secondary data sources, such as systematic reviews or clinical practice 'grey' literature, so there are no or minimal additional resources required apart from researcher time.

All universities and many healthcare organisations, including ambulance services, will have research departments that can help you identify potential funders, and may also be able to help you prepare your funding application. In the UK, the National Institute for Health and Care Research (NIHR) Research Support Service (National Institute for Health and Care Research, 2024) offers individuals free and confidential advice to develop funding applications. Be aware, it can take *at least* six months, and often much longer, to prepare and submit a competitive application for research funding. Preparation and responding to feedback are key! There are always more people applying for grant money than can be funded, and success rates can be below 10%; you may need to apply two (or more) times to receive a successful funding outcome.

More tips for funding are provided in Chapter 21.

Step 8: Obtain ethics, governance and approvals

For participant safety, organisational reputation and quality reasons, a study cannot commence until the appropriate permissions and approvals are in place. In the UK, healthcare research involving human participants may require Health Research Authority (HRA) approval prior to commencement. Research involving humans, or

Chapter 3 — Making sense of the research process

that uses information from humans including biological samples, may also require approval from a research ethics committee or board. Certain types of research designs, such as where informed consent cannot be obtained from the study participants due to incapacity or being unconscious, will undergo additional scrutiny and approval processes.

Governance refers to oversight of how a study is run. As part of good governance, some funders will require the inclusion of a study or trial steering committee, which comprises independent researchers and experts who will provide oversight in study delivery on behalf of the funder. They will meet regularly with the research team during the course of the study.

All research also needs some form of approval from the institutional body and sponsor that has oversight of the research. As a study sponsor, an organisation takes overall responsibility for proportionate, effective arrangements being in place to set up, run and report a research project (Health Research Authority, 2023a).

Further details on ethics and governance are provided in Chapter 16.

Step 9: Data collection

Whatever type of study you are planning, a rigorous approach to designing data collection is essential to promote participant engagement and collection of reliable and valid data, and to ensure the research question/s are answered. The methods of data collection need to be acceptable to participants, not unduly burdensome and should use the best available measures that are feasible for the scope and budget of the project.

Primary data

Data types may include interviews, observations or surveys, in addition to clinical measures such as physiological, cognitive, neurological and biological assessments. Each data collection approach will require a careful process of selection to understand best practice for each measure, which considers your study context and resources. For example, it may be best practice to physically measure height and weight to estimate body mass index, but this is frequently self-reported by participants in studies that do not have any direct participant contact due to budget or other constraints. Your study protocol will need to detail handling of collected data before the data are processed for analysis. For biological samples, this may include procedures for collection, transport, storage, processing and then disposal at study end. For self-reported data, such as from online surveys or interviews, the protocol needs to specify how and when the data are collected, by whom, how data are stored or shared with other organisations, and methods of disposal at study end.

Secondary data

Your study may be using existing datasets, such as a trauma registry (see Mansour et al., 2022) or population survey (see Stevelink et al., 2020), so there are no new data to be collected. You still have to justify in your study protocol why these existing data sources are fit for purpose and that they include appropriate measures of your constructs of interest. For data collection for a systematic review, where the data are sourced from existing publications such as journal articles and grey literature reports, a data extraction tool will be developed and applied to standardise what data are extracted and how they are coded. The Cochrane Collaboration and Joanna Briggs Institute (JBI) provide examples of data extraction templates for systematic reviews of quantitative and qualitative studies.

Further detail on data collection considerations is provided in Section 2.

Step 10: Analysis

Once you have collected or collated your data, it is time to analyse the data and test your hypotheses (if applicable). The first step is cleaning, which is a term referring to the process of preparing a dataset for analysis. It may involve checking missing data and data integrity and combining different sources of data into a single database ready for analysis.

Depending on the nature of your study, you may conduct the analysis yourself, often with support and supervision of more experienced researchers, or with a specialist data analyst. In writing your protocol, you will have already detailed the type of quantitative (i.e. statistical) or qualitative (i.e. thematic) analysis techniques you intend to use and, where relevant, any computer software you will be using. There are a variety of software packages available; those commonly used are NVivo, Qualtrics, Stata, SPSS, ATLAS.ti and MAXQDA.

It is good practice to involve all research team members in data analysis and interpretation where feasible. This is particularly so for patient and public members of the team, who can provide unique insights into data patterns and meaning and help make the results more real for people with lived experience.

Further detail is provided in Chapters 11, 14 and 15.

Step 11: Write-up

Knowing the findings of your study which, hopefully, have answered your research questions, it is time to finalise the write-up of your study. Often, study funders will have requested an interim or annual report, which aids the writing of the final report or dissertation and subsequent publications. The research protocol can be very useful here; it detailed what was planned, so can be amended to describe what actually did occur and form part of your paper/report/dissertation.

The typical format for research reports is:

- background/rationale/introduction
- aims and objectives

Chapter 3 — Making sense of the research process

- methods
- results
- discussion and conclusion
- implications for policy and practice (if appropriate).

Step 12: Dissemination and impact activities

Preparing a journal article and report to funder are important steps in getting your findings out to research end-users, but these formats are not readily accessible to all the potential stakeholders interested in your study. Not everyone has the time or interest to read detailed, academic, scientific journal articles. Lay summaries can be useful resources for wide dissemination; involving patient and public research team members in their production can ensure they have the desired impact and facilitate practice or policy change.

Funding bodies increasingly expect researchers to detail in advance how they will communicate their findings to diverse audiences. Currently, approaches being used include social and general media, blogs or vlogs, podcasts, easy-read guides and visual depictions of results (infographics). Follow-on activities such as hosting a stakeholder panel and undertaking a Delphi study (Barrett and Heale, 2020) can aid dissemination and prioritisation of study findings.

Additional activities, also called impact activities, can increase the likelihood of your findings being adopted in practice or by policy makers. These could include meeting with policy makers or commissioners to share how your findings could be implemented in practice, and the funding needed to achieve this. It could be by making a submission to government inquiries to advocate for change. You may wish to help charities and other advocacy bodies communicate your findings to stakeholders.

Further detail is provided in Chapter 19.

These steps in the research process are repeated as needed. For example, a study might have two phases: intervention refinement and tailoring to specific groups, and then being tested in a randomised controlled trial. The two phases of the study might have different stakeholders, different methodologies, separate ethics and governance applications, and separate data collection, analysis and write-up.

Summary

This chapter has provided an overview of the steps in the research process, from study conceptualisation to dissemination to research end-users. For some studies the steps will be linear and in sequence, for others the steps may progress in parallel or are repeated as needed for different stages of the study. Careful consideration of each step will help you design research that is a priority for patients, the public and services, and is rigorous and valid. A well-executed research process helps produce new research evidence that is more likely to be translated into practice and policy.

Useful resources

- Library and Knowledge Service for NHS Ambulance Services in England: https://ambulance.libguides.com/home1/partners
- National Ambulance Research Steering Group: https://narsg.uk/

Chapter 4

Clinical audit, quality improvement, service evaluation and innovation: what are they?

Duncan Robertson and Mary Peters

> **Purpose of this chapter**
>
> Completion of this chapter will help you to:
> - understand the differences and similarities between clinical audit, service evaluation, quality improvement and innovation
> - understand the roles these activities have in healthcare
> - identify the key characteristics of these different approaches.

Introduction

Research, clinical audit, quality improvement, service evaluation and innovation all drive progress in healthcare, but in different ways. They are concepts that represent activities with specific applications, which produce different outcomes. Each is characterised by a multiplicity of techniques, methods and theories, yet all are aimed at making improvements in patient outcomes via direct changes to clinical practice or indirectly through systems changes. While meanings and purpose may differ, each concept exists within, and is defined through the application of, a set of rules which govern the nature of the specific enquiry. Such rules provide further insights into the individual strengths and weaknesses.

To the uninitiated, there may appear to be methodological overlaps between the different activities, and the terminology can often be confusing. In addition, some aspects may appear in different organisational or academic silos, with philosophical distance between practitioners of their respective arts, each championing their school of thought and quick to point out the flaws in the other. However, a detailed understanding of the techniques enables individual clinicians and organisations to critically understand the place that each approach occupies, to make the best use and understand the inherent limitations of each to inform practice and policy.

It is important to recognise that none of the approaches discussed in this chapter sits in isolation. Each is strengthened by a deeper appreciation of the other and as

Chapter 4 — Clinical audit, quality improvement, service evaluation and innovation

health systems increase in their complexity, understanding these methods enables greater focus on the delivery of better quality care. This does not always mean the implementation of something new, as it is equally important to recognise when to de-implement or withdraw a technique, procedure or treatment according to the evidence base.

Determining which of the techniques described in this chapter is the most appropriate to deploy is guided by the nature and design of the question being asked (see Chapter 7). A soundly structured line of inquiry linked to a well-written question will enable the selection of the approach most suited to efficiently seek the answer. The curious individual will begin by making fundamental choices, such as are they after assurance or do they seek new knowledge? Are they looking to make an improvement, are they wanting to evaluate something that exists already or are they applying something into a new operational context? These choices are bound by a series of unconscious and conscious biases linked to personal ontologies and preferred epistemological approaches (see Chapters 3 and 5).

This is a textbook for paramedics, and while we recognise that many paramedics practise outside ambulance services, it is important that concepts are tied to readily-recognised clinical scenarios. World Health Organization data (2021a) indicate that cardiovascular diseases are the leading cause of deaths globally, of which 85% were due to heart attack or stroke. The treatment of S-T segment myocardial infarction (STEMI) over the last 20 years of ambulance and paramedic practice has been driven by innovation, research, audit, service evaluation and quality improvement. Using STEMI as a focus, the purpose of this chapter is to provide an overview of clinical audit, quality improvement and service evaluation to enable them to be considered in context through published studies. Clearly, research is the main focus of this book and so, to avoid repetition, it will not be addressed in this chapter.

Clinical audit

NHS England defines clinical audit as follows.

> *Clinical audit is a way to find out if healthcare is being provided in line with standards and lets care providers and patients know where their service is doing well, and where there could be improvements.*
>
> (NHS England, n.d.)

One of the earliest documented clinical audits is accepted as that of King Hammurabi (1810–1750 BCE) who instructed his war surgeons to measure the effectiveness of their care (Modayil et al., 2009). Florence Nightingale measured care using polar area diagrams which led to key changes, changing mortality from 40% to 20%; she believed that 'to understand God's thoughts we must study statistics' (Short, 1999). Donabedian, one of the forefathers of modern clinical audit, divided the quality of healthcare measures into structure, process and outcomes in his publication 'Evaluating the quality of medical care' (1966) and by 1985 he published the trilogy 'Explorations in quality and assessment and monitoring'. Arguably, this laid the foundations for modern-day clinical audit.

Clinical audit

> ### Box 4.1
>
> **Brief history of clinical audit in the NHS**
>
> **1989** 'Working for Patients' White Paper – aimed at doctors, described local audit teams and medical audit advisory groups as well as reflective practice using the process to improve the quality of patient care.
>
> **1997** 'The New NHS: Modern, Dependable' introduced the concept of clinical governance, identifying clinical audit as a key mechanism to measure quality of care and extended clinical audit to be undertaken by nurses and other healthcare professionals.
>
> **2002** 'Principles for Best Practice in Clinical Audit' was published by the National Institute for Clinical Excellence which formalised best practice in clinical audit.
>
> **2008** Department of Health reinvigorated local and national clinical audit.
>
> **2012** Department of Health awarded the local and national clinical audit contract to the Health Quality and Improvement Partnership (HQIP).

Box 4.1 describes the growth and development of clinical audit in the NHS, the key feature of which being that it is a cyclical process enabling clinicians to review their own clinical practice and organisations to review quality. It has a systematic quality improvement intent that directly engages those involved in the care process by comparing actual practice to agreed standards which are linked to good outcomes.

Clinical audit data are used to benchmark and improve patient care, and clinical audit seeks to improve multidisciplinary working within and across clinical teams and should be an integral part of clinical practice. The clinical audit process measures whether patients are receiving the best clinical care possible (as recognised within the evidence base) by assessing clinical interventions against those standards, identifying any gaps and considering how to improve compliance against the recognised standards if needed. It is a cyclical process, which links in with the quality improvement methodology 'Plan, Do, Study, Act' (PDSA).

Clinical audit relies on the existence of evidence-based standards, identified through research evidence such as those of the National Institute for Health and Care Excellence (NICE) in England and Wales and Health Improvement Scotland (SIGN) in Scotland. NICE has developed a clinical audit tool based on the standards for the management of chest pain of suspected cardiac origin. Not all elements are applicable for use by UK ambulance services, but the immediate management of a suspected acute coronary syndrome contains standards which are relevant and set out in Box 4.2.

Unlike some research studies, clinical audit does not seek to test a hypothesis and is driven by data standards that are at once defined and measurable. As there is no change in the patient pathway, there is no requirement for ethical approval, although the use of data must comply with data protection standards.

Chapter 4 — Clinical audit, quality improvement, service evaluation and innovation

> **Box 4.2**
>
> **Clinical guidelines for management of chest pain of suspected cardiac origin**
>
> NICE NG 185 (NICE, 2020)
>
> - Offer pain relief as soon as possible. This may be achieved with GTN (sublingual or buccal), but offer intravenous opioids such as morphine, particularly if an acute myocardial infarction (MI) is suspected.
> - Offer people a single loading dose of 300 mg aspirin as soon as possible unless there is clear evidence that they are allergic to it. If aspirin is given before arrival at hospital, send a written record that it has been given with the person.
> - Do not routinely administer oxygen, but monitor oxygen saturation using pulse oximetry as soon as possible, ideally before hospital admission. Only offer supplemental oxygen to:
>   - people with oxygen saturation (SpO_2) of less than 94% who are not at risk of hypercapnic respiratory failure, aiming for SpO_2 of 94–98%
>   - people with chronic obstructive pulmonary disease who are at risk of hypercapnic respiratory failure, to achieve a target SpO_2 of 88–92% until blood gas analysis is available.
>
> SIGN guidance 148 (SIGN, 2016) supports a number of similar clinical interventions and has referenced them directly with the research evidence.
>
> - Patients with acute coronary syndrome should have continuous cardiac rhythm monitoring.
> - There is no evidence that routine administration of oxygen to all patients with the broad spectrum of ACS improves clinical outcome or reduces infarction size.
> - Aspirin halves (absolute risk reduction (RR) 5.3%, relative RR 46%) the rate of vascular events (cardiovascular death, non-fatal MI and non-fatal stroke) in patients with unstable angina and reduces it by nearly a third (absolute RR 3.8%, relative RR 30%) in those with acute MI.
> - Nitrates should be used in patients with acute coronary syndrome to relieve cardiac pain due to continuing myocardial ischaemia or to treat acute heart failure.
>
> 1+: Well-conducted meta-analyses, systematic reviews or RCTs with a low risk of bias.

The largest UK clinical audit project related to STEMI is managed through the National Institute for Cardiovascular Outcomes Research, and is known by the acronym MINAP (Myocardial Ischaemia National Audit Project). This large-scale audit requires engagement across the whole of the healthcare system, and includes information from ambulance services through to patient discharge. The latest report (NICOR, 2024) refers to the audit (measurement) outcomes and then links across into quality improvement and is a good example of how clinical audit and quality improvement are entwined.

Quality improvement

Quality improvement (QI) refers to the systematic use of methods and tools to try to continuously improve quality of care and outcomes for patients. There are a range of different methods and tools, such as Lean, Six Sigma and the Institute for Healthcare Improvement's Model for Improvement. There is no clear evidence that one technique is superior to others; rather, it is the process of having a systematic approach to quality improvement and applying this consistently that is important (Ross and Naylor, 2017).

All NHS organisations in England are required to improve the quality of the care they deliver. The NHS Next Stage Review (Department of Health, 2008) defined quality based on three criteria:

- *Safety*: doing no harm to patients.
- *Experience of care*: this should be characterised by compassion, dignity and respect.
- *Effectiveness of care*: including preventing people from dying prematurely, enhancing quality of life and helping people to recover following episodes of ill health.

The Health Foundation (2021) refers to the same criteria and adds a further three dimensions for those providing services which should be:

- *Well-led*: open and collaborate internally and externally and committed to learning and improvement.
- *Sustainable*: use resources responsibly and efficiently, providing fair access to all and according to the need of their populations.
- *Equitable*: provide care that does not vary in quality because of a person's characteristics.

Quality improvement is a creative process and requires several factors to be addressed before an improvement intervention can be developed, including the following:

- *Understand the problem*: understand how and why the problem has arisen. It is important to use data from a number of sources, staff, patients and

Chapter 4 — Clinical audit, quality improvement, service evaluation and innovation

service users to avoid treating the symptoms rather than the root cause of the problem. Consider capacity, flow and backlog.

- *Design an improvement and delivery plan*: to design a specific aim with measurable targets, aligning the aim of the intervention with the organisation's goals. Learning from others is key here to avoid repeating mistakes made previously.

- *Data measurement*: in order to measure the impact of the change the intervention has brought, it is necessary to undertake a baseline measurement of the current situation without intervention. Quality improvement requires regular measurements that may take the form of process as well as outcome measures. Invariably the data are processed using statistical process control methodology which enables the 'ruling out' of common cause variation that we would expect to take place regardless of the improvement intervention.

- *Reliability*: the improvement of system and process reliability, reducing variation through staff willingness to identify hazards and safety problems by investing in identifying and learning from errors.

Foreshadowing quality improvement in healthcare are the methods of quality control used in industry. There are many quality improvement techniques, and the challenge is in selecting the best tool for improvement. One of the most commonly used QI tools is the Model for Improvement which uses the familiar PDSA cycle (Langley et al., 2009). Here, instead of measuring against recognised standards as in clinical audit, in QI an idea for a change that may lead to improvement is tested. The impact of the idea is measured and the data are studied, which may generate a new idea or iteration, and the cycle is repeated.

The small tests of change in QI are linked to three questions:

- What are we trying to accomplish?
- How will we know that a change is an improvement?
- What changes can we make that will result in an improvement?

Quality improvement collaboration is a QI mechanism which engages multidisciplinary teams within a single organisation or, more usually, teams from across multiple organisations. In using a structured approach, setting targets and undertaking rapid cycles of change and sharing the learning across the teams, a healthcare system can be improved. The Health Foundation (2014) paper 'Improvement collaboratives in healthcare' addresses the questions about the effectiveness of collaboratives in healthcare. Four key factors were identified that need to be present to promote successful outcomes:

- Focus on who should be included.
- Consider the topic focus.
- Consider how to run activities.
- Provide appropriate resources.

One example of a successful QI collaborative is the longitudinal study by Scholz et al. (2020) which describes how, by using QI methodology over time, the team were able to provide evidence that supported the cardiology guidelines. In short, the guidelines, based on research evidence, recommended that repetitive monitoring and feedback are key in the management of STEMI patients. The team instituted a ten-year programme collaborating with local STEMI management teams across six primary percutaneous coronary intervention (PPCI) centres in Germany. This QI methodology can be described as a QI collaborative. In addition, Howard et al. (2019) described the sustained success of a national QI initiative aimed at improving the care received by STEMI patients in Qatar. They were aware of the standards they were reporting against in their clinical audit and deployed QI methods to make improvements to the documented care, therefore demonstrating the importance of linking audit and improvement together for the benefit of patients.

While some QI activity can be scalable, it cannot be said to be generalisable across systems in the same way that the results of research studies might be. While research seeks to control variables, the iterative deployment and refinement of QI in an operational context mean that solutions will be dependent on such variables to work optimally and often seek to alter the behaviour of actors within a system to provide a measurable improvement.

Service evaluation

The Health Foundation (2015) uses three definitions for service evaluation:

- The process of determining the merit, worth or value of something.
- Using systematic, data-based inquiries about whatever is being evaluated.
- A process undertaken for the purposes of improvement, decision making, enlightenment and persuasion.

Service evaluation is concerned with providing data to support decision making. Often, evaluation will use data readily available from clinical audit and performance management and triangulate these with other data to support the evaluation.

Evaluations take several forms and the form selected should be the one that best suits your desired outcome and will depend on factors including what you hope to learn, the length of time and budget available and what the stakeholders need from the exercise.

A formative evaluation is a parallel process that occurs during the lifetime of the intervention and can generate data that are used to modify the original intervention premise. The data (quantitative and qualitative) are combined to inform judgements about the effectiveness of the intervention. Alternatively, a summative evaluation is traditionally carried out at the end of an intervention process when all the data are available to determine if it was successful or not – whether the intervention worked and the objective was met. Summative evaluation is best used when the intervention and the environment in which it is being used are unlikely to change during the

Chapter 4 — Clinical audit, quality improvement, service evaluation and innovation

evaluation period. The value of a summative evaluation is that the stakeholders are provided with all the information to consider if the intervention was valuable and if it should continue, be modified or rolled out across a wider intervention footprint.

A widely-used technique is the developmental evaluation — a methodology used in collaborative change QI processes, which is best employed in complex and/or unstable environments. A modification of formative evaluation, it relies on mutual collaboration between the intervention team and those doing the evaluation work, trying out new ideas, recording and assessing their impact as the data emerge. This means the intervention and its original aims may change, requiring the teams to be open to responsive methods of working.

While service evaluation may be argued to lack rigour, successful evaluations use research methods as a known framework. In addition, as they evaluate something that is in operation, rather than a novel intervention, they do not require the same level of ethical approval to proceed as they are not considered to be research.

Platt (2020) neatly described the process of a service evaluation in practice where the 'golden question' was to determine the factors that affected the transport destination, hospital characteristics and survival rates. The question could not be answered through audit methodology, as there are no standards to measure against, nor could it be immediately, addressed through QI methodology, as the 'issue' was not identified. Therefore, in the absence of standards, and clarity of the issue, service evaluation methodology was the most appropriate.

Hsia et al. (2020) explored through evaluation, using a cohort study methodology, whether regionalisation of services was associated with widened or narrowed disparities in access to treatment and outcomes for patients with STEMI. They concluded that patients in minority communities derived significantly smaller improvements relative to non-minority communities. This opened a conversation regarding equity of access to STEMI care.

Innovation

The core definition of innovation depends on the lens through which it is observed. Greenhalgh et al. (2004) define innovation in service delivery as:

> *... a novel set of behaviours, routines, and ways of working that are directed at improving health outcomes, administrative efficiency, cost effectiveness, or users' experience and that are implemented by planned and coordinated actions.*

The attributes of a successful healthcare innovation are further described by Greenhalgh (2019) as displaying a relative advantage, low complexity, compatibility, observability, trialability, potential for reinvention and, for technologies, ease of use. The Royal College of Nursing (RCN) uses West and Farr's definition (1990) as a purposeful change to realise specific benefits, without the need for the idea to be brand new, but new within a specific context. However, innovation is a term that can be applied at a series of scales, from the individual to the system (West et al., 2017).

Some innovations are small-scale and align more closely to QI through creating measurable efficiencies (Health Foundation, 2021). Larger-scale innovations require the application of the scientific method and rigour to ensure that they are ethically the right thing to do. Pacifico Silva et al. (2018) argue that within innovation, there needs to be an ethical framework that acknowledges the growth of new technologies in health that raise complex policy challenges. Their integrated approach aims to address what they describe as the distinct goals of health and innovation policies to better articulate the supply of innovation to the demand of health systems. Innovation is not just technology, and the King's Fund (Collins, 2018) describes entrepreneurs and innovators within health who enable better care by mobilising low-cost therapies to marginalised groups or break down traditional siloed thinking.

A particular challenge within innovation described by Collins (2018) is that of scale and spread. Greenhalgh et al. (2004) recognised that for an innovation to be a success, it is the relative advantage that stimulates this. Collins (2018) likewise acknowledges that traditional methods of communicating innovation do not lend themselves to ensuring adoption, leading to only the most 'sticky' innovations getting adopted.

Dixon-Woods et al. (2011) identify three paradoxes within innovation; the first describes the uptake and diffusion of innovations with limited or no benefit while others which might be more beneficial don't make it into practice. The second paradox is the death of innovation delivered through democratic processes while the third is that with the pace of innovation, there is limited capacity for whole systems to keep up with the pace of change. Within the paper, they argue that a critical lens needs to be applied to ensure that there is recognition of innovation that steps into the realms of a clinical experiment, as opposed to the normal experiential learning that continually improves healthcare. For the former, they acknowledge the requirement to then use the same level of evidence and oversight as other clinical interventions, that is, the basis of research methodologies.

Current treatments for STEMI are based on a culmination of multiple innovative practices and thoughts that have driven large-scale, population-based improvements through the novel application of technologies. Agich (2001) identified limitations within the model of medical ethics deployed in the USA when innovation was required, arguing that the rigid structure of the scientific research method may not enable the iterations required for innovation to occur. Nevertheless, he acknowledges that the aim is to protect the patient from harm, which is the essence of ethics in studies. In some cases, he states, significant developmental processes must occur first to bring a procedure to the point at which formal research is possible. He uses the example of coronary artery bypass grafting (CABG), the 'procedures for which evolved against a background of no or poor therapeutic options, underwent technical alterations as they were employed and were dependent on analogous advances in imaging, anaesthesia and postoperative care'.

Innovation is therefore a looser term that takes into consideration a range of methodologies, from the iterative approaches of quality improvement to the rigorous

Chapter 4 — Clinical audit, quality improvement, service evaluation and innovation

approach of controlled trials. Innovation is naturally disruptive and may require the redefinition and reframing of ethical constructs to be applied safely in health.

From the perspective of STEMI care, innovations were driven by treatments delivered in hospital. Over time, with the introduction of thrombolytic therapies, there was the realisation that to be more effective, administration as close to the point of infarct, or call, would improve mortality and was feasible (Myers, 1998; Pedley et al., 2003). Studies such as Pitt (2002) provided evidence that paramedics could select cases suitable for thrombolysis. With the additional training and the deployment of reliable portable 12-lead ECGs, it became possible for thrombolysis to be part of the paramedic's skill set. Further innovations within the hospital driven by technology enabled the widespread use of balloon angioplasty to recanalise occluded coronary arteries, and multiple studies demonstrated the superiority of PPCI over thrombolytic therapies. In addition, the realisation that centralised services offered a safer (through more practised) application of PPCI required further technological innovation to support paramedics to bypass the nearest ED to take the patient to definitive care. Innovations included telemetry on the 12-lead ECG to transmit the diagnostic trace to the specialist team, as well as advances in communications technologies to enable greater coverage of mobile phone signals.

As an emerging profession, the opportunities for innovation within paramedic practice are broad. As Newton et al. (2020) proposed, the paramedic profession itself resulted from disruptive innovation, and practice, as it continues to evolve from a focus on emergency to unscheduled care, lends itself to further disruptive innovations as the profession shifts from its early roots. Nevertheless, innovation in paramedic practice has to be safe for patients, and delivered within a rigorous ethical framework. The challenge is not only deciding with clarity on the definition of innovation and its scope, but also to perhaps resist, through critical thought, the temptation to innovate solely through the application of new technology when lower-cost innovations may confer more benefit to the patients we treat.

Summary

As detailed above, not all questions relating to clinical care, services and improvements can be answered by research alone. Clinical audit is a safe endeavour as long as the data are used as designed and in line with legislation. However, quality improvement, service evaluation and innovation may require the use of the rigorous standards required by research in terms of ethical considerations and protection of the participant, which may be largely dependent on the scale and nature of the enquiry. Therefore, the choice of method to use should be undertaken with knowledge of the strengths and limitations inherent in each approach as outlined in the chapter.

As we can see, research may only take patient care so far. The other techniques described here can often be applied faster and gain results sooner. Within modern healthcare, with its associated pressures in terms of time, expectation and the need to develop rapidly under funding constraints, this confers an advantage, as detailed research trials often take many years to set up, for the results to be analysed and subsequently published. However, characteristics of research and of the other techniques should be recognised and Table 4.1 outlines the comparative aspects of each.

Table 4.1 Summary of characteristics of the different activities.

	Research	Clinical audit	Service evaluation	Quality improvement	Innovation
Designed to:	Generate new knowledge	Determine if the quality of a service meets a defined standard through systematic measurement against explicit criteria to enable focused change for improvement	Explore what is happening in a service as well as outcomes and experiences for patients	Improve patient care and experience through testing changes	Create or apply something new or something existing within a novel context
Nature	Tests a predicted but not necessarily proven hypothesis. Explores relationships between variables such as clinical processes and outcomes	Compares actual patient care to the type of care that represents best practice (explicit standards) and acts on the findings to improve the delivery of best practice	Considers the cumulative effectiveness of a service following evaluation of a service against expected outcomes	Uses data to identify problems in the delivery of care and their causes, and acts to achieve improvement through tests of change	Creates something that is new in order to grow a new process, service or product. Almost all innovation is improvement, but not all improvement is innovation. Has three components: novelty, application and intended benefit
Ethics	Requires research ethics committee review	Should have oversight of projects to identify and address any ethical issues	Should have oversight of projects to identify and address any ethical issues	Should have oversight of projects to identify and address any ethical issues	Should have oversight of projects to identify and address any ethical issues

(*Continued*)

Chapter 4 — Clinical audit, quality improvement, service evaluation and innovation

Table 4.1 (Continued).

	Research	Clinical audit	Service evaluation	Quality improvement	Innovation
Data	Uses secondary and primary data sources. Secondary: research already published. Selecting data using certain criteria adds to increasing levels of research validity and reliability. Criteria to be considered include date of publication, author credentials, depth of analysis, and quality of discussions and extent of the contribution to the area of interest. Primary data are those derived from the activity of research. They may be quantitative in nature and rely on mathematical interpretation through correlation and regression as well as mean, median and mode analysis. Qualitative data analysis is used extensively in research	Quality of data is embedded in all stages of clinical audit. The data must be fit for purpose, unbiased, complete, valid, timely and reliable. Audit relies on sampling. It may be representative: simple, stratified and systematic random sampling. It may be non-representative: purposive, convenience and quota sampling. Requires adherence to data collection protocols: cleansing, triangulation, identification of auditor fatigue. Uses: control charts to display data	Qualitative and quantitative and described as a balanced scorecard. May be summative evaluation: makes a judgement. May be formative: evaluation ongoing. Outcome evaluations look at the impact of the project and are explicitly summative. Process evaluations look at the internal operation and may be summative and formative. May be unitary, from a single organisation or profession perspective, or pluralistic, from multiple stakeholders, and will include the unintended consequences	Important to capture the baseline prior to the intervention. Measurement at regular intervals to gauge impact of the intervention. Uses statistical process control (SPC) to examine the difference between common cause and special cause variation. May be unitary, from a single organisation or profession perspective, or pluralistic, from multiple stakeholders, and will include the unintended consequences	Data-driven innovation – use of data and analytics to improve new products. Data motivate ideation, development, execution and evaluation Big data – large-volume data structured and unstructured which are analysed for insights. Caution: big data analysis can create bias, e.g. digital race recognition issues for people of colour as unintended consequence of big data analysis by white analysts

Chapter 5

Research paradigms

Cheryl Cameron, Adam Greene and Alan M. Batt

> **Purpose of this chapter**
>
> Completion of this chapter will help you to:
> - outline the benefits of engaging with elements of a research paradigm, and the risks of not doing so
> - describe the main components of a research paradigm
> - describe common research paradigms and their characteristics
> - identify methodological approaches and methods used within paradigms
> - describe the role of conceptual frameworks in conducting research.

Introduction

Research in paramedicine (and more broadly) is about answering questions such as the following:

- How do people perceive the care they receive from paramedics?
- What are the experiences of paramedic students on placement?
- How safe is paramedic-delivered care?
- What do we know about the role paramedics play in primary care?
- What is the clinical and cost-effectiveness of ambulance clinician administration of peripheral nerve blocks in adult patients over 65 years of age with a hip fracture?

Researchers answer these (and many other) questions using various research paradigms – knowingly or unknowingly. Philosophical assumptions underpin every research approach, and considering these in advance will help to provide clarity (and promote alignment) between your worldview, your questions and the conclusions you come to from your analysis of data.

Writing a chapter on research paradigms is a risky undertaking for several reasons. First, philosophers and epistemologists disagree on many definitions and elements of paradigms. Keep this in mind if you access other resources describing research paradigms, as they may present this material from differing perspectives. Second, researchers in paramedicine have historically avoided meaningful engagement with concepts related to paradigms, theories and frameworks despite their foundational importance to every research question asked. This may be due to a biomedical foundation and evolution that revered gold-standard 'objective evidence'. Paramedicine did not (and some would argue still does not) place the same value on more subjective ways of knowing. Finally, the mere mention of philosophy or epistemology to undergraduate (and graduate!) paramedic students often results in 'research avoidance syndrome', posing a challenge to developing future researchers in the discipline.

This chapter seeks to demystify and dispel anxiety related to philosophical perspectives by providing accessible descriptions and encouraging you to take time to delve into and grapple with these concepts. There is no rule about where you 'sit' or 'should sit' on the spectrum of paradigms. Much like political views, you may align with distinct positions based on the question you are investigating. You also have permission to not really know and evolve as you go.

What is a research paradigm?

Paradigms, theories and frameworks guide how research is conducted and how knowledge is conceptualised (Kuhn, 1994). At the highest level, research paradigms are a shared mental model – a set of beliefs, assumptions and principles that guide the way researchers understand and approach problems (Brown and Dueñas, 2020).

When a researcher adopts a set of beliefs about what they value (axiology), what they believe (doxology), how they see reality (ontology) and how they understand knowledge (epistemology), they are said to have adopted a research philosophy. These philosophical positions form some of the elements of a research paradigm (see Figure 5.1).

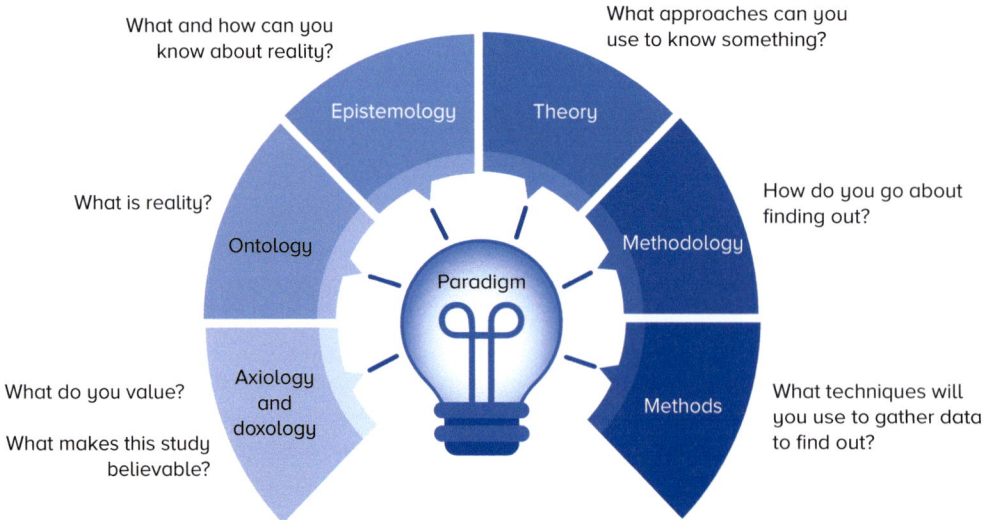

Figure 5.1 The elements of a research paradigm.
Source: Alan M. Batt, Creative Commons CC-BY 4.0 International Licence.

Informed by this philosophical position, an appropriate research methodology can then be identified, which will often determine the methods that are subsequently used to collect and analyse data. Combined, your research philosophy and methodology make up a research paradigm. Beginning to build an understanding of the philosophical underpinnings of research (through your own reading or course work) can be a useful skill to improve your research.

How will research paradigms improve my research?

As paramedicine evolves as a profession, there is a growing need for high-quality research to inform our next steps. Engaging with the elements of a research paradigm (see Figure 5.1) from the outset of your research will strengthen the trustworthiness of your work to others (thereby increasing quality) and will help inform choices throughout the project. It also allows those undertaking research in the paramedic discipline to consider and debate the very nature of knowledge they seek to create. You should understand how your research philosophy impacts your approach to the questions you want to answer. Then, guided by theory, conceptual and methodological choices, you will seek to answer these questions by collecting and analysing data. Your research will benefit from your understanding of these elements and their alignment, and this insight will help you clarify your message to your readers.

What if I do not engage with research paradigms?

Not engaging with research paradigms may result in misalignments – for example, between your own mental model and the ontological and epistemological perspectives employed (don't worry, these are explained shortly), or between your research aims and the answers you seek.

Let's assume you're interested in staff retention in the paramedic profession. If you are looking to confirm whether paramedics are leaving the profession, this is an objective truth ('Are paramedics leaving the profession?') that you can observe and measure. Therefore, an objectivist approach would best answer this problem. If instead you want to know *why* paramedics are leaving the profession, using a subjectivist approach ('Why are paramedics leaving the profession?') will help you gain insight (subjective truth). Depending on your interest, or what remains unknown about a topic, different approaches may be more appropriate or helpful.

What about other ways of knowing?

Considering the international readership of a text such as this, it seems prudent to offer some points to consider and reflect on. The very nature of knowledge, and the power to decide what counts as 'real' knowledge, are at the core of colonialism (Smith, 2021). Many of the concepts and paradigms outlined in this chapter are based on Western perspectives of truth and knowledge, and many can trace their roots back to 'old white man' scientific perspectives. There are diverse languages and cultures throughout the world and as a result, a multitude of other ways of knowing truth and approaching knowledge. Some of these ways of knowing are contextual, with deep connections to the land, water and places, and between people. Depending on the question asked

Chapter 5 — Research paradigms

and the people involved, readers may find value in learning about and engaging with decolonised and/or Black methodologies, Māori, Indigenous or Aboriginal methodologies, and culturally aware perspectives on truth and knowledge. Additional resources are outlined at the end of the chapter, but this is by no means an exhaustive list.

What are the elements of a research paradigm?

There are multiple elements that make up a research paradigm which will be explained in the pages that follow. You can refer to figure 5.2 as you read this section.

Axiology – what do you value?

Axiology is the science of inquiring into values (Bahm, 1993). A key consideration in clarifying your research paradigm is to determine (a) what you value within the research (for example, informed by ethical considerations) and (b) what values the research seeks to align with. You may find it helpful to consider who the research is targeting, and why they would value it.

This concept of value can mean different things depending on the audience. You should consider whether the research offers a societal or economic value. Perhaps you are committed to person-centred research as a value? Or maybe the primary value of the research team is cultural competence or social justice? An example that may resonate with paramedic researchers is valuing evidence-based practice. However, policy makers may value research with economic or health programming implications more than they value that with paramedic practice implications.

Next you should consider what values the research seeks to align with. Does it seek to explain or predict events or outcomes? Or does it seek to contribute to understanding an issue (contextually bound)? These value commitments will guide your choices during the research process.

Doxology – what makes this study believable?

Doxology is the study of belief-forming processes (Goldman, 2001). As a component of the research process, you should consider what actions you need to take to make the research 'believable'. This requires clear alignment between the elements of your paradigm and your methods, findings and claims. It also means maintaining an awareness of your audience. For example, paramedics may only 'believe' the findings if they relate to their own experiences. On the other hand, policy makers may only 'believe' the research findings if they consider the study design to be dependable and the claims justifiable. Audiences will consider elements of your research differently, and this is something you must address when designing your research approach.

Ontology – what is reality?

Ontology is the branch of philosophy concerned with the nature of reality and answers the fundamental question: 'What is reality?'. For example, does your research exist within the framework of a single reality? Ontological perspectives vary on a spectrum from naïve realism (there is only one reality) to relativism (reality is constructed by people and groups based on experiences). What you believe 'reality' to be has implications for

What are the elements of a research paradigm?

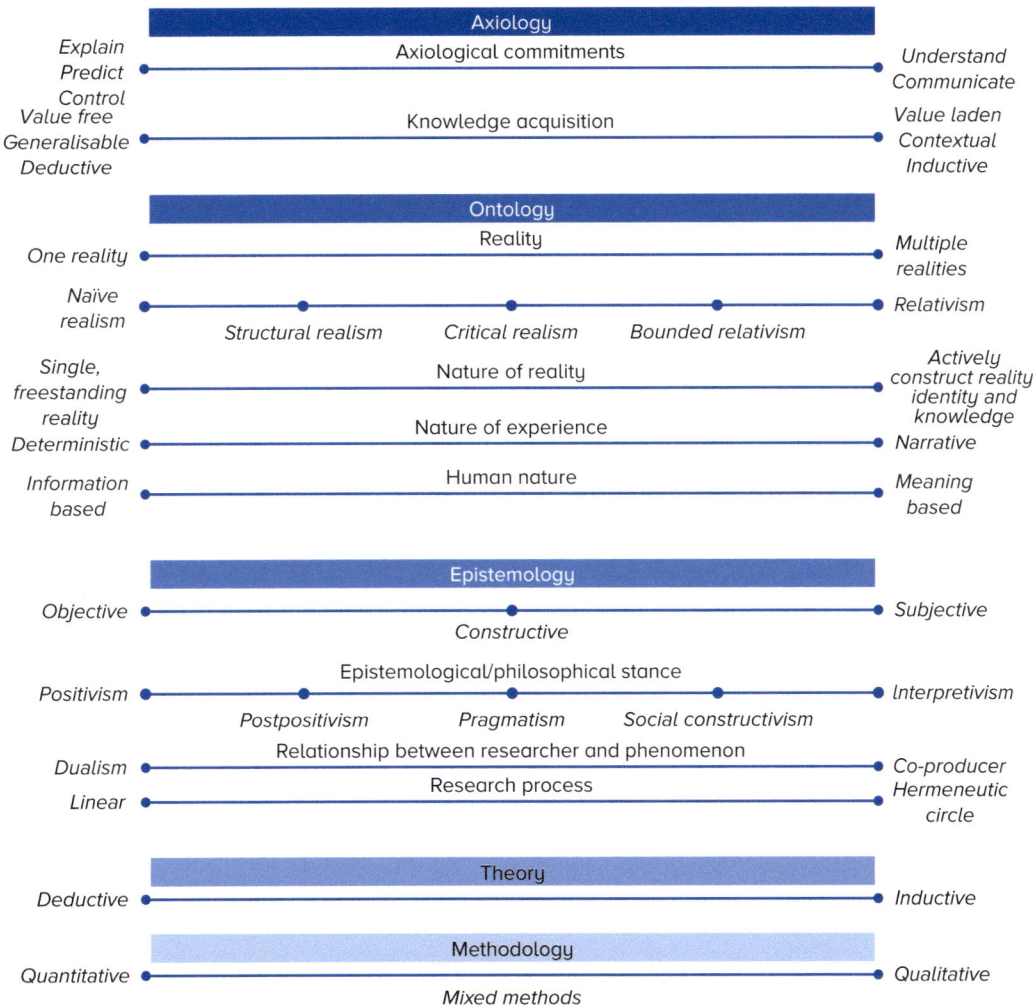

Figure 5.2 The research paradigm spectrum.
Source: Alan M. Batt, Creative Commons CC-BY 4.0 International Licence.

your position as a researcher relative to the phenomenon you are studying (including the types of questions you might be interested in and your intent). This can range from proving that something exists, through to exploring the experience of something existing or not (see Figure 5.2). An example of an ontological question would be: 'Do humans feel pain?'. There are several possible realities (or ontologies) in response to this question, such as: 'Yes, humans feel pain', 'No, humans do not feel pain' or 'The perception of pain can vary and be influenced by a variety of factors, beliefs or realities'.

Epistemology – what and how can you know about reality?

Epistemology is the branch of philosophy concerned with the nature of knowledge, and answers the theoretical question: 'How is it possible to know reality?'. Epistemology incorporates the validity, parameters and methods of acquiring knowledge. Epistemological stances vary on a spectrum from objective (we can

45

know through observation) to subjective (we may know through interpretation). What you believe about how we can know reality has implications for your position as a researcher relative to the phenomenon you are studying. This can range from that of a pure observer of a phenomenon (aligned with the positivist tradition), through to co-production with the study population (interpretivist tradition) (see Figure 5.2).

An example of an epistemological question would be: 'How is it possible to know whether a human feels pain or not?'. There are many responses to this question along a spectrum, from 'We can know pain by measuring it objectively with a scale' through to 'Pain is a complex, personal and subjective experience that must be explored from within'. Epistemological assumptions reflect what is meaningful and valid knowledge, as well as how knowledge can and should be generated.

Theory – what approaches can you use to know something?

Theories describe how concepts are related in a logically interconnected way that explains the situation or phenomenon (Varpio et al., 2020). Theories can be descriptive, explanatory, emancipatory, disruptive or predictive, and can explain broad social patterns or individual-level phenomena. All research is framed by theory, whether explicitly stated or not (Green and Thorogood, 2018), and there can be multiple theories that inform our understanding of a single phenomenon. Theories will vary along the spectrum from being deductively derived (where conclusions follow logically from premises or measurements) to inductively informed (where principles or generalised conclusions are informed by observations) (see Figure 5.2).

The use of theory can strengthen the rationale for conducting research, and is useful to place new research within broader fields of knowledge, thereby increasing transferability and principles-based approaches (Green and Thorogood, 2018).

Methodology – how do you go about finding out?

Methodology is the overarching strategy governing how you will approach your research project or question. It involves developing an approach using theories, principles and methods that align with your objectives. Your research methodology should outline how you plan to conduct your research, including the process of data collection and analysis, and demonstrate that the findings are valid. This requires the researcher to make active decisions on how they will collect and analyse data and draw conclusions. Your methodological choices guide the activities required to produce knowledge, including the research problem and questions, the approach to analysis, and the selection of methods for data collection and analysis.

Methodological approaches include qualitative, quantitative and mixed methods approaches to data collection and analysis (see Figure 5.2). For further details on quantitative research designs, please refer to Chapter 8. Qualitative research designs are discussed in more detail in Chapter 12 and mixed methods research designs in Chapter 15.

Methods – what techniques will you use to gather data?

Methods are specific procedures for collecting and analysing data in your research project. Developing your research methods is an integral part of your research design. These are often informed by your methodological choices, and require you to consider the type of data that you need to collect. For example, will your data be in the form of words, recordings, media or numbers? Will you collect the data yourself or will you use data that have already been collected for another purpose? Do you need to measure something as it occurs or do you plan to perform a controlled experiment? Will you need to combine several types of data to answer your question appropriately? For example, experimental design research methods are considered inadequate for studying complex, non-linear social issues, and therefore using such methods in this context would be inappropriate (Berwick, 2008). Methods of data collection are discussed in more detail in Chapter 9 (observational), Chapter 10 (experimental) and Chapter 13 (qualitative).

Exploring the paradigms

Research paradigms exist across an epistemological spectrum from positivism to interpretivism (Guba and Lincoln, 1994). In the descriptions of common research paradigms and their characteristics that follow, remember that others might present paradigms differently or indeed present different paradigms. In Table 5.1 you will find a brief overview of research paradigms in several paramedic-led research projects.

Positivism (objectivism) – there is only one truth and I will find it

Positivism suggests that there is a single objective reality, or truth, that exists outside the researcher (Park, Konge and Artino, 2020). This approach seeks to explain what is 'out there'. Ontologically, this is naïve realism or objectivism. Positivists believe that reality can be observed in a purely objective manner, free from culture, personal beliefs and assumptions. The researcher must be separate from the subject of research, thereby reducing bias. A useful visualisation of positivism is that of a scientist looking through a microscope – this represents the distance between the observer and the observed and the exclusion of all surrounding context (Alderson, 1998). Positivists argue that reality can be objectively observed and measured through valid and reliable tools. Positivism uses deductive reasoning to produce theories, whereby a theory is formed based on observation – derived by reason and logic from sensory experience – and this theory can then be proved or disproved with further observation or experiment. Methodological choices are often quantitative in nature to test hypotheses, for example experimental or observational studies. This often involves quantitative methods of data collection including measurement, statistical analysis and the use of scales.

Postpositivism – there is only one truth but I can never really know it

In recent years, positivism has largely been replaced by postpositivism, which relies more on critical realism and modified objectivism than naïve realism and objectivity (Guba and Lincoln, 1994). Now the dominant framework underpinning scientific research, in postpositivism objective knowledge is still the goal, but it acknowledges that one can never have a fully objective view. All observations are partial and selective, offering only an imperfect perspective, which is inherently influenced by the researcher's values and culture (Guba and Lincoln, 1994). Postpositivists understand that we can never fully observe or experience or understand reality, but still believe

Chapter 5 — Research paradigms

that one truth/reality is 'there' — we just cannot ever see it. The researcher is still an observer but there is recognition that all observations are partial and selective.

Postpositivist researchers may engage with multiple theories to inform their understanding of phenomena. They seek multiple perspectives to reduce subjectivity and improve objectivity, and thus methodological choices are often mixed methods. There is a particular alignment with sequential explanatory mixed methods designs, which tend to place more emphasis on quantitative data collection and analysis.

Realism – reality exists whether I think it does or not

Philosophical realism is the view that entities exist independently of our perception or our theories about them (Burrell and Morgan, 2019). While realist philosophy underpins much of modern health and social science, it is only recently that this philosophical approach has been popularised within mainstream health and social science literature.

Ontologically, realists may believe that there is no perfectly observable and describable reality (direct realism) or that reality is perceived through experience (sensations and images) of real objects or processes (critical realism). Things (whether they exist naturally or are social creations) are independent of whether they are recorded or perceived to exist. Realist researchers seek to explain the underlying cause or mechanisms that generate observed phenomena. Realists also view the world as consisting of strata or layers of reality which may interact with other layers to produce new mechanisms. Realists view extremes of objectivity and subjectivity as limited in their ability to answer questions. This approach is proving useful for studying and developing theory about complex health and social care systems, and then designing and evaluating interventions. Realists often use meta-theories (theories about other theories) including critical realist feminism, and social theories with realist ontologies. Realism promotes methodological plurality (using multiple or not valuing one over others) and may use methodologies such as critical discourse analysis and constructivist case studies, and can disrupt long-standing qualitative–quantitative divides between disciplinary traditions (Wiltshire, 2018).

Researchers often use a combination of quantitative and qualitative data collection methods that are deemed most appropriate to get as close as possible to understanding what is real. Realist research methodology is increasingly being described in research areas that are relevant to the study of integrated care, namely organisational management, information science, social epidemiology, economics and health services evaluation. Importantly, realist approaches are increasingly used in mixed method research designs and to explore the processes at play in experimental and quasi-experimental studies.

Pragmatism – what matters is that it works

Pragmatism seeks to avoid debates about 'truth' and 'reality' and instead focuses on providing insights and answers to 'real-world' practical issues. Pragmatists ascertain the value of objective and subjective understandings of issues by assessing the practical consequences of such insights. Pragmatists contend that knowledge is constructed, continually interpreted and renegotiated based on interactions between people and their environments (Biesta and Burbules, 2004). As a result, pragmatic research uses human experience as the primary means for building knowledge and understanding the world, as opposed to relying on absolute truths (Hildebrand, 2011).

This approach can be useful for exploring organisational issues, societal advances and complex dynamic processes. Because action can be experienced differently by individuals, pragmatic inquiry encourages and supports multiple and flexible methodologies, whereby the choice of methodology is the one (or more) that best answers the question. Pragmatic researchers focus on answers that can be implemented in a real-world setting. Pragmatists recognise that methodologies are tools used to aid in understanding the world – some have suggested that pragmatism itself is a set of philosophical tools rather than a specific paradigm due to its lack of ontological and epistemological positioning (Tashakkori and Teddlie, 2010).

Pragmatists often combine positivist and constructivist principles in the same research project, using both qualitative and quantitative methodologies and data collection methods to investigate different components of a research question. Pragmatic approaches offer a flexible and reflexive guide to research design and grounded research (Feilzer, 2010).

Radical/critical paradigm – I will change the world

Research under a critical or radical paradigm is focused on inciting action and social change by adopting the interests of those who have not historically been prioritised or heard (Crotty, 2020). Ontologically aligned with relativism, there is no single reality. Reality is a product constructed through power relations in, with and between groups. These power relations are often unjust, where inequity follows social attributes (gender, race, age, sexual orientation, ability).

Research under a radical/critical paradigm is overtly political, with a core aim of 'emancipat[ing] people from unjust or oppressive social structures through radical transformation' (Grant and Giddings, 2002 p. 19). Therefore, critical researchers are interested in investigating social phenomena that are the direct result of power relations, and they take on a moral obligation and action-oriented approach to address injustices through their research and change the way things are. Often informed by theoretical perspectives including queer theory, feminism, critical race theory and intersectionality theory, the focus of radical/critical methodologies is usually on collaboration or co-creation approaches that attempt to enact power sharing. The approaches usually seek to represent and engage with diverse and under-represented views, with an active focus on action and emancipation.

Methodologies under a radical/critical paradigm include participatory research, emancipatory action research, critical discourse analysis, co-operative or co-designed research, and many (but not all) types of feminist research. The methods employed are often qualitative, including gathering open-ended perspectives through non-structured interviews and focus groups, journalling or art-based methods. Quantitative methods may also be used, with a focus on iterative and participatory design.

Chapter 5 — Research paradigms

Interpretivism (subjectivism) — I will listen to you

Often known as the 'qualitative paradigm', the interpretivist paradigm seeks to understand human experience and meanings that people attach to events that occur in their lives (Crotty, 2020). Ontologically, interpretivism reflects a relativist worldview, in that there is no one singular 'truth' but rather the truth is created by and between individuals and groups. Reality needs to be interpreted, not just described. The researcher takes on an active role (versus passive or 'objective') in interpreting what they see. The researcher cannot separate themselves from knowledge creation and their position is a key factor in how the data are interpreted.

Bias is not a 'bad thing' in the interpretivist paradigm; in fact, questions about researcher bias are not relevant, as the researcher's position and perspective are integral to the creation of knowledge. Researchers overtly identify their position in relation to the data, including where they sit in society and in relation to their participants or other people, and actively reflect on how their position informs their view and interpretation of the data. This active and overt identification of the researcher's position and interaction with the data is known as reflexivity, and it is of the utmost importance in an interpretivist paradigm. This act of interpretation creates new meaning and knowledge. The focus is on understanding and using inductive reasoning. Knowledge is therefore subjective and situated between individuals and groups.

Interpretive approaches are supported by theories or theoretical perspectives that align with an interpretivist paradigm, such as phenomenology, hermeneutics, critical inquiry feminism and symbolic interaction. Interpretivist methodologies will share basic philosophical assumptions and commitments, but different theoretical perspectives can be enacted. Ethnography, grounded theory, discourse analysis, phenomenological and heuristic inquiry are all interpretive methodologies. Case studies and narrative approaches are commonly used methods. Data collection methods used under an interpretivist paradigm are usually qualitative in nature, including observations, interviews and focus groups.

Paramedic researcher engagement with paradigms

Where possible, in Table 5.1 the authors' own words are used to describe their ontological, epistemological, theoretical and methodological positions. Engagement with the elements of a research paradigm is noted as either explicitly addressed or implicitly inferred.

Avoiding methodologism

Moving from a research paradigm to specific data collection methods can be challenging. In practice, this will often involve balancing elements of data collection and analysis. While some suggest that research methods are not intrinsically linked to specific philosophical positions (Tashakkori and Teddlie, 2010), a central consideration should be alignment between the methods used and the research questions. A common obstacle for novice and experienced researchers alike is overly focusing

Table 5.1 Paramedic researcher engagement with paradigms.

Author and year	Focus of research	Ontology and epistemology	Theory and methodology (as applicable)
Brydges, 2022	Professionalisation	Interpretivism – reflexive epistemological stance (explicit)	Neo-Weberianism and neo-institutional theories Qualitative constructivist case-study design
Mausz, 2022	Mental health among paramedics	Realism – flexible epistemological stance (explicit)	Role identity theory Mixed methods design
MacQuarrie, 2018	Health status of paramedics	Postpositivism – objectivist epistemology (implicit)	Multiple quantitative methods including survey and biometric data collection
Eaton, 2024	Paramedics in primary care	Realism (explicit)	Realist methodology Mixed methods design
Goldstein, 2013	Frailty assessment	Postpositivism – objectivist epistemology (implicit)	Multiple quantitative methods including survey and epidemiological data
Shannon, 2023	Community paramedicine	Critical realism (explicit)	Complexity theory Multiple methods design
Ford-Jones, 2019	Mental health calls	Critical (implicit)	Feminist political economy Qualitative case-study design
Reed, 2023	Professionalisation	Interpretivism – social constructivism (explicit)	Hermeneutic phenomenology Mixed methods design
Whitley, 2020	Pain management	Postpositivism – critical realism, modified objectivist epistemology (explicit)	Sequential explanatory mixed methods design
Cormack, 2022	Non-technical skills	Pragmatism (explicit)	Human factors theory Multiphase sequentially timed mixed methods design

Chapter 5 — Research paradigms

on methods without considering the philosophical and axiological components of the research. Researchers need to 'slow down' and take the time to consider the ontological, epistemological, practical and political dimensions of their research. In doing so, you can engage with the work on a deeper, more meaningful level (Bressers, Brydges and Paradis, 2020). That means you must resist the urge to jump straight to a known or proposed method(s).

This is not at all to say that methods are not important. Rather, developing a connection between the proposed area of study, the research problem or question, and the philosophical foundations will help create a strong alignment to methodological choices and subsequent methods.

Conceptual frameworks

Finally, it would be a missed opportunity to not speak to the value of conceptual frameworks in this chapter. Conceptual frameworks represent ways of thinking about a topic — they help to illuminate and magnify (Bordage, 2009). Using conceptual frameworks provides you with a clear outline of the problem, how you think about it, and your approach to it. They should be considered both a process — aligning literature, design and methodology — and a product — grounding your work and situating it for readers and other researchers who wish to build upon it.

Conceptual frameworks represent the way we think about a problem (Brydges and Batt, 2023). A conceptual framework aims to justify why the research should be undertaken by describing the state of known knowledge, identifying any gaps in our understanding of a phenomenon or problem and outlining the methodological underpinnings of the research. Conceptual frameworks are constructed to answer two fundamental questions: 'Why is this research important?' and 'How will this research contribute to the larger body of knowledge?'. An example would be thinking about the roles that paramedics enact when they are practising (Tavares et al., 2016).

Some final thoughts

Is your brain exploding? Do not expect to 'get it' immediately when it comes to some of these philosophical considerations. This stuff is hard! Take time away and come back another time. Consider reading other sources, talking to researchers from diverse paradigmatic backgrounds, and revisiting these concepts regularly throughout your research journey.

Summary

Research paradigms are frameworks comprising sets of beliefs and values, which guide how research is conducted and how knowledge is conceptualised within the paramedic research community. They guide research through their assumptions and principles, and engaging with them will help to align elements of your research design and inform theoretical and methodological choices. Understanding paradigm-specific assumptions along a spectrum will help illuminate the quality of findings that support studies and identify gaps in generating answers to the questions posed by paramedics and researchers.

Acknowledgements

The authors would like to thank Dr Madison Brydges for earlier work with Alan Batt that was incorporated into this chapter, and Paige Mason and William Johnston for their reviews of drafts of the chapter.

Useful resources

- Chilisa B (2012). *Indigenous Research Methodologies*. Thousand Oaks: Sage.
- Collins P (2000). *Black Feminist Thought: Knowledge, Consciousness, and the Politics of Empowerment*. New York: Routledge.
- Kovach M (2021). *Indigenous Methodologies: Characteristics, Conversations, and Contexts*, 2nd edn. Toronto: University of Toronto Press.
- Martin D (2012). Two-eyed seeing: a framework for understanding indigenous and non-indigenous approaches to indigenous health research. *Canadian Journal of Nursing Research*, 44(2): 20–42.
- Rameka L (2017). Whakapapa: a Māori way of knowing and being in the world. In: Peters, M. (ed.) *Encyclopaedia of Educational Philosophy and Theory*. Singapore: Springer.
- Wilson S (2020). *Research is Ceremony: Indigenous Research Methods*. Nova Scotia: Fernwood Publishing.

Chapter 6

The role of existing literature in research: searching, retrieving and evaluation

William Broughton and Ian Maconochie

Purpose of this chapter

Completion of this chapter will help you to:

- understand the importance of reviewing existing literature in paramedicine
- describe the different types of review methodology informing paramedic research and development
- explore topic identification and creation of a robust search strategy
- consider various approaches to quality assessment and critical appraisal in evaluation of published work.

Introduction

While undertaking research and the creation of new knowledge will remain important, paramedics and other clinicians must not ignore the vast amounts of existing literature which has the potential to inform or change their practice. Critical to the successful use of existing literature is the ability to find it, retrieve it and evaluate it — conclusions can then be written up and implications for practice considered. This chapter provides the reader with the information and resources to complete those three core activities and embark on understanding the role that existing literature has to play in clinical practice.

Why is the existing literature important?

If you search for the word 'paramedic' in an online database (such as PubMed), it will return thousands of results, linking you to existing literature which is matched to that keyword. In fact, you will probably see tens of thousands of results from national and international sources, some dating back more than 80 years and others which are yet to be published (pre-print).

You will see from the results shown in brackets in Box 6.1 that the volume of existing literature linked to the term 'paramedic' is far less than that of our nursing and

Chapter 6 — The role of existing literature in research

physician colleagues. However, existing literature does not have to be profession-specific to be useful. Literature produced from other disciplines can still be relevant for paramedic practice and while a search strategy might choose to focus on 'paramedics', always be prepared to remove the setting or discipline from your search to increase the range of your results.

> **Box 6.1**
>
> **Quick search task**
>
> Open a browser window and search for PubMed.
>
> Search for the following terms and see how many results you get (the result on 20 October 2024 in brackets):
>
> - Paramedic (21,330)
> - Nurse (473,276)
> - Doctor (787,903).

Within these large volumes of existing literature is information that may hold the answer to your problem or question. There will also be large amounts of information that is not relevant to your topic of interest, which is why a comprehensive search strategy is crucial to locating the information that will inform your work. The existing literature is important, not only because of those answers that you may find, but because there is knowledge waiting for translation to clinical practice (Grimshaw et al., 2012), that could be of real benefit to patients and healthcare systems all over the world.

Researchers wishing to conduct a review should check the PROSPERO register of systematic reviews to see if something similar has already been registered, and it would be good practice to register your review there as well. Once all the relevant literature is found, authors can use a variety of publication types to present their discussion and evaluation of the existing literature, which is described in the next section.

Reporting guidelines

When determining what should be included in a paper — or indeed what should be included in a review — authors should follow reporting guidelines. The Equator Network provides reporting guidelines and extensions for a significant number of study types. All authors should be utilising this information to inform the production of their publications, and it is often a requirement of a journal to confirm the use of, or include a copy of, the reporting guideline checklist. The PRISMA guideline is designed for systematic reviews and meta-analyses, but it also includes extensions for different types of review, including scoping reviews and diagnostic studies (McInnes et al., 2018; Tricco et al., 2018; Page et al., 2021).

What is the difference between a systematic literature review, rapid review, scoping review, evidence mapping and narrative literature review?

A paramedic interested in using evidence to inform their clinical practice should never consider the findings of a single study to be conclusive, robust and ready for immediate translation to practice or policy. Publications, including those which are subject to peer review, have potential to:

- be at risk of bias
- contain methodological flaws
- be time or context dependent
- be misunderstood or misinterpreted (by author or reader) (Wilson and Petticrew, 2008).

For those reasons, and many others, it is considered best practice to combine the results of a search for evidence into a review which evaluates and synthesises the published findings, highlighting any limitations and creating the opportunity for better-informed translation of knowledge.

There are different review types (Table 6.1), which are chosen depending on the question, available literature, timeframe, resources and expertise available/expertise of the author.

Table 6.1 Different types of literature review.

Systematic literature review	A comprehensive review, with a detailed search strategy aiming to reduce the risk of bias by finding, selecting, appraising and synthesising all relevant literature on a topic (Uman, 2011). Systematic reviews may incorporate a meta-analysis, which involves using statistical methods to synthesise the data from several studies into a single quantitative estimate or summary effect size.
Example (without meta-analysis): Contribution of paramedics in primary and urgent care: a systematic review (Eaton et al., 2020)	
Example (with meta-analysis): Mechanical chest compression for out of hospital cardiac arrest: systematic review and meta-analysis (Gates et al., 2015)	
Rapid review	Like a systematic review, but components of the review process can be streamlined or removed to produce the information in a timely manner (Tricco et al., 2015).
Example: How do paramedics learn and maintain the skill of tracheal intubation? A rapid evidence review (Pilbery, 2018)	

(Continued)

Chapter 6 — The role of existing literature in research

Table 6.1 (*Continued*).

Scoping review	Aims to *scope* the key concepts underpinning a research area, locating the main sources and types of evidence which are available (Arksey and O'Malley, 2007).
Example: A scoping review of out-of-hospital research in Ireland from 2000 to 2022 (Bowles et al., 2024).	
Evidence mapping	An evidence map is a systematic search of a broad field to identify gaps in knowledge and/or future research needs that presents results in a user-friendly format, often a visual figure or graph, or a searchable database (Miake-Lye et al., 2016).
Example: Mental health, well-being and support interventions for UK ambulance services staff: an evidence map, 2000 to 2020 (Clark et al., 2021)	
Narrative literature review	The author will present findings on a topic of interest, but typically the search strategy will not be systematic and there will be no protocol. Findings are presented, but a comprehensive and reliable understanding is not achieved by this method (Bourhis, 2017).
Example: Right ventricular myocardial infarction and adverse events from nitrates: a narrative review (Wilkinson-Stokes, 2021)	

Understanding the differences between each type of review will help you select the one most appropriate for your circumstances. Doing a comprehensive systematic review can take a long time, and will usually require the input of others to ensure it is methodologically sound. You might consider using an information specialist (librarian) to support your search strategy; you could enlist others to complete screening for inclusion/exclusion; you may need specialist support to perform the meta-analysis correctly.

There are several resources (Table 6.2) available to guide the development of different types of review or evidence synthesis.

Table 6.2 Guides to development of review or evidence synthesis.

Joanna Briggs Institute (JBI) Manual for Evidence Synthesis	https://jbi-global-wiki.refined.site/space/MANUAL
Centre for Reviews and Dissemination (CRD)	www.york.ac.uk/crd/guidance/
Cochrane Collaboration	www.cochrane.org/
Centre for Evidence-based Medicine	www.cebm.ox.ac.uk/resources

Defining the problem and developing a search strategy

Developing a problem/topic into a review question

To build an effective search strategy, the problem or topic area must be developed into a review (or research) question. A question that is too broad risks creating an unmanageable number of search results, many of which will be irrelevant to the topic or problem you wish to explore (for example, how to treat cardiac arrests). A question that is too narrow risks the opposite – too few results or none that help to address the problem or topic area (for example, how to treat cardiac arrests in males called Gary aged 34–37 caused by food poisoning in Sunderland). Concept mapping is a useful exercise to take a topic and begin to narrow the focus towards something manageable, while identifying important keywords for your search.

Once some key words are identified and the broad topic has some focus, it is time to develop the question. Several different question formulation structures exist to support this activity which are explored with three common examples in Table 6.3.

Table 6.3 Structures for development of research questions.

Topic	Method	Example
Paramedic pain management in paediatric trauma	**PICO** 1. **P**opulation or **P**roblem 2. **I**ntervention 3. **C**omparison 4. **O**utcome	In [**1.** children aged 0–18 with open fractures], does [**2.** intranasal fentanyl] provide [**4.** more effective analgesia] when compared with [**3.** intravenous morphine]?
Ambulance care for patients with substance misuse	**PEO** 1. **P**opulation 2. **E**xposure 3. **O**utcome	What are the [**2.** attitudes] of [**1.** frontline ambulance paramedics] towards [**3.** caring for patients who disclose substance misuse]?
Paramedics' experience of or confidence in managing life-threatening asthma	**SPIDER** 1. **S**ample 2. **P**henomenon of **I**nterest 3. **D**esign 4. **E**valuation 5. **R**esearch Type	What [**4.** factors influence] [**1.** paramedics'] [**2.** confidence levels in handling life-threatening asthma emergencies]? [**3.** Questionnaires, surveys, interviews, focus groups, case studies, observational studies] [**5.** Qualitative and mixed methods)

The PICO format is more commonly used to develop quantitative review questions, while PEO and SPIDER are more commonly used for qualitative review questions. Variations and alternative formats exist, which can include adding the 'setting' to a search (such as UK ambulance services) but that carries a risk of excluding relevant literature from non-UK ambulance settings or important evidence from other settings.

Chapter 6 — The role of existing literature in research

With a well-developed question, search terms can be compiled and a search strategy formulated. While preparing to complete the search, think carefully about the types of evidence that will be required to answer the question effectively. Remember the hierarchy of evidence and which evidence types will be most relevant to the question. Importantly, the desired evidence type may not always be available; this does not mean a review question cannot be answered, but it may affect the reliability or quality of the discussion, or a lack of evidence may highlight a gap in the evidence.

Developing the search strategy

Without a thorough and effective search strategy, the review question may not be answered or may not incorporate the best available evidence. A systematic approach will ensure that key evidence is identified related to the topic under review. Developing an effective search strategy will include defining the types of evidence sought, the inclusion and exclusion criteria, defining search terms, building and carrying out the search and recording the search. Once results are identified, further evidence can be located by searching the reference lists of those articles (sometimes called 'backward chaining') and identifying more recent literature that references already-identified papers (forward citation chaining).

Where possible, there should be multiple members of a review team and all should contribute to development of the search strategy. If specific expertise does not exist within the review team, or reviewer, consider working with a librarian or search specialist on this aspect of the review. Their expertise will be invaluable for designing a search that is relevant to the question – they can also assist with use of Medical Subject Headings (MeSH), choosing appropriate databases and using software to collate and deduplicate the results.

MeSH terms are useful to ensure maximum coverage of relevant terminology within your search, but they may also introduce non-relevant results. For example, the MeSH term 'Allied Health Personnel' in PubMed would be relevant for a search considering paramedic practice. However, within that MeSH tree structure there will be irrelevant terms (as seen in Figure 6.1). Selecting the heading 'Allied Health Personnel' will also incorporate 'Pharmacy Technicians'. You could restrict it further and include only 'Emergency Medical Technicians' but this risks limiting the search. It might be appropriate to step back up the 'tree' to 'Health Personnel' and then build a specific search which excludes those professions which are less relevant.

Defining search terms

Using the PICO example from the previous section, a set of search terms will need to be defined before an effective search can commence. It is useful to create a table for each element of the PICO question and add relevant search terms to each column (Table 6.4). Olaussen et al. (2017) developed a set of paramedic literature search filters, which should be reviewed to help build a specific search.

Building the search and doing it effectively

Once ready to build the search, it will be important to identify the databases that will be used and understand how they work. Common databases used in health include

Defining the problem and developing a search strategy

All MeSH Categories
    Persons Category
        Persons
            Occupational Groups
                Health Personnel
                    Allied Health Personnel
                        Animal Technicians
                        Community Health Workers
                        Dental Auxiliaries
                            Dental Assistants
                            Dental Hygienists
                            Dental Technicians
                            Denturists
                        Emergency Medical Technicians
                            Combat Medics
                        Home Health Aides
                        Licensed Practical Nurses
                        Medical Record Administrators
                        Medical Secretaries
                            Medical Receptionists
                        Nursing Assistants
                            Psychiatric Aides
                        Operating Room Technicians
                        Paramedics
                        Pharmacy Technicians
                        Physical Therapist Assistants
                        Physician Assistants
                            Ophthalmic Assistants
                            Pediatric Assistants

Figure 6.1 Example of PubMed MESH tree structure (accessed 10 June 2024).

Table 6.4 Example of developing search terms to answer a PICO question.

Population	Intervention	Comparison	Outcome
Children Child Paediatric Pediatric Infant Adolescent Teenager	Fentanyl Intranasal	Morphine Intravenous	Pain Pain score Analgesia Pain rating Pain rating scale Pain measurement Pain intensity Pain reduction

PubMed, CINAHL, EBSCO and Cochrane. It is advisable to create an account with each of the databases used, so that searches can be saved as they are performed. This will help later when downloading and recording the search for the final write-up.

Begin by building a search for each heading, using the 'OR' function to maximise the number of results returned and the 'AND' function to make a search more specific.

Chapter 6 — The role of existing literature in research

The 'AND', 'OR' and 'NOT' functions are termed Boolean operators, and some databases will provide advanced searching tools which allow a combination of these terms to be included within a search. Table 6.5 uses PubMed to illustrate the results.

Table 6.5 Illustration of results from PubMed search.

#	Search terms	Results
1	P – children OR child OR paediatric OR pediatric OR infant OR adolescent OR toddler	4,701,365
2	I – fentanyl AND intranasal	381
3	C – morphine AND intravenous	8032
4	O – pain OR pain score OR analgesia OR pain rating OR pain rating scale OR pain measurement OR pain intensity OR pain reduction	949,217

There are obviously too many results above to start screening for relevant studies and so the search must be narrowed further, using the 'AND' function again. Building a search which combines 1 AND 2 AND 3 AND 4 should provide a more manageable number of studies to review (Table 6.6).

Table 6.6 Example of combining searches in PubMed.

#	Search terms	Results
5	#1 AND #2 AND #3 AND #4	25

This example demonstrates how building an effective search around the PICO criteria can return a focused search with 25 results to review. Depending on the purpose of the review, this might be a very sensible number of results to work with. Initial title and abstract screening should identify how valid and reliable the search is. If key articles that you already know about do not come back in the focused search, then it may have been too narrow.

Of course, a focused search might only produce a small number of results if the topic area is not yet widely researched. One option for this is to revise the search, removing some keywords. For Table 6.7, we will remove the route of administration (intranasal and intravenous) to show how that could affect the return.

If screening the initial result of 25 did not produce suitable articles for inclusion, the steps taken above to expand the search to 610 papers create an opportunity to identify missing articles that may still be relevant. With enough time, or a small team, 610 articles is still a manageable number to complete title and abstract screening against the agreed inclusion and exclusion criteria.

Table 6.7 Example of widening a search strategy.

#	Search terms	Results
1	P – children OR child OR paediatric OR pediatric OR infant OR adolescent OR toddler	4,701,365
2	I – fentanyl	26,260
3	C – morphine	72,614
4	O – pain OR pain score OR analgesia OR pain rating OR pain rating scale OR pain measurement OR pain intensity OR pain reduction	949,217
#	Search terms	Results
5	#1 AND #2 AND #3 AND #4	610

For a systematic review, the searches would then need to be completed in other relevant databases. Searches should also be performed on relevant systematic review databases such as Cochrane. Each search should be recorded in tables like those used in the examples so that it can be repeated. Most databases also provide a download function to take a record of the completed search. As mentioned previously, creating an account in each database also allows searches to be saved and therefore documented and repeated more easily.

Screening

Even with a very systematic and effective search, some results may not be relevant or suitable. This is where screening comes in – the reviewer normally starts with title and abstract screening, which means reading the titles and abstracts of all papers returned in the search.

When building the review, it is best practice to produce a protocol which will guide the review team from start to finish. Within that protocol will be inclusion and exclusion criteria, determined in advance of the searches and used to screen results identified from each search. This step is crucial as the searches may have produced hundreds or thousands of articles, but the review team is only interested in those which are relevant. Use of software, such as EPPI-reviewer or Covidence, can save a great deal of time during the screening phase.

Results from all searches are uploaded into the review management software which can then remove any duplicates (step 1). At each step, note the numbers removed as this will all be included in a PRISMA (or similar) flow diagram.

Once duplicates are removed, step 2 is title and abstract screening. That means reading the title and abstract of each paper against the inclusion and exclusion criteria. Best practice would see this completed by at least two reviewers, with a third available to resolve any conflicts. Record the results of this step (ready for the PRISMA

Chapter 6 — The role of existing literature in research

diagram) and move to step 3 – full text review. Of the papers left, it is now time to read each included paper in full against the set criteria. Only those which meet the criteria for inclusion will be taken forward to the final review.

Reference management software, such as Mendeley or EndNote, can integrate with software such as Covidence. Of course, for smaller reviews or where access to software is not possible, review teams can use spreadsheets or collate results directly into word-processing software.

The Centre for Reviews and Dissemination, based at the University of York, produces a handbook with detailed chapters on each stage of the review process (Centre for Reviews and Dissemination, 2009). A reviewer or team of reviewers should decide how each stage of screening will be undertaken and be systematic in their approach. The result should be production of a PRISMA (or similar) flow diagram which clearly charts how the initial results became the final number for inclusion. An example of a PRISMA flow diagram can be seen in Figure 6.2.

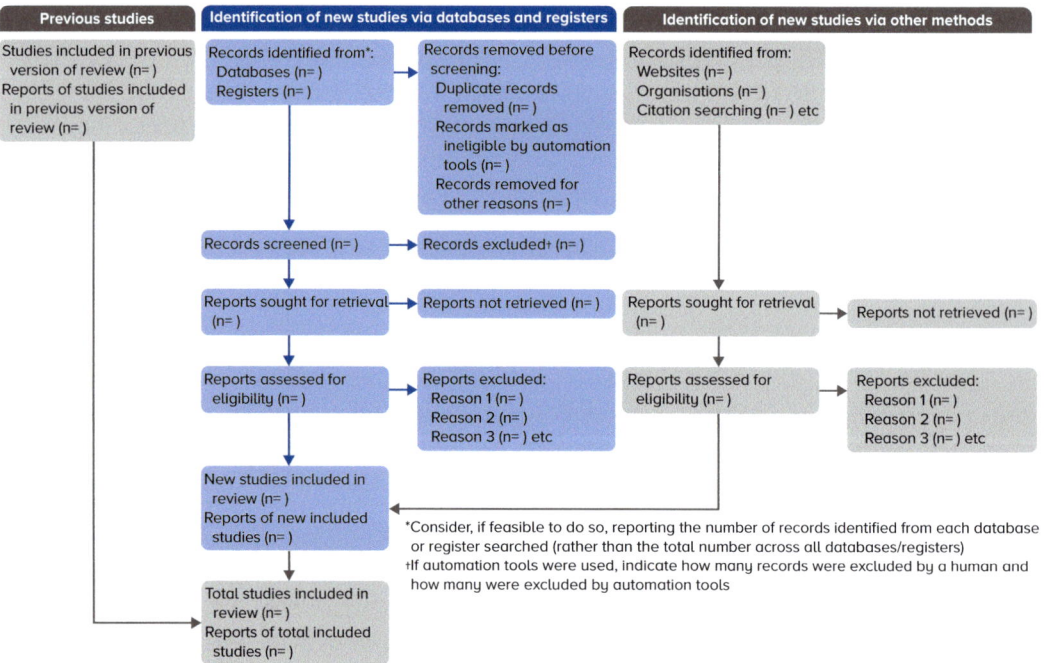

Figure 6.2 Example of a PRISMA flow diagram.
Source: Page et al. (2021). Adapted from Boers, Mayo-Wilson et al., and Stovold et al. Published by BMJ under CC BY 4.0 (https://creativecommons.org/licenses/by/4.0/).

Data extraction

Once the included studies are identified, the next stage is data extraction. The results from the included studies should be summarised into a table for inclusion in the final report. There are several templates which can help guide data extraction, or the review team may adapt these or create their own. Data extraction should feed into other elements of the review, where relevant, such as risk of bias assessment and meta-analysis. Importantly, not every review type will include every aspect of data extraction or synthesis, so it is for the reviewer to determine what is to be extracted and presented in the review.

Summarising all the included studies in this way allows the reviewer to examine for homogeneity and heterogeneity within the results. This may permit the grouping of studies for analysis or it may demonstrate complete heterogeneity (or clinical/methodological diversity) across the included papers, meaning that direct comparison or meta-analysis will be less useful and not a reliable method of data synthesis.

How to critically appraise the literature – use of critiquing frameworks

Screening of articles using predetermined inclusion and exclusion criteria will certainly narrow the results and go some way to ensuring that relevant articles will be included in the final review. However, depending on the topic area, there may still be a significant number of results, and the quality of those results could vary significantly. It is at this point that critical appraisal and quality assessment of the included studies must begin, to allow the review to focus on reliable evidence when attempting to answer the review question. A review which utilises high-quality evidence will carry more weight than one which simply focuses on the quantity of included studies. Quality assessment will provide the review with greater internal validity and will highlight the potential for bias introduced by poor methodology within the included studies.

> **Top tip:** Before embarking on critical appraisal, be sure to understand how to navigate published papers. Look at 'How to read a paper' by Trisha Greenhalgh for a step-by-step guide (Greenhalgh, 2019).

There are several tools and checklists available to guide reviewers on critical appraisal for almost any publication type. Greenhalgh (2019) recommends three 'preliminary' questions, before embarking on detailed appraisal of any paper.

1. What was the research question – and why was this study needed?
2. What was the research design?
3. Was the research design appropriate to the question?

Armed with the answers to these three questions, a reviewer can then be certain which appraisal tool they should be using.

Before starting on critical appraisal, a decision should be made on how the results of the appraisal will be reported and used to inform the review. In the context of a review, it may be appropriate to exclude a paper if the answers to these questions are unclear or suggest that the research design was not in fact suitable. Alternatively, the paper can be included but will be discussed in relation to its poor methodological

Chapter 6 — The role of existing literature in research

quality. Not every type of review will require detailed critical appraisal. Scoping reviews are not intended to produce recommendations based on the quality of the evidence (Arksey and O'Malley, 2007). Rapid reviews are time-bound but will still need to demonstrate a critical and rigorous approach to quality assessment. A systematic approach to data extraction will provide some structure to assessing methodological quality, albeit not in a formal way such as use of a checklist.

Critical appraisal tools and checklists are published by reputable sources, but still require the user to be able to interpret and apply the content of the paper to the checklist questions. Table 6.8 lists some commonly-used critical appraisal frameworks.

Table 6.8 Examples of critical appraisal frameworks.

Critical appraisal framework	Link
Joanna Briggs Institute (JBI)	https://jbi.global/critical-appraisal-tools
Centre for Evidence-based Medicine (CEBM)	www.cebm.ox.ac.uk/resources/ebm-tools/critical-appraisal-tools
Critical Appraisal Skills Programme (CASP)	https://casp-uk.net/casp-tools-checklists/
BestBETs	https://bestbets.org/links/BET-CA-worksheets.php

Whichever method is chosen to undertake the critical appraisal, care should be taken not to introduce further bias at this stage. If two independent reviewers are unable to perform critical appraisal on the included papers, there should be a moderator or someone who can review the results of reviewer one. The output of critical appraisal can be recorded in a table, either combined with the characteristics of included studies or presented separately. Where relevant, reviewers may also choose to include an overall assessment of the risk of bias for each included paper. This can provide a useful visual summary for the reader, as this is often colour coded.

Summary

There are vast quantities of existing literature out there just waiting to be found and included in a review (of any type) which may then produce recommendations or implications for practice. The methods one chooses to undertake this review will determine the strengths of its conclusions and, in acknowledging that every paramedic could not keep up with, nor read, all the publications relevant to their practice, the review will remain an important element of knowledge translation and changes in practice guidance. Reviews are best conducted in a team or with the help of people with specific expertise (such as information specialists) to assure the methods and contribute to the quality assessment of included papers.

This chapter has provided an overview of the role of existing literature in research, including searching, retrieving and evaluation of information. From these foundations, paramedics should use the plethora of resources available to design robust review protocols, carry out high-quality reviews and evidence syntheses and contribute to the ever-growing evidence base for paramedic practice.

Useful resources

Guidance on the creation and publication of review protocols:

- Centre for Reviews and Dissemination Handbook: www.york.ac.uk/crd/guidance/
- PROSPERO International Prospective Register of Systematic Reviews: www.crd.york.ac.uk/prospero/
- PRISMA-P Checklist for Protocol Development: https://www.prisma-statement.org/protocols

For further development of critical appraisal skills, consider these resources:

- The Resus Room – Critical Appraisal Lowdown Course: www.criticalappraisallowdown.co.uk/
- Online courses from CASP: https://casp-uk.net/online-learning/

General information:

- Equator network (reporting guidelines): www.equator-network.org/
- Library and Knowledge Service for NHS Ambulance Services in England (LKS ASE): https://ambulance.libguides.com/home1

Chapter 7

Developing research questions: avoiding the 'so what' factor

Scott Devenish and Julia Williams

> **Purpose of this chapter**
>
> Completion of this chapter will help you to:
> - identify the difference between a research problem and a research question
> - understand the differences between a research aim, objective and hypothesis
> - discuss the processes of refining a research question
> - look at how to construct different types of research question.

Introduction

This chapter explores how to develop a good research question for paramedic research. It begins by identifying the research problem and then explores how to create a research question for both quantitative and qualitative research. Furthermore, terms such as aim, objective and hypothesis are examined, and the important role of the research question in driving the research study is discussed.

The skill of building a good research question is of paramount importance to developing a robust study (Laine, 2009). It is possibly the most important step to bring everything in the research project into alignment. Forming research questions can be a difficult and challenging process (White, 2017). A common mistake for many new researchers, and some experienced ones, is to develop a research question to suit a given methodology. Instead, it is the research question that should drive the choice of methodology (Williams, 2012).

What is the difference between the research problem and the research question?

The research problem is the overall broad concept to be researched. It usually starts with a curious interest such as 'I wonder',' What is' or possibly 'Why ...' and

Chapter 7 — Developing research questions: avoiding the 'so what' factor

maybe 'How ...' (Agee, 2009; O'Leary, 2018). Transitioning from the research problem to a well-articulated research question can be a challenging and time-consuming process, but giving this stage the time it needs is vital to ensure the study is achievable and valid. When selecting a research problem, choosing a topic area of significant interest is key to maintaining your engagement with the research and the motivation to continue, as research can be a process likened to a rollercoaster ride with both highs and lows.

A hypothetical example of a research problem is given in Box 7.1.

> **Box 7.1**
>
> ### Hypothetical example of a research problem
>
> - *Research problem*: 'How can paramedics remain alert during shift work?'
> - *Significance*: The significance of the research problem may be to improve alertness, reduce clinical errors and improve staff well-being. It may be transferable to other types of shift workers.
> - *What is known*: The role of energy drinks/diet/exercise, circadian rhythms, adequate sleep, settling routines and environmental aspects such as noise may impact staying alert during shift work. Imagine the issue chosen focuses on 'the benefits of energy drinks for paramedics working shift work'.
> - *Specific issues*: Figure 7.1 highlights many of the possible aspects of the problem to consider when constructing a research question and possible aims and objectives of the study.

The research question also needs to address the 'so what' factor; that is, the research should be significant to the paramedic body of knowledge, and possibly transferable to other fields or disciplines (Selwyn, 2014) so that at the end of it, people do not question what the point of the research was.

Research problem, aims, objectives and the research question

While the research problem is a broad conceptual view, a literature review (except in some types of grounded theory) is a very useful step in constructing aims, objectives and the research question. The literature review (see Chapter 6) identifies gaps in the body of knowledge or highlights existing findings that can be tested in a different setting (O'Leary, 2018; White, 2017). Narrowing the research problem helps to identify possible aims and objectives and provides a clearer description of the study's proposed outcomes. The research aims and objectives are then further refined into a clear and specific research question or research questions likened to a funnel (Figure 7.2).

Research problem, aims, objectives and the research question

Are there any benefits of energy drinks to maintain alertness for paramedics on shift work?

- Which shift, i.e. first night shift or second in a row?
- What sort of energy drink and how often?
- What, if any, benefits?
- What, if any, limitations?
- What volume of drink over what time period?
- Mgs of caffeine or other ingredients?
- Current usage of energy drinks
- Comparisons, e.g. other interventions like coffee/tea
- How to measure the benefits, e.g. over what period of time, is there a control group?
- Circumstances affecting sleep and normal routines between night shifts
- Research confounders (Laine, 2009), e.g. participants who also smoke while having an energy drink

Figure 7.1 Example of narrowing down a research problem into a specific focus area.

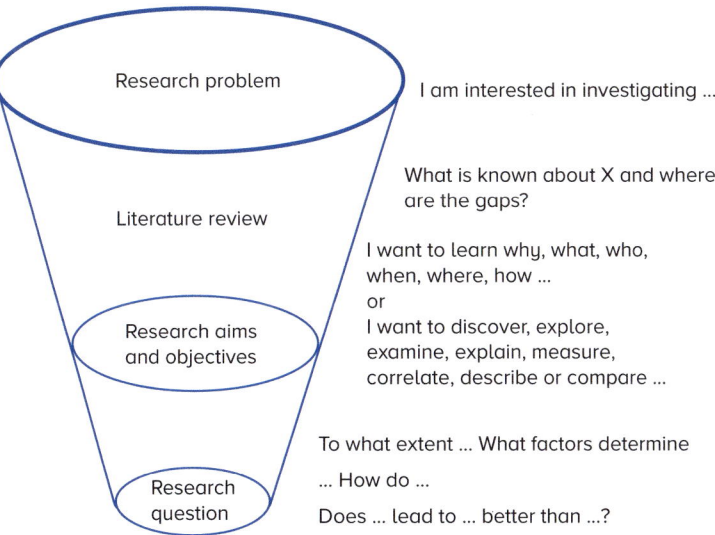

Figure 7.2 Refining the research problem into a question.
Source: Adapted from O'Leary (2018).

The research aim indicates the problem to be researched in a short succinct statement, usually within a sentence or two. The research objectives highlight in more detail how the research aim is to be achieved; they are smaller mini-steps and if you add them all together, they should enable you to achieve the aim, and if you achieve the aim then you should be able to answer the research question. An example of how you could use the funnel model is shown in Table 7.1.

In the context of paramedic research, it is crucial to differentiate between the research aim, objectives and hypothesis. Each component plays a distinct role in shaping the study, guiding the research process and ensuring clarity in what the research seeks to achieve. Understanding these differences enhances the effectiveness of the research design and the quality of the findings.

Research aim

The research aim is the broad, overarching goal that outlines the general intent of the study without specifying the methods or steps for achievement.

Example: The aim of the study might be to enhance the safety and outcomes of childbirth in ambulance settings. This general goal sets the direction for a more detailed investigation into improving maternal and neonatal outcomes and/or experiences during emergency deliveries.

Research objectives

Research objectives break down the aim into specific, measurable actions that the study will undertake to achieve the broader goal. Objectives are clear and focused, usually framed in a way that they can be directly acted upon and evaluated.

Example: Objectives for the study focused on childbirth in ambulance settings might include:

- assessing the effectiveness of specialised training programmes for paramedics in managing births before arrival at hospital
- evaluating the impact of prehospital interventions on maternal and neonatal outcomes during births occurring in ambulance settings
- exploring the experiences and satisfaction levels of mothers who give birth in emergency situations while in the care of ambulance service staff.

These objectives specify the areas the study will explore, providing clear metrics and/or targets that contribute directly to achieving the broader aim.

Each objective is specific, providing clear steps towards achieving the overall aim of the study.

Research hypothesis

It is important to remember that not all research studies are appropriate for hypotheses. A research hypothesis is a specific, testable prediction about the

Table 7.1 Example of using the funnel model.

Research problem	Is paramedic education and training adequate to meet the demands of our expanding scope of practice?
Literature review	Literature found on: • in-house training versus university education for paramedics • clinical placements • paramedic internship and mentoring • ambulance culture • professionalism and paramedicine • organisational socialisation and professional socialisation in allied health, nursing and medicine • expanding scope of practice and working in different settings other than ambulance services. Gap: • Transition to professional practice, i.e. the professional socialisation of university-educated paramedics
Research aim	To assess the adequacy of current education and training programmes for paramedics in addressing the evolving demands of their professional roles. *This aim is focused on evaluating the sufficiency and appropriateness of existing paramedic training and education frameworks as they relate to the changing and expanding requirements of the paramedic role.*

Objectives	1. To identify the key competencies and skills that paramedics currently require to perform safely in their expanding roles.
	
	    This objective involves mapping out the essential skills needed in the profession today, which may include advanced medical procedures, crisis management and the use of new technologies, to see if current training/education adequately covers these areas.
	
	2. To evaluate the content and delivery of existing paramedic training programmes against the identified competencies and skills.
	
	    This objective focuses on a detailed analysis of current educational curricula and training methods to determine if they align with and effectively impart the necessary competencies.
	
	3. To gather feedback from practising paramedics and their supervisors/mentors on the effectiveness of their initial and ongoing training in preparing them for real-world challenges.
	
	    This objective aims to collect qualitative data from both new and experienced paramedics, as well as their direct supervisors/placement educators, to assess their views on the sufficiency of their training/education and any gaps that may exist in their preparedness.

Research question(s)	Does the current education and training provided to paramedics enable them to meet the expanding demands of their scope of practice?

relationship between two or more variables. It is formulated based on existing knowledge, theories or observations and is used in studies that seek to prove or disprove these relationships through empirical data.

Example: A hypothesis in this study might be: 'Women who give birth in ambulance service settings with paramedics who have had additional training in maternal care report better outcomes than those attended by paramedics without such training'.

This hypothesis provides a specific expectation that can be empirically tested through the study, offering evidence to either support or refute the effectiveness of specialised obstetric training for paramedics.

While a hypothesis is more common in quantitative studies, it does not mean that it is completely absent from qualitative studies (White, 2017). Qualitative inquiry methodology traditionally involves the researcher seeking to generate knowledge about a phenomenon from the findings (Meinefeld, 2004). However, by using reflexivity (Finlay, 2003; Maso, 2003), researchers are increasingly bringing previous lived experience and assumptions into the data analysis process, findings and discussion, possibly developing hypotheses through theories and theoretical models but not necessarily testing them (Malterud, 2001). Some qualitative studies might involve developing what could be seen as a form of preliminary hypotheses known as 'research assumptions' or 'theoretical ideas'. These ideas are not intended for hypothesis testing but serve as starting points for exploration. They can guide initial data collection and analysis, but researchers remain open to adapting their focus as they engage with the data.

Putting it all together

In paramedic research, these components form a hierarchy of planning and delivery:

- The aim sets the broad, overarching goal of the study.
- The objectives outline the specific steps that will be taken to achieve this aim.
- The hypothesis (if appropriate) provides a focused prediction that can be tested to validate or invalidate the assumptions underlying the objectives.

By clearly defining these elements, paramedic research can be methodically structured to not only address specific gaps in knowledge or practice but also contribute substantively to improving urgent unplanned and/or emergency care.

How to develop a research question

Is it achievable?

The research question needs to equate to an achievable project. It is common for new researchers to present such broad research questions that the study could be divided into multiple studies, and is therefore not achievable given the budget, resources and timeline allocated to the project.

Significant consideration needs to be given to resources required to undertake the study. For example:

- What sort of equipment (if any) is necessary? Are there sufficient funds/grants to purchase necessary equipment?
- What sort of training is required to use the equipment?
- Is specific software required?
- Is lab space required?
- Is there sufficient time to complete the study? For example, a 10-year longitudinal study would be outside the time allotted for a PhD (White, 2017).

In relation to higher degrees, the supervisory team can guide the research candidate when developing a study to make sure it is achievable. However, not all researchers are undertaking higher degree research. When starting out, or if less experienced in developing research questions and study design, it is always advisable to consult a trusted colleague with significant research experience (O'Leary, 2018). Talking to research representatives from a professional body (for example, College of Paramedics or equivalent association), experienced clinical researchers and/or university academics with established track records can be a good start.

Constructing quantitative research questions

Developing a quantitative research question involves research which aims to critique, evaluate, forecast, retrospectively evaluate, test or involve statistical observation (Higgs and Llewellyn, 1998). Quantitative research is discussed in detail in Chapters 8–11.

The PICO method is well utilised in the evidence-based research space when developing clinical research questions, and is frequently used in quantitative studies. PICO stands for Problem/Population, Intervention, Comparison and Outcomes (Booth, 2017). For example, using the topic 'Are energy drinks useful for maintaining the alertness of paramedics working shift work', a PICO could look like this.

- *P (Population/Problem)*: Tiredness and fatigue felt by paramedics (non-smokers) during night clinical shift work.
- *I (Intervention)*: Consumption of energy drinks.
- *C (Comparison):* Consumption of coffee (fully caffeinated).
- *O (Outcome)*: Improved alertness during shift; reduced tiredness and fatigue.

Based on the PICO elements, the research question could be formulated as:

'Does the ingestion of energy drinks improve the alertness and reduce fatigue in paramedics aged 20–25 who do not smoke, compared to ingestion of coffee, during frontline clinical shifts at night in an ambulance service?'

Chapter 7 — Developing research questions: avoiding the 'so what' factor

With the addition of detail such as which brand of energy drinks and coffee, and how much volume is needed, this research question is specific and measurable, allowing for a focused study on the effects of energy drinks compared to other common stimulants like coffee, specifically targeting the age group most likely to consume them and under conditions (night shifts) where alertness and levels of fatigue can be critical.

There are often different ways to answer a research question but, based on this research question, it would be appropriate to design a randomised control trial (see Chapter 10) comparing the benefits (or otherwise) of drinking energy drinks as opposed to caffeinated coffee for paramedics (between the ages of 20 and 25 years) who do not smoke, to see which (if any) is more beneficial in increasing alertness and reducing tiredness and fatigue.

This randomised controlled trial design allows for a clear comparison between the effects of energy drinks versus coffee on the alertness of young paramedics (who do not smoke) during night shifts, potentially providing evidence that can influence policy and practice in paramedic services regarding consumption of stimulants during shifts.

Using the PICO framework to structure a research question helps clarify and focus the study by systematically identifying the population/problem, intervention, comparison group and outcomes, which enhances the precision and relevance of the research.

Constructing qualitative research questions

In qualitative research, the research question also informs the methodology and research methods to be used. Often qualitative researchers are required to justify the use of methods and methodology based on the study's purpose (Crotty, 1998), framed against philosophical approaches, theoretical frameworks and other sensitising concepts (Agee, 2009; Higgs and Llewellyn, 1998). Using traditional qualitative methods, new knowledge and theories emerge from the data (Williams, 2012) or are built on existing frameworks or paradigms investigating states of being and processes which are specific to a field of study or discipline (Agee, 2009). Qualitative research is addressed in greater detail in Chapters 12–14.

Unlike a quantitative question using the PICO method, qualitative questions are frequently more open in design (Higgs and Llewellyn, 1998). Qualitative research questions about a topic are driven by a desire to know or understand the concerns, problems or lived experiences of others, or interactions between people. It is common for qualitative questions to evolve through a reflective and integrative process before they become set (Agee, 2009). That is, the initial question may undergo several iterations, with the final question being very different from the original one proposed (Higgs and Llewellyn, 1998).

When forming a qualitative research question, it is important to consider first what knowledge or understanding about a phenomenon is to be investigated (except for traditional grounded theory). By first narrowing down the topic to be investigated into a short statement of a sentence or two, a precise description of the research is formed, which can then determine how and even if the phenomenon can be researched (Agee, 2009; Higgs and Llewellyn, 1998). It can be common for qualitative questions to be written as broad aims or research statements (Williams, 2012) with several subquestions. Subquestions are particularly useful in guiding the study when a research statement is used instead of an overarching question.

There are many models that you can use to help you structure a qualitative question, such as PICo or SPIDER (addressed in Chapter 6). PICo is an acronym for Population, Interest and Context, and is a framework specifically designed for constructing qualitative research questions. This model assists researchers in clearly identifying the key components of their study, which is essential for conducting focused and relevant qualitative research.

Imagine a research scenario where we aim to understand the experiences of paramedics in managing individuals in mental health crisis presenting to the emergency ambulance services. This topic is of particular interest due to the increasing number of mental health-related calls presenting to ambulance services.

Using the PICo framework, the research question can be broken down as follows.

- *P (Population)*: Paramedics.
- *I (Phenomenon of interest)*: Experiences in managing individuals with mental health emergencies.
- *Co (Context):* Ambulance service setting.

Based on the PICo elements, the research question could be formulated as:

What are the experiences of ambulance paramedics when managing patients with mental health emergencies presenting to ambulance services?

To explore this question, a qualitative study design would be suitable. A phenomenological approach could be employed to understand the lived experiences of paramedics in this context or alternatively, a generic qualitative approach might be considered (see Chapters 12–14).

By framing the research question with the PICo model, the study ensures that the inquiry is directly relevant to the needs and experiences of the target population, leading to more impactful and applicable research outcomes.

What if PICO and PICo do not fit?

While PICO and PICo are well known in health disciplines when researching to establish best practice, they may not be suitable for all types of studies, so you might want to consider other methods, for example the five-step research method (Table 7.2) outlined by O'Leary (2018).

Just remember that there are many different structures to use, and you should explore alternatives and practise using a range of models and frameworks. Do not try to make

Chapter 7 — Developing research questions: avoiding the 'so what' factor

Table 7.2 Example of a research question structured using O'Leary's framework.

1. Topic – What is the topic to be researched?	Benefits of energy drinks for tired night shift workers
2. Context – What is the research context, e.g. ambulance service, management, education	On-road paramedics between the ages of 20–25 who do not smoke working night shift in an ambulance service
3. Goal – What do you hope to achieve by doing the research?	Identify the benefits (or drawbacks) of energy drinks for paramedics aged 20–25 who do not smoke working night shifts in a patient-facing capacity compared to a control, e.g. coffee
4. Nature of the question – What, who, where, how, when or why?	What are the benefits or limitations of energy drinks in staying alert on night shift for paramedics aged 20–25 who do not smoke?
5. Relationships – Potential relationships such as decreases, increases, comparisons, causes, impacting factors	Relationship between alertness and drinking energy drinks as opposed to drinking coffee

your research question 'fit' a framework. These models are there to help rather than hinder. Collaborating with other researchers, clinicians, academics, patients or service users helps to develop succinct, clear and relevant research questions.

Role of the research question in driving the research

This chapter has explored the processes involved in developing a research question. It is clear that the research question should guide the methodology, and not the other way around. The research question is key to converting the research problem into a study process and deciding whether in fact the question is researchable. While the question should come first, researchers may tend to favour a particular research design, such as qualitative or quantitative methods, and that can be self-limiting. Linking a study to a philosophical viewpoint or methodology before developing the research question may limit the effectiveness and outcome of the study (White, 2017).

The development of an effective research question is paramount, shaping the trajectory and impact of the study. This process is crucial as it ensures that the research is directly relevant to clinical practices, operational procedures and patient outcomes in paramedic practice.

Defining the research question

For paramedic researchers, a well-crafted research question must directly address the specific challenges or gaps in knowledge that affect paramedicine. It should clarify the scope of the study, whether it is exploring new techniques for managing cardiac arrests, assessing the efficacy of prehospital treatments, managing patients with chronic illness or understanding the psychological impact of the job on paramedics' health and well-being. This clarity guides all subsequent methodological choices, ensuring that the study can achieve meaningful results that enhance the effectiveness and efficiency of paramedic practice.

Impact on methodological choices

The specificity of the research question in paramedic research determines the selection of the most appropriate methodological approach. If the question pertains to the effectiveness of a new drug administration protocol, a quantitative, possibly experimental, approach might be necessary. Conversely, questions about paramedic experiences or clinical decision-making processes may be better explored through qualitative methods like interviews or focus groups. The research question ensures that the chosen methodology aligns with the objectives, facilitating accurate and relevant findings.

Role in data collection

In paramedic research, the research question defines who the participants should be (e.g. paramedics, patients, healthcare professionals), what data should be collected (e.g. patient outcomes, paramedic feedback), and where and when the data collection should occur (e.g. during shifts, in different environments where paramedics work). For instance, a study investigating the impact of fatigue on paramedic performance will guide the researcher to collect data on shift patterns, sleep schedules and error rates during long shifts, to name but a few areas.

Informing data analysis

The research question helps paramedic researchers determine how to analyse collected data. In studies investigating paramedic response times, statistical analysis might be used to identify factors that significantly affect speed and efficiency. For research exploring paramedic perceptions of new communication tools, thematic analysis would help reveal common themes and feelings about the tool's usability and effectiveness.

Ensuring relevance and feasibility

By focusing the research on specific, relevant questions, paramedic research remains directly applicable to the field. This relevance is crucial for engaging stakeholders, such as emergency departments, community health practices, other health and care organisations and healthcare policy makers, who rely on evidence-based data to make informed decisions about training, procedures and equipment. Moreover, a clear and focused research question helps manage the scope of the study, preventing unnecessary diversions and ensuring that resources are efficiently used to explore the most pertinent issues affecting paramedic services.

Summary

This chapter demonstrates that the research question in paramedic research is not just an early step, but is the basis upon which the entire study is structured.

Chapter 7 — Developing research questions: avoiding the 'so what' factor

A crucial point is that the research question should drive the methodology, not the other way around. This helps avoid the common pitfall where researchers choose a methodology first and then shape the research question to fit it, which can limit the study's scope and relevance. The chapter further discusses how the research question influences every aspect of the study – from selecting the methodology and designing the study to data collection and analysis – ensuring that the research is methodologically sound and directly relevant.

Please remember there is not just one single way to construct a research question, and never underestimate how long developing effective research questions can take. By meticulously defining research questions, aim(s), objectives and hypotheses (if relevant), paramedic research can make substantive contributions to improving the quality and effectiveness of the services we provide, thereby benefiting both paramedics and their patients.

Useful resources

- Developing a research question, presented by Steve Campitelli, University of Melbourne: https://www.youtube.com/watch?v=mrWeLJZydUU
- EQUATOR Network: www.equator-network.org/
- Crilly J et al. (2022). Research priority setting in emergency care: a scoping review. *Journal of the American College of Emergency Physicians Open*, 3(6): e12852.

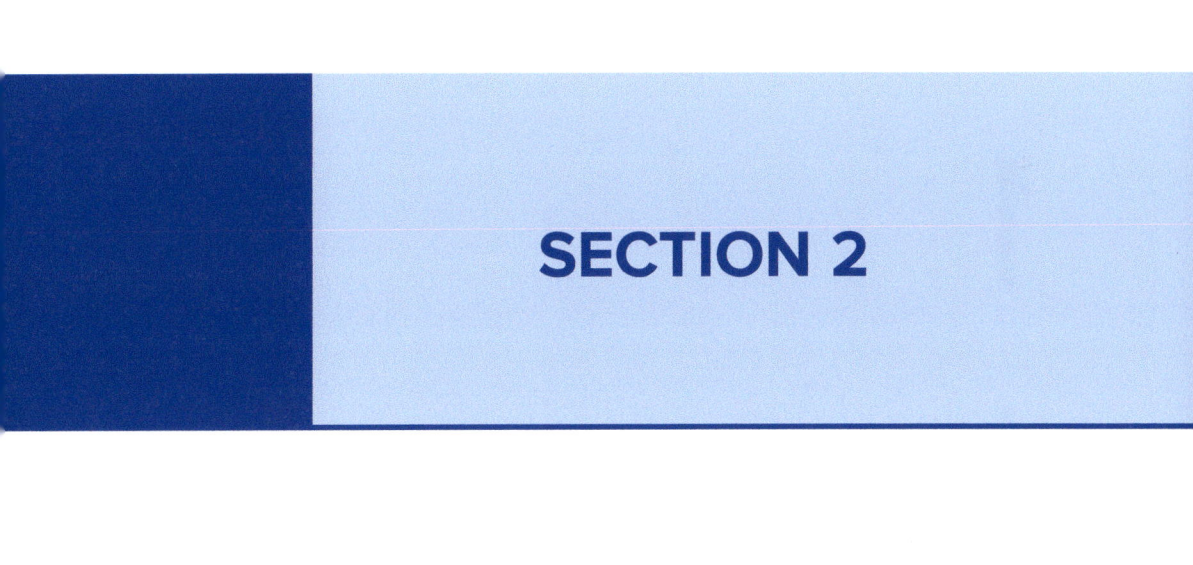

SECTION 2

Chapter 8

Quantitative research design

Helen Snooks and Christopher Stein

Purpose of this chapter

Completion of this chapter will help you to:
- understand the role of quantitative research in paramedicine
- discuss different approaches to quantitative research, including experimental and observational designs
- recognise challenges to undertaking quantitative research and be able to suggest solutions to address these
- understand sampling techniques and their applications.

Introduction

This chapter deals with research designs commonly used in quantitative research. Research design refers to a set of logical decisions or choices that are made with respect to the high-level plan required to answer a specific research question or questions. A research design can be thought of as a framework for how the research will be conducted, which takes into consideration selection of a sample, comparisons to be made, allocation of participants to groups or treatments, collection and analysis of data. Quantitative research is a wide term used to describe research conducted to answer questions through collection and analysis of numerical data.

Broadly speaking, quantitative research designs can be thought of as either observational (non-interventional) or experimental (interventional). In observational designs, experiences and outcomes of research participants are observed and recorded in a healthcare setting without any intervention or change in care. Participants are selected for inclusion by meeting defined criteria, such as diagnosis with a particular disease or disorder, or exposure to a risk factor for a particular disease or disorder. In experimental designs, participants meeting defined inclusion criteria are placed in groups for the purposes of receipt of care and later analysis by the researchers.

Chapter 8 — Quantitative research design

Participants may be randomly allocated to study groups – individually or in some situations by another factor, such as clusters or time blocks. However, it may not be possible or appropriate to randomly allocate participants to groups in an experimental design. In such situations, while group comparisons may still be made, they are not between groups of randomly assigned participants but between groups where the assignment has been made some other way, or where the groups represent observations made on the same participants at different times, rather than independent participant groups. Research designs of this nature, which involve manipulation of a variable but without random assignment to groups being compared, form a third type of research design called quasi-experimental.

Observational designs

The main feature of observational research designs is that data are collected without any attempt to change practice. Within this broad group of research designs, there is a further distinction between observational designs that employ the use of a control group and those that do not. Observational research designs without a control group are referred to as descriptive designs, while those that employ a control group are referred to as analytical or comparative designs.

Descriptive observational designs

Case series

What is it?

A case series research design involves the description of one (case report) or a number (case series) of clinical cases sharing a common condition. The common condition can be a disease or syndrome, or a particular treatment. Data collected could be related to clinical or pathophysiological features, diagnosis or treatment and are descriptively analysed.

When is it best used?

Case series research is normally used when little is known about a condition or treatment and, as a preliminary step, an attempt is made to simply describe some aspects of its basic characteristics. A case series may be useful when a condition is very rare or an intervention is rarely performed.

Appropriate sampling strategies/methods of recruitment

Use is typically made of convenience sampling, often consecutive cases.

Most common data collection methods

Data are typically extracted from routine patient care records. Some case reports include the patient voice or experience within the report.

Strategies to enhance rigour

A case series is very simple but quite limited. Consequently, it is situated low on the traditional evidence hierarchy as it contributes only a characterisation of cases with little inferential or comparative value. It is necessary to ensure that the series of cases is complete, according to case selection criteria, and that missing cases (and case data) are minimised to control biases and transparently reported to enhance rigour. Involvement of the patients described may enhance the presentation of the cases.

Overall strengths and limitations

The key strength of a case series is its simplicity and accessibility. It thus can serve as the basis for generating hypotheses about causal relationships, to be tested with more sophisticated research designs and analysis. A case series is limited because it may utilise a small sample from one location and makes no comparisons which, along with selection bias and confounding, make the assessment of causation and wider applicability difficult.

Significant challenges in this type of research

Data quality is typically the greatest challenge with this type of research, as it is often routine clinical data stored in a registry or database. Consequently, there may be missing data or cases; it is often not known exactly how specific variables were measured and with what validity.

Retrospective record review

What is it?

In a retrospective record review, the researcher describes a set of existing clinical cases, to answer a specific research question. The main difference between a case series and a retrospective record review is that the case series aims to describe aspects of clinical cases that are new or novel in some way. Retrospective record reviews do not necessarily involve new or novel clinical cases, but rather new research questions that can be answered by analysis of data from existing cases.

When is it best used?

A retrospective record review is an effective way of answering simple research questions about current volume, case mix or care, when high-quality data exist and particularly when time or research funding is limited. They can also be used in situations where prospective designs are either ethically or practically not feasible. Retrospective record reviews may be conducted as pilot studies that precede a larger prospective study (Worster and Haines, 2004).

Appropriate sampling strategies/methods of recruitment

If few cases are available, or the clinical condition studied is rare, all cases are typically included in the analysis. If the number of clinical cases is larger, then a random sampling strategy to identify a representative subset of the available cases is preferred.

Most common data collection methods

Typically, the same method is used as for a case series; data are extracted from existing routine clinical or patient care records.

Chapter 8 — Quantitative research design

Strategies to enhance rigour

These include stating carefully thought-out and structured research questions, setting explicit inclusion and exclusion criteria for records, including a power calculation to understand precision and generalisability of any results, a robust sampling strategy (random sampling if possible), ensuring reliable data extraction and performing a pilot study (Vassar and Mathew, 2013).

Overall strengths and limitations

Retrospective record reviews can usually be done quickly and at low cost because the data already exist. This study design is appropriate for answering descriptive epidemiological questions. Like a case series, though, this research design does not include randomised group comparison, and can therefore not be used to demonstrate causal relationships. Sampling bias, particularly if non-random samples are used, and poor data quality or missing data are two further limitations.

Significant challenges in this type of research

The quality and pertinence of data to research questions set.

Survey

What is it?

A survey is a method used to describe and draw inferences about people, organisations, current practice and social phenomena. Surveys work well when there is a well-defined population to target. In most cases, a sample will be drawn from the population of interest, from which inferences are made. Surveys can be designed to obtain information from respondents about opinions, attitudes, behaviours or knowledge related to experiences, practices or events that respondents have been exposed to or know of. Surveys make use of a questionnaire that may comprise closed or open-ended questions or both. Questionnaires can be distributed by post, online or in person.

When is it best used?

A survey should be used when the aim of research is to describe or draw inferences about the opinions, attitudes or knowledge of people or current practice. Survey questionnaires typically make use of closed questions, meaning that they are less suited to investigate the kind of research questions of interest to qualitative researchers, which require more detailed, open and rich data. While it is possible to include open questions in survey questionnaires, these usually have quite a limited scope and rarely provide rich data supporting qualitative forms of inquiry (LaDonna et al., 2018).

Appropriate sampling strategies/methods of recruitment

Broadly speaking, survey sampling may be either probability or non-probability. Probability sampling means that every unit of analysis has an equal and non-zero probability of being included. Simple random sampling is the most commonly used type of probability sampling. While probability sampling generally may yield a representative sample, it requires a complete list of the population – the sampling frame – that can be difficult or impossible to obtain.

Non-probability sampling means that another strategy is used for sample selection based on either researcher judgement or convenience. Sampling strategies based on researcher judgement include purposive sampling (where participants are targeted because they possess a characteristic relevant to your question) and quota sampling. Convenience sampling is determined by ease of access to participants, which may be geographical or based on access to another source such as a list of employees. Convenience sampling differs in principle from purposive sampling in that researcher judgement is not used to determine inclusion or exclusion from the sample. It is also not considered representative of a specific population.

Most common data collection methods

Internet sites or emailed questionnaires are frequently used for data collection. While the use of web surveys is easy and cost-effective, it introduces sampling bias as it depends on access to devices and the internet, which is typically not equally distributed across the population.

Strategies to enhance rigour

Lack of rigour is a criticism often levelled against surveys. This can be addressed in four areas: sampling, delivery and data collection, questionnaire design and analysis:

- *Sampling*: If the intention is to generalise survey results from a sample to a population, then a sampling frame should be available that represents features of the target population and sampling should be probabilistic. Purposive and convenience sampling are not necessarily suitable for surveys wishing to make generalisations to a wider population.

- *Delivery and data collection*: Non-response is a risk with surveys and may introduce significant bias. Several strategies can reduce unit (i.e. lack of response at the level of a whole questionnaire) and item (i.e. lack of response to one or more items in a questionnaire) non-response. A good overview of these is given by Phillips et al. (2016).

- *Questionnaire design*: Choices made regarding the length of survey questionnaires, the types of questions (closed or open), the response scales used and the order of questions, among others, can influence the validity and reliability of data collected and the degree of non-response. The survey checklist (Gehlbach and Artino, 2018) and development guide (Gehlbach et al., 2010) offer a good starting point for questionnaire design. Questionnaires should be piloted on a small number of relevant people before use, if possible.

- *Analysis*: Transparent reporting of completed responses, missing data items and missing cases is crucial. Analysis of non-responses can strengthen the validity of results.

Chapter 8 — Quantitative research design

Overall strengths and limitations

The strengths of a survey include its ability to reach a large sample and to produce a 'snapshot' at relatively low cost. Limitations of a survey include the inability to generalise results to a larger population if sampling has not been carefully conducted and lack of validity of custom-developed questionnaires.

Significant challenges in this type of research

Obtaining a sampling frame for surveys can be challenging, depending on the aim of the research and the type of respondent sought. Low response rates can be a challenge, especially if only one survey distribution method is used or if the population targeted is frequently surveyed and has survey fatigue. Design and development of well-crafted questionnaires can be technically difficult and time-consuming.

Analytical/comparative observational designs

Case–control

What is it?

A case–control study design is one in which patients with a well-defined outcome (cases) are compared to patients without the outcome but who are similar in other respects (controls) with regard to possible risk factor exposure. Because case–control studies begin with an outcome, they are retrospective designs. Due to their retrospective nature, case–control studies cannot produce incidence rates. Rather, they produce odds ratios which are a reasonable estimate of relative risk provided the incidence rate of the outcome studied is low (typically <5% in either exposed and unexposed groups) (Schulz and Grimes, 2002).

When is it best used?

A case–control design could be used when researchers have a question about the causation of outcomes and a more rigorous design is impractical. The reasons for this may be that it is unethical to manipulate an independent variable to study its effect, complexity or cost. Case–control designs are also utilised when more hypothesis-generating research is required prior to the application of more complex research such as a clinical trial. Case–control studies are relatively easy to conduct, at low cost. However, selection of cases and unbiased controls can be challenging (Newman et al., 2013).

Appropriate sampling strategies/methods of recruitment

Inclusion and exclusion criteria should be clearly defined to guide case selection. It is important to clearly describe where cases are sampled from, along with a clear description of criteria used to diagnose or identify them. Correctly sampling controls is essential to prevent bias. Controls should be free of the outcome, but otherwise be representative of the population from which cases were selected and independent of the exposure under investigation.

Most common data collection methods

Being retrospective in nature, case–control studies tend to rely heavily on existing clinical data. This may be in the form of routine clinical records or data in registries or databases created for the purpose of conducting future research. Data on exposure can also be obtained from patients by interview or questionnaire.

Strategies to enhance rigour

Care should be taken to clearly identify and apply diagnostic criteria when sampling cases to ensure that all those identified as cases meet the criteria. If cases are available from records spanning a long period of time, it is recommended to sample more recently-diagnosed cases as these are more likely to be accurate and less likely to be subject to variation of diagnostic accuracy or coding over time (Schulz and Grimes, 2002). Three approaches can be used to reduce control sampling bias:

- *Convenience sampling*: This approach uses a non-probability sampling strategy, but one that focuses on selecting controls in the same way as cases. While this avoids selection of controls from clinical contexts that are different from those from which cases are sampled, the ability to generalise to a broader population may be negatively affected (Mann, 2003).

- *Matching*: Using various patient characteristics (age range, gender, co-morbidities) to match randomly selected cases and controls can minimise confounding bias. However, there are several potential problems associated with matching including reduced external validity and underestimation of differences between the two groups. Matching should be limited to a few known confounders (Mann, 2003; Mansournia, 2018).

- *Population-based sampling*: In this approach, cases are sampled randomly from either a defined geographic area or a registry. Controls are then also sampled randomly from the same area or registry and matched. This approach may not be feasible if well-defined sampling frames are not available.

Overall strengths and limitations

Case–control studies are well suited to research involving uncommon outcomes or when there is a long delay between exposure and outcome. They may offer a potentially large amount of data at relatively low cost. Limitations of these studies include the various biases that may complicate selection of cases and controls. In addition to sampling bias, there may also be observation bias (on the part of the researcher or clinician) and recall bias (on the part of the patient or participant) due to the retrospective nature of case–control studies. In some cases, data from the clinical record or in registries may be incomplete or of uncertain validity.

Significant challenges in this type of research

Gaining access to high-quality data for both the identification of cases and the valid and reliable determination of exposure can be a challenge. However, the single greatest challenge in case–control studies is the selection of appropriate, unbiased controls.

Cohort (prospective and retrospective)

What is it?

A cohort study design involves following a group or groups (cohorts) of patients, or sometimes two groups – one that has been exposed to a factor and one that has not. Following patients from exposure to a specified outcome implies that the cohort design is prospective. In the case of retrospective data collection, the cohorts and outcomes are assembled from existing data at the time of the study. In some cases, where researchers might be interested in a mix of short- and long-term outcomes, data collection may be a combination of retrospective (for the short-term outcome) and prospective (for the long-term outcome) (Hulley et al., 2013).

When is it best used?

A cohort design could be used where it is not possible to conduct more rigorously designed research to answer a clinical question. It could also be used in the early stages of clinical research to generate hypotheses that may be tested with more rigorous designs. Retrospective cohort designs are often used where time or cost limitations preclude a prospective approach.

Appropriate sampling strategies

Sampling of the exposed cohort is based predominantly on accurate identification of the exposure variable. The unexposed cohort should be as similar as possible to the exposed cohort in all respects except for the exposure factor. This can be accomplished by selecting the unexposed cohort from the same data source as the exposed cohort.

Although matching is uncommon in cohort studies, it can be used, particularly where the unexposed cohort are to be sampled from a very diverse population with respect to important exposure-related variables such as age (Schulz and Grimes, 2002). If it is not possible to sample the unexposed cohort internally (i.e. from the same data source as the exposed cohort), then an external data source might be used. This could be in the form of a population judged to be similar to the exposed population, either concurrent or already existing (e.g. from a registry or clinical database of cases). The risk of bias tends to be greater when the unexposed cohort is sampled externally.

Most common data collection methods

Data collection methods may vary, depending on whether a cohort study is prospective, retrospective or both. Prospective (concurrent) studies rely on access to current clinical data for identification of the exposed cohort and future identification of outcomes. As with data collection methods in case–control studies, retrospective cohort studies make use of existing data.

Strategies to enhance rigour

Generally, prospective designs tend to be better than retrospective mainly because it is possible to put measures in place to collect better-quality or customised data. Regardless of which is chosen, researchers should very carefully and unambiguously define the exposure and outcomes of interest across cohorts in advance of data collection and analysis. Those responsible for assessing and recording outcomes should be blinded to the exposure status of individual patients.

Overall strengths and limitations

The main strength of prospective cohort studies lies in their ability to provide a more valid picture of association due to the time order of inquiry and the fact that identification of exposure cannot be influenced by knowledge of outcomes at the time of documentation (Schulz and Grimes, 2002). While the time ordering effect still applies to retrospective cohort studies, the availability of data on exposure and outcomes at the time of the research may introduce bias.

In general, cohort studies have other strengths: they can be used to study multiple outcomes from a single exposure, they are less susceptible to survivor bias (patients that are not included in analysis because they die before documentation) than case–control studies, and they are effective in studying rare exposures because data can be accessed from places where such rare exposures are more common (Schulz and Grimes, 2002). Limitations of cohort studies include that they are prone to bias and confounding and loss to follow-up can be a problem, particularly for prospective studies conducted over longer periods of time (Deeks et al., 2003). Although association can be demonstrated, causality cannot be definitively demonstrated due to the danger of confounding.

Significant challenges in this type of research

In the case of prospective cohort studies, the greatest challenges are the time and cost involved and the possible loss to follow-up which can limit sample size and statistical power. Significant challenges in retrospective cohort studies are mainly related to the quality of existing data.

Quasi-experimental designs

A quasi-experimental study design is one in which groups of participants for comparative analysis of outcomes are assigned without any randomisation. Quasi-experimental studies aim to determine causality, not just association, so it is important to define groups that are as similar to each other in every way at baseline (preintervention).

Non-randomised experimental

What is it?

In a non-randomised experimental study design, the researcher uses preset criteria to assign participants to different groups for the purpose of studying effects of an intervention without randomisation.

When is it best used?

Non-randomised experimental research designs may be used when the intervention of interest has already been implemented in some settings and not others, or when randomisation of patients is not feasible for any other reason (e.g. cost, complexity, willingness of care provider). Non-randomised experimental research designs are prone to selection bias, meaning that patient characteristics

Chapter 8 — Quantitative research design

tend to be different in different groups at baseline (Grady et al., 2013). In addition, non-randomised allocation is usually non-blinded — a weakness that can lead to further bias (e.g. detection bias) and overestimation of intervention effects (Grady et al., 2013).

Appropriate sampling strategies/methods of recruitment

Researchers define inclusion and exclusion criteria specific to the aim of the study and to optimise external validity. A sample size calculation, based on estimates of a clinically meaningful effect size, should guide the decision of how many participants to include.

Most common data collection methods

Data collection methods include accessing and extracting data from the clinical record. Data may include text or numerical data recorded by clinicians, data downloaded directly from devices, images or laboratory results. Typically, both predictor and outcome data are recorded at baseline, with further measurements and recording of predictor data over time.

Strategies to enhance rigour

It may be possible to adjust statistically for known factors that are responsible for differences between groups (Grady et al., 2013). However, there may be unknown confounders that influence outcomes between groups.

Overall strengths and limitations

The strength of a non-randomised experimental research design is that it is simpler and less costly due to omission of the randomisation process. This study design provides a real-world pragmatic option when randomisation is not possible. However, findings can be affected by bias and confounding.

Significant challenges in this type of research

In cases where it is not possible to assign participants to intervention groups randomly and there is a desire for an experimental approach, such a design may be the only option. Where this is the case, every effort should be made to adjust for factor differences between groups as outlined above.

Externally-controlled experimental

What is it?

Externally-controlled experimental research collects control group data that are not obtained from the same sample as the experimental group. The researcher treats the entire sample as the experimental group, meaning that all participants receive the new or experimental intervention. To obtain a control group for comparison, the researcher accesses clinical data from another source, taking care to match the data as closely as possible to those contained in the sample that has received the intervention.

When is it best used?

The use of external controls is seen as weakening internal validity because of the difficulty in controlling selection bias, and thus comparing an experimental intervention with a control group that is in some way systematically different. This approach may be used when a randomised controlled trial (RCT) is not feasible due to cost, complexity or in rare diseases, where randomisation may not be practical. In other situations, ethical concerns related to control group randomisation, particularly in the case of a placebo control, may preclude an RCT. Participants themselves may be more willing to participate in a study without randomisation, as there is often some possibility of benefit in experimental studies (Burger et al., 2021). Externally-controlled experimental studies may have a more compelling ethical justification in trials involving diseases with patients at significant risk of mortality and trials involving children because randomisation is avoided.

Appropriate sampling strategies/methods of recruitment

Sampling is conducted in a similar way to that described above for research with a non-randomised experimental design for the experimental group, which in this case is the entire sample. For the control group, sampling takes place from another data source, which might be a clinical registry, database or existing data from a previous study. Various options exist for sampling from an external data source, ranging from application of inclusion and exclusion criteria and simpler forms of matching through to more advanced approaches such as propensity score matching and Bayesian methods (Thorlund et al., 2020).

Most common data collection methods

Data collection methods for the experimental group are like those described above for research with a non-randomised experimental design.

Strategies to enhance rigour

The most important strategies to enhance rigour are those aimed at eliminating the biases that may be introduced by comparing data derived from different populations. Other forms of possible bias include calendar, regional, assessment and study bias, among others. Burger et al. (2021) provide a useful overview of these and steps that may be taken to minimise them.

Overall strengths and limitations

Externally-controlled experimental research designs offer an opportunity to obtain experimental evidence in situations where an RCT is not possible. Using external data for control purposes can be less time-intensive and more cost-effective than running an RCT. There are also ethical advantages to using this research design in select situations, as outlined above. The most significant limitation is the possibility of biased results due to differences between the experimental group and the external controls.

Significant challenges in this type of research

The most significant challenges in this kind of research are finding a suitable external control data source and controlling bias in the external control group.

Chapter 8 — Quantitative research design

Before–after (pre-test post-test, paired)

What is it?

A before–after research design involves the selection of one sample or group based on a set of inclusion and exclusion criteria. Baseline measurement of the variables of interest is made, followed by an intervention, followed again at some time interval by repeated measurement of the same variables of interest. Depending on the aim of the research, there may be more than one postintervention set of measurements.

A variation of the before–after design is the interrupted time-series design which can be used where outcome data are repeatedly measured over time, often at population level. The objective is to use these time-series data to investigate the effect of an 'interruption' – an event representing a change in the intervention that is hypothesised to influence the outcome or, even stronger, multiple interruptions across sites (Bernal et al., 2017). For example, a public health intervention may be launched at a particular time to raise awareness of pedestrian accidents in a population. An interrupted time-series analysis may then compare the number of pedestrian emergency department admissions in the population over time before the intervention with the number of admissions for a period after the intervention. Statistical methods including regression analysis are used to analyse the data and results are produced in the form of relative risk for the outcome after the intervention compared to before the intervention.

When is it best used?

A before–after design is best used to investigate the effect of an intervention. The intervention is typically one that has a rapid onset and relatively short duration. For an interrupted time-series, the intervention should be one that is associated with a well-defined period of implementation, and for which there exist adequate pre- and post-implementation data.

Appropriate sampling strategies/methods of recruitment

Inclusion and exclusion criteria must be clearly defined at the outset of a before–after study to identify participants. For an interrupted time-series, data will typically be collected from existing clinical or other public health records.

Most common data collection methods

Case selection and variables to be collected must be defined at the outset. In the case of an interrupted time-series, data collection will most often be from an existing clinical or public health database or registry. Self-reported outcomes may be gathered through questionnaires.

Strategies to enhance rigour

Careful management and early strategies can mitigate effects over time of learned behaviour and regression towards the mean, where initial high or low measurements tend to be closer to mean values after the intervention. This change can be taken as having been caused by the intervention when it may not have been. Regression towards the mean can be corrected for at the design and data collection stage, by taking multiple baseline measurements instead of just one, and at the data analysis stage with the use of statistical procedures such as analysis of co-variance (Grady et al., 2013).

In the case of interrupted time-series, several features of time-series data such as seasonal variation, other time-varying confounders and autocorrelation may negatively affect inferences drawn from the data. These factors can generally be dealt with by statistical adjustments (Bernal et al., 2017).

Overall strengths and limitations

The main strength of a before–after research design is that each participant is their own control and thus variation due to personal factors is eliminated. This can increase the statistical power for a given sample size and thus reduce the required sample size compared to the use of two independent samples. The main limitation of before–after studies relates to wider changes over time that may have occurred and caused differences in outcomes.

The strength of an interrupted time-series design is its ability to provide evidence of the effect of population-level interventions when this would otherwise be very difficult to do, and often with the use of routinely-collected historical data. The use of historical data has its own limitations due to missing data and unknown validity of measurements which should be borne in mind.

Significant challenges in this type of research

The most significant challenges in before–after research designs are dealing adequately with time-dependent confounding and, in the case of interrupted time-series, obtaining high-quality data for analysis.

Experimental designs

Randomised controlled trials (RCTs) are acknowledged as providing the best evidence of effectiveness of treatments, if they are planned, carried out and reported with a high degree of rigour. RCTs can directly inform policy and practice through inclusion in guidelines and protocols. RCTs must follow strict guidance for all aspects of implementation, patient recruitment and reporting, as specified in the CONSORT statement and checklists (Schulz et al., 2010) defined and agreed by medical and methodological specialists, in response to problems in interpreting the results of inadequately reported studies.

Randomised controlled trials should address important areas of uncertainty – indeed, an RCT is only ethically justified in the case of equipoise (true uncertainty) about effectiveness of the intervention. The research question, primary and secondary outcomes and analysis plans must be prespecified in protocols which must receive ethical approval. RCTs must include enough participants with outcomes to detect clinically meaningful differences between groups.

In an RCT, participants who meet clearly defined criteria for inclusion are prospectively randomly assigned to different groups, usually experimental (intervention) or control (placebo or usual care) although there can be more than one experimental group, such as different drugs, doses or routes of administration. In a pragmatic (real-world) trial, with results intended to inform clinical practice, participants are analysed in the group to which they were randomly allocated, whether or not they received the treatment, for comparison of outcomes (known as per protocol analysis). Sometimes adherence to treatment allocation may be low, but as this is judged to be likely to reflect what would happen in real-life practice should the intervention be routinely implemented, standard practice is to carry out analysis in studies of effectiveness in this way – referred to as 'intention to treat' analysis or analysis 'by treatment allocated' (Gupta et al., 2011).

Randomised controlled trial design may be at individual or cluster level, and with parallel or staggered points of recruitment. These designs are discussed below in more detail.

Individually randomised designs

What is it?

This is the strongest randomised trial design as it is least open to selection bias. Each individual person who meets the inclusion criteria is allocated at random to a treatment arm. Various methods are used for random allocation, but reliable options are limited in the prehospital setting. Drug or treatment packs can be randomly allocated to intervention or placebo, as in the PARAMEDIC2 adrenaline trial (Perkins et al., 2016); envelopes are sometimes used, although this method has some critics as allocation may be subverted; scratch cards have been successfully used at the scene of hip fractures in the RAPID trial of fascia iliaca compartment block (Keen et al., 2018).

When is it best used?

Where there is equipoise about effectiveness, and where the new treatment has not been previously available or rigorously tested; when practitioners are able to randomly allocate patients at individual level (Perkins et al., 2018).

Appropriate sampling strategies/methods of recruitment

Each person who meets predefined inclusion criteria should be assessed for inclusion and recruitment to the trial, consented and randomly allocated to a trial arm, using trial protocols.

Most common data collection methods

Data collection in an RCT is prospective and can be gathered from routine clinical records, specifically designed data collection forms if new data items are required, patient questionnaires and centrally-held records. Subject to appropriate ethical and information governance permissions, data can be linked across sources so that identifiers are not included and can be analysed in a secure environment with participants anonymised.

Strategies to enhance rigour

Researchers should adhere to widely-accepted standards for carrying out and reporting randomised trials (CONSORT). Demonstrating adherence to these standards helps assure the quality and rigour of the trial. Inclusion of patient/ public representatives with experience of the condition being studied can help to define important aspects of the trial, including outcomes to measure, ways to reach participants to gather self-reported outcomes and interpretation of findings (see Chapter 17).

An RCT to determine effectiveness needs to be adequately powered, based on a sample size calculation to establish how many participants with the primary outcome need to be included in analyses to have a strong chance of detecting a clinically important difference. It is also good practice to undertake an RCT across several sites, to ensure that results are transferable.

Overall strengths and limitations

Randomised controlled trials with individual randomisation are the highest study design in the traditional hierarchy of evidence. They provide clear evidence of effects which are attributable to the intervention, as all other aspects of groups compared should be similar, and any small differences described. Limitations of RCTs are often related to restrictions on participant recruitment, such as exclusion of patients with co-morbidities; failure to reach recruitment target, leaving the study underpowered; or clinically-focused outcomes which do not reflect the priorities of patients.

Significant challenges in this type of research

Challenges include gaining funding and permissions to undertake a trial while equipoise exists, and services are willing but have not yet introduced the intervention. In other words, there is a window of opportunity that can disappear if practice changes. Once new interventions have been introduced, based on clinical consensus rather than evidence, it becomes increasingly difficult to carry out a randomised evaluation, although not impossible (McDonnell et al., 2006). One example of a trial in this situation was the PARAMEDIC2 RCT to establish an evidence base for adrenaline, which was already routinely used in prehospital care of cardiac arrest patients. In this case, the active intervention was non-administration of adrenaline, with standard practice being administration of adrenaline when existing protocols were met. Significant resistance to withdrawal of adrenaline was encountered from patients and paramedics, but the trial was successfully completed.

Cluster randomised designs

What is it?

In some circumstances, it is not feasible or appropriate to randomly allocate interventions at individual level, in which case groups (clusters) can be randomly allocated.

When is it best used?

When the intervention is introduced at site level or requires training which cannot be unlearned, it may be impossible to individually randomly allocate participants to treatment groups. In this situation, it is possible to still use a randomised design but at cluster or group level. In this case, the cluster – by which analysis will take place

Chapter 8 — Quantitative research design

– must be defined prior to the commencement of recruitment. Prehospital trials have used clustering at the level of ambulance station (Snooks et al., 2017), responding vehicle (Perkins et al., 2015) and week of year (Mason et al., 2007).

Appropriate sampling/method of recruitment

As for individually randomised trials, inclusion and exclusion criteria must be clearly defined prior to the start of patient recruitment. A method of flagging cases who should be included in the trial needs to be designed so that recruitment is clear, and any attrition described clearly in the CONSORT flowchart.

Strategies to enhance rigour

CONSORT checklists have been developed for the reporting of cluster randomised trials. If CONSORT standards and checklists are adhered to then a high level of rigour is assured. Training in trial methods can help to improve adherence to protocols for randomisation, treatment and data collection. There is always a possibility of clustering effects, such as unanticipated differences between groups based, by chance, on similarities within groups. If clustering effects are recognised, then allowances can be made in the power calculation and/or analysis of results (Mason et al., 2007).

Overall strengths and limitations

When clustering is introduced it will reduce the certainty with which effects can be attributed to the intervention. However, using a randomised design at any level is preferable in terms of the reliability of the attribution of effects to intervention compared to a non-randomised design.

Randomised stepped wedge designs

What is it?

This study design is like a cluster randomised trial, but the intervention is introduced over time, so that all participants recruited at the start of the trial are in the control group but increasing numbers are recruited to the intervention group as the recruitment period progresses, with all participants recruited to the intervention arm by the end of the recruitment period.

When is it best used?

This design can be used in a situation where an intervention is due to be implemented across an area, and for evaluation purposes it is arranged to stagger the intervention across an implementation period, and further, to randomly allocate practitioners or sites to implementation across that period. This study design has been used in the prehospital setting to encourage participation of paramedics who all had the opportunity to be trained and to offer the experimental treatment (take-home naloxone) (Moore et al., 2014).

Appropriate sampling/method of recruitment

As for cluster RCTs.

Strategies for improving rigour

As for cluster RCTs.

Strengths and limitations

Every step further away from individual randomisation compromises reliability of study findings. However, whenever randomisation is successfully used, study validity is stronger than for non-randomised designs. Differences between groups should be adjusted for, as far as possible, in predefined analysis plans.

Summary

Quantitative research designs cover a broad spectrum mainly divided by whether they are observational, quasi-experimental or experimental in nature. Observational designs, both descriptive and analytical, are generally cost-effective and easy to perform. However, they are typically constrained by the quality of data available. While in some instances using a prospective design may improve this situation, the potential for bias in observational designs limits the inferences that can be drawn from them.

Quasi-experimental designs, including non-randomised designs, externally controlled and before–after designs, are aimed at going beyond association and determining causality when stronger designs are not feasible. While preferable to observational designs, the quasi-experimental designs all suffer to some degree from bias due to the way treatment and control groups are allocated.

To overcome bias, experimental designs – such as individual RCTs, cluster and stepped wedge designs – offer the most rigorous evidence for the effectiveness of prehospital treatments. These designs are also the most complex and expensive to deploy.

Understanding of the fundamental differences between the categories of quantitative research designs described above along with their strengths, weaknesses and limitations will allow researchers to use the most appropriate research design for their purpose, whether this is well-resourced or constrained. While experimental designs occupy the apex of the evidence hierarchy, all designs have a place in contributing some value to the practice of prehospital emergency care if interpreted in context.

Chapter 9

Data collection in observational studies

Tim Edwards and Jack Barrett

Purpose of this chapter

Completion of this chapter will help you to:
- define the difference between retrospective and prospective data collection
- identify sources of data
- appreciate legal and ethical issues associated with data collection
- describe common types of observational study.

Introduction

Observational methodologies employ non-experimental and non-randomised approaches to collect data and identify associations between variables, such as smoking status and cardiovascular disease. Historically, the use of observational data in paramedic practice has been commonplace for research, service evaluation and audit. Observational studies are broadly defined as either retrospective or prospective. Retrospective studies rely on extracting data from pre-existing records. Such data can only be used to study past events, and will not usually have been collected for the primary purpose of undertaking research. In contrast, prospective data collection is undertaken on a preplanned basis to study an intervention or outcome of interest in the future over a predefined period. Prospective data collection strategies are therefore normally undertaken for the express purpose of research activity. For this reason, prospective observational studies tend to occupy a higher position than retrospective approaches in the hierarchy of evidence.

Retrospective data collection

What is it?

A retrospective chart or medical record review is one of the most straightforward methods for collecting data in routine practice and is frequently used for audit and research purposes. In its simplest form, an audit may involve scrutinising clinical records to extract data to compare the standard of care against predefined audit criteria based on established standards. In ambulance services globally, clinical performance indicators are frequently based on chart review of specified cases compared with protocols or guidelines. Such reviews may be used to determine compliance with standards of care and benchmark performance against other services or individuals.

In retrospective observational studies, a researcher may compare or evaluate clinical practice within or between a cohort of patients. While the data collection methods should be identical, an observational study is interested in comparing and contrasting two or more groups based on an intervention or outcome, which may influence future practice. For example, retrospective observational studies demonstrated a relationship between adrenaline administration in out-of-hospital cardiac arrest (OHCA) and worse patient outcomes (Dumas et al., 2014). This association informed the development of a randomised controlled drug trial, PARAMEDIC2. An audit would only inform whether clinicians adhered to guidelines, whereas observational research suggests whether the clinical practice had a potential benefit or harm to a patient.

Overview of data extraction in retrospective observational research

The ease with which data may be extracted from charts varies. It depends on factors such as the structure or design of the clinical record, legibility of handwritten notes and comprehensiveness of the clinician's information. Clinical records were historically handwritten and paper-based but are increasingly electronic and typed. The form of the record may range from entirely free-text notes to very structured documents with predetermined response options and limited free-text options. Records may be accessed electronically or require the researcher to obtain scanned or hard copies.

Consideration must be given to the data extraction methods, the environment in which this will take place and meeting information governance and patient confidentiality requirements. Similarly, adequate arrangements must be in place for the secure storage of both electronic and paper-based records.

Approach to data extraction in retrospective research

The methods through which data extraction is undertaken will vary according to the nature of the records used. Highly-structured clinical records with limited opportunity for free-text entry will be relatively straightforward to extract data from due to the presence of predefined fields. Still, they may lack the detail required in some circumstances. Retrospective records may contain incomplete data; however, the use of electronic systems with the option to prompt the clinician to complete a field may, to some extent, alleviate this.

In all cases, it is essential that the information required and extraction methods used are clearly defined and understood, especially where multiple researchers are involved in the process, to reduce inter-rater variation. This often requires that a standardised data extraction tool be developed and piloted before use in practice. This may include definitions of variables and procedures for handling missing records or data fields. These measures are important in reducing the potential for measurement and interpretation bias during data extraction. Where electronic records are available, it may be possible to obtain some or all data automatically without the need for manual review and extraction.

In observational research, some degree of missing data will inevitably be encountered, especially in retrospective studies where records were not completed for research purposes.

Case–control studies in retrospective research

Case–control studies are a more complex form of retrospective observational research in which cases (patients who have the outcome or exposure of interest) are compared with a control group of patients who do not. Conditions commonly encountered in paramedic research to date include OHCA (Egly et al., 2011; Gahan, Studnek and Vandeventer, 2011; Hanif, Kaji and Niemann, 2010; Woodall et al., 2007) and brain injury (Fouche et al., 2019; Sloane et al., 2000) where exposure to various interventions such as different airway management strategies or drug therapies have been compared between groups. Equally, groups of patients may be exposed to a different type of method of service delivery, for example, by a paramedic with an advanced level of training in a specialist area of practice.

Of note, patients in these studies are not randomised to different treatments or interventions; rather, they report outcomes from historical data based on comparisons between groups with different characteristics.

Although chart review frequently forms part of the data collection in case–control studies, there is often a requirement to extract data from various sources involving multiple organisations. This may necessitate establishing data-sharing agreements, for example between an ambulance service and hospital. Processes for identifying cases and controls will also be required according to predefined criteria. In some studies, patients will be matched according to established criteria to ensure that key demographics and characteristics between the two groups are comparable.

Role of retrospective methods in paramedic research

Retrospective methods have often been used to examine the impact of paramedics in ambulance services and other settings. Early evaluation of paramedics often concentrated on their impact on survival from OHCA. Data were retrospectively extracted from ambulance records and hospital notes to determine survival for patients treated by advanced life support paramedics versus other ambulance staff restricted to basic life support and defibrillation. A common theme encountered was the number of missing records, highlighting one limitation of retrospective data collection.

More recently, retrospective observational studies have been used to evaluate paramedics with additional education and training in the assessment and management of lower acuity patients in the community and other clinical settings compared with standard ambulance or other clinical responses (Eaton-Williams et al. 2020). While these studies have generally concluded that such initiatives are

Chapter 9 — Data collection in observational studies

associated with positive patient outcomes, retrospective data collection limits the extent to which long-term outcomes can be assessed.

Prospective data collection

What is it?

The most common requirement for prospective observational data collection is as part of a cohort study whereby a group of individuals are followed over time to determine the consequences of exposure to a variable of interest. Although cohort studies may be conducted retrospectively, prospective approaches tend to be regarded as more reliable, in part due to data being collected in real time for the purpose of conducting research. Unlike retrospective approaches, where historical data are usually accessed at a single point in time, prospective cohort studies require that data are collected on multiple occasions over a defined period.

Approach to data extraction in prospective research

The same requirement for standardised data extraction remains; however, there is increased potential for the researcher to obtain data via direct contact with patients either face to face or remotely, depending on the nature of the study. Under these circumstances, researchers may require further training and support both in obtaining data in a standardised way and responding to queries and concerns raised by participants. Depending on the time over which the study is conducted, participants may be lost to follow-up due to a host of factors such as relocation, withdrawal from the study or ill health.

Data collection costs are generally appreciably higher than those associated with retrospective approaches, although this depends on the study's scale and duration.

Role of prospective methodologies in paramedic research

Prospective cohort studies relating to paramedics tend to concentrate on specific conditions and/or interventions. One study investigating the impact of paramedic rapid sequence intubation of patients with severe traumatic brain injury prospectively enrolled patients over a two-year period (Davis et al., 2003). Ambulance and hospital data were extracted, and researchers monitored the in-hospital course for patients until death or discharge. To compare outcomes, prospectively enrolled patients were then matched to non-intubated retrospective cases drawn from an established trauma registry. While the study was in progress, data monitoring identified worrying trends in patients arriving in hospitals after prehospital intubation and increased mortality compared with matched historical controls. In this instance, monitoring of the prospective data collection facilitated the early identification of concerns, resulting in the trial being suspended.

Of note, a more recent randomised controlled trial found that paramedic rapid sequence intubation in traumatic brain injury was associated with improved neurological outcomes at six months (Bernard et al., 2010), potentially highlighting the limitations of studies of prospective research and studies which are stopped early.

Sources of observational data

Multiple sources of observational data are often available in ambulance services and other healthcare settings. In traditional ambulance settings, this may include patient care records, internal registries for specific conditions such as ST-elevation myocardial infarction or stroke, especially when required for national reporting requirements, and data downloads from devices such as defibrillators or vehicle management systems. Where paramedics are employed in other settings, further data may be available, including diagnostic imaging and laboratory tests alongside standard clinical records.

On a national and international basis, several other observational data sources may be available to paramedics, especially when working as part of established research teams. Examples from UK practice include the Trauma Audit and Research Network (TARN); the Myocardial Infarction National Audit Project (MINAP) and the Warwick Out of Hospital Cardiac Arrest Outcomes (OHCAO) data registries. Given the costs associated with establishing and maintaining these registries, there are frequently costs associated with data extraction that need to be accounted for at the outset of any observational research project.

As electronic access to patient records evolves, paramedics will probably have the ability to access more observational data relating to longer periods regardless of the settings where they work. While this is an attractive proposition in facilitating more profession-specific observational research, including cohort approaches, the use of such data will be subject to stringent ethical and information governance regulations (see Chapter 16).

Surveys

This section outlines where a researcher may want to use a survey, how they could design it, its strengths and limitations, and the ethical considerations one should take into account when conducting survey-based research.

Purposes of a survey

The purposes of a survey (also known as a questionnaire) can be categorised into three areas: 'breaking ground', 'drawing comparisons' and 'providing context', and these areas may overlap in a stand-alone survey or over multiple (repeated) surveys.

Surveys allow a researcher to ask a population questions about a particular subject and generate a wealth of data from a single point in time or time series. Surveys are not without their weaknesses, and conducting a successful one is challenging. If done correctly, the data are invaluable, but a poorly-designed survey or an inappropriate recruitment strategy could undermine its findings. While surveys are typically considered to be prospective cohort studies, they have a lower position on the hierarchy of evidence than other prospective approaches due to several limitations and inherent biases in their design, and researchers should be aware of the implications for their findings.

Chapter 9 — Data collection in observational studies

Breaking ground

Surveys can be used as a 'fact-finding' exercise. Knowledge and understanding may be lacking in clinical practice or patient experience, and little or no relevant research has been conducted in this area. For example, it was recognised that end-of-life care (EoLC) was a growing area in the ambulance service. A nationwide survey of paramedics in England explored the current level of exposure they had with patients with unmet EoLC needs. This study was used to understand what was happening in paramedic practice to inform future research and development (Eaton-Williams et al., 2020).

Drawing comparisons

A survey can allow a researcher to draw comparisons within and between groups. Emond, Furness, and Deacon-Crouch (2015) evaluated final-year student paramedics' perceptions and attitudes towards mental health patients presenting to the ambulance service. Participants completed a questionnaire about their views on mental health patients, undertook a mental health module and then repeated the same questionnaire once the module was completed. There was a notable difference in students' perceptions towards mental health patients following a teaching intervention. Repeating the same survey twice (pre- and post-intervention) allows the researcher to evaluate the impact such an intervention has on a group.

Surveys can also evaluate differences between groups. Khan et al (2020) explored the sleep quality and mental health differences between paramedics in Australia and Saudi Arabia. A group of paramedics from both countries were given the same survey, which included standardised self-reported assessment tools to evaluate their mental health and sleep quality. This survey reported that paramedics in Saudi Arabia had worse mental and physical health than their Australian counterparts. However, while this survey noted a difference between groups, it could not empirically explain why.

Providing context to concurrent data collection or data collected

The randomised controlled drug trial PARAMEDIC2 compared adrenaline to a placebo administered by paramedics to OHCA patients (Perkins et al., 2018). Within UK ambulance research, few trials have relied on ambulance paramedics to enrol incapacitated, critically unwell patients. The trial was unable to detect how paramedics felt about this or whether it may have influenced the trial's running.

A survey by Lazarus, Iyer, and Fothergill (2019) explored the attitudes and experiences of paramedics participating in the study. Recruiting incapacitated patients into a drug trial has several ethical issues. The paramedic profession has limited exposure to this form of patient recruitment although, arguably has a wealth of experience of acting in the patient's best interest under 'normal' circumstances. This piece of work considered what part the paramedic plays as the recruiter in these types of trials. A primary focus was on how the paramedic dealt with the controversy that surrounded the PARAMEDIC2 trial. This is an example of how surveys can provide context to a study's findings.

How to design a survey

Who is the target population and why does it matter?

It is essential to clarify the target population for a survey. The research question will generally dictate this, but it is necessary to define it.

For example, both Eaton-Williams et al. (2020) and Lazarus et al. (2019) wanted paramedics' views. However, where the former study was recruiting all paramedics who work for the ambulance service, the latter study recruited paramedics who had participated in the PARAMEDIC2 trial. Had Eaton-Williams et al. (2020) included all ambulance clinicians who met EoLC patients, then their results could have been different. The assessment and co-ordination of EoLC should be performed by a paramedic but not an ambulance technician. Therefore, one group of clinicians' views in a study may not have been as relevant as others' opinions. Likewise, had Lazarus et al. (2019) sought the views of paramedics who were not involved with PARAMEDIC2, then the study's context would have changed.

Once the target sample population is identified, several considerations will depend on who the survey is written for.

Language of the survey

Is the survey targeting a specific group of people, for example advanced paramedic practitioners working in the primary care setting, or a broad group of people, such as patients who call 999 for non-life-threatening presentations? The target audience must easily understand the language used. Jargon and specific medical terms may be familiar to a paramedic but not a layperson. Limit abbreviations to only the essentials.

The language of the survey should also be unbiased. Consider these two fictional questions below asking a patient about their perceptions of an ambulance crew:

- On a scale of 1–10, how would you rate the hostility of the ambulance crew that attended you? (1 – no hostility, 10 – very hostile)
- How would you describe the behaviour of the ambulance crew that attended you? (Professional, unprofessional, neither professional nor unprofessional).

The first question implies that ambulance crews were hostile and may introduce a bias in the participant's response, whereas the second question is comparatively neutral.

Finally, if conducting an international survey, does it need to be translated? If a survey is translated, ensure that the questions' meanings are not lost in translation. Otherwise, participants may interpret the same question differently depending on the language in which they view it. Khan et al. (2020) used standardised reporting tools translated (and validated) from English to Arabic to resolve this issue.

Length of the survey

There is no defined number of questions to ask in a survey, but long surveys should be avoided if possible. Asking a participant to answer questions can be time-consuming. While participants may be enthusiastic about sharing their views, they may tire and not complete the survey or rush through it, diminishing the data's quality.

Testing/piloting

Processes of survey validation are beyond the scope of this book, but it is essential to understand that surveys should be tested on the target population. Testing allows the researcher to see how long the survey would take a participant to complete and whether participants understand the wording of the questions. Feedback here will contribute to the success of the survey. However, it may be appropriate to reuse a survey that is already validated. For example, Khan et al. (2020) used the General Health Questionnaire SF-36 because it is a validated survey used in different settings and cultures to measure a population's physical and mental health.

Use of closed and open-ended questions

Closed questions

These questions provide the researcher with a level of control over the response a participant can provide. The participant can only provide an answer available to them in the survey as single or multiple-choice answers. Scales, such as Likert scales, can also be used to measure the level of agreement a participant may have with a question or statement. However, the question must be precise. If a question is ambiguous, the participant's interpretation of the question could differ from the researcher's intention, meaning their answer may not be appropriate.

Closed questions allow for descriptive analysis and provide a general overview of how participants feel about a particular issue. However, they do not provide the context around that answer. For example, the survey conducted by Eaton-Williams et al., (2020) reported that 62% of their participants did not use EoLC guidelines when referring their patients to primary care. While these results perhaps highlight that most participants do not refer to EoLC guidelines, it does not explain what clinicians are using to guide the care they provide.

To encourage completion of the survey, it can be good to give participants a neutral/don't remember/not relevant option as well, so they are not forced to answer a question that is not relevant to them.

Open-ended questions

These questions allow the participant to share their views, opinions and feelings on a subject and provide a rich context for the research. However, these questions also need to be precise so that a participant knows what the question is asking.

The answers provided in open-ended questions do not lend themselves to the same global descriptive perspective that closed questions offer and can pose a challenge during analysis (O'Cathain and Thomas, 2004). Their generalisability is limited but appropriate analysis allows the survey responses to be contextualised.

Eaton-Williams et al., (2020) asked participants if they felt that paramedics should be identifying patients at the end of their life; 97% thought that they should. An open-ended question was used to invite participants to add comments to their response. This highlighted that while participants felt they should be identifying these patients, there needed to be an improvement in clinical training and referral pathways because paramedics are in a unique position to identify patients with unmet EoLC needs.

Paper or electronic survey?

Historically, surveys were printed on paper and respondents would complete and return it. However, it is more common now to find surveys online on digital platforms. Technology has allowed versatility in how the survey is displayed and how the data are collected. For example, with an electronic survey, functions such as 'Skip Logic' enable the survey to populate questions based on a respondent's answer, allowing for a better flow through the survey.

When paper surveys are used, they will need to be manually uploaded for analysis. There is a risk of human error in this process, and quality assurance measures (i.e. a second or third reviewer) will be needed to check the recorded data's accuracy; this can be time-consuming. Electronic systems are favoured as the dataset can be easily copied over from the survey platform to the software package being used for analysis.

How to distribute a survey

Paper surveys need to be handed out, emailed or posted to participants. This means a distributor must be in a location where the surveys can be distributed by hand or they have to be sent to sites where they can be shared with the target population, for example an ambulance station, hospital ward or primary care practice. Permissions will be needed before the surveys can be sent. Postal surveys will need a return envelope enclosed so that the participant can return the survey.

If the survey is electronic, it can be distributed via electronic mailing lists, electronic bulletins and posters (with QR codes), or social media. The more public the survey, the more likely it is that inappropriate participants may be enrolled.

Ethical considerations – participant anonymity

An advantage of a survey is that a participant can provide information to a study without disclosing their identity. Anonymity may allow the participant to provide honest and truthful answers without the risk of prejudice. However, this is dependent on a survey not collecting information that identifies the participant. It would be unusual to ask participants to disclose personal information such as their name, date of birth or home address. Confidential information should be avoided. However, if a follow-up survey is required, participants may be asked to volunteer their preferred contact details. However, it would be best to work within the principles of the researcher's employer data protection policies. It should be clearly stated how personal information such as email addresses are used.

Chapter 9 — Data collection in observational studies

There are other ways in which participants could identify themselves or other people. For example, age, job role, length of service in a study could identify a clinician if the population sample was taken from a small ambulance station. Likewise, asking participants to give open-ended, free-text answers introduces a risk where an individual could be named or disclose an inappropriate clinical practice. It is important to remind participants not to reveal names or other identifiable information. It may be appropriate for the survey to highlight where clinical practice, for example, could be improved. A risk management plan should be developed in the design stage of the study, and in place in case a concerning disclosure is made by a participant.

Design of data collection tools

Should you use a validated data collection tool or a bespoke one?

Data collection tool design and implementation methods can significantly influence a study's results, reliability and validity. It is important to consider whether an established, validated data collection tool may be used or whether a bespoke version will be designed and who will use it. Consideration must also be given to the costs and resource requirements associated with the chosen approach.

Use of an existing tool avoids the need for a design phase but may incur licensing costs and require investment in processing software or other materials. Conversely, a bespoke tool specifically designed for a study will not have these direct costs but will incur indirect costs in development and production time. Use of an existing validated tool provides the opportunity to easily compare results with other studies using the same tool. Development of a bespoke tool will probably necessitate a pilot phase, which may delay data collection, especially if further modifications and additional pilots are required.

Regardless of the approach taken, any requirements relating to training in the use of the tool, quality assurance arrangements, information governance and data processing need to be factored into the study plan.

The clinical specialisms and environments in which paramedics work can be unpredictable and geographically dispersed. Where the use of an established data collection tool is contemplated, the practicalities of its use in the specific patient group or practice environment of interest must be considered. For example, data collection tools designed for use in general practice or an acute hospital may be impractical in out-of-hospital or emergency settings.

A systematic review reported wide variation in data collection tools developed for use in humanitarian emergencies, in part due to the differing target populations and types of emergencies, as well as the degree of infrastructure failure present and availability of resources such as power and telecommunications (Pyone et al., 2015). The tools reviewed consisted of a range of pre-existing and bespoke designs, although data collection methods were poorly described in some studies.

Concluding remarks cautioned against the development of further data collection tools, favouring evaluation and standardisation of existing versions based on a sound understanding of the populations of interest, clinical requirements and operating environments.

Considerations in data collection tool design

As part of the selection or development of a data collection tool, consideration must be given to the environment in which it will be used and the numbers and needs of those who will administer it in practice. While a poorly-designed tool may affect the validity of study results, inappropriate administration or application in practice may result in incomplete or inconsistent data collection, adversely impacting reliability. Researchers must be mindful of the professional backgrounds of staff expected to use the tool in clinical practice, and any associated training requirements. This may be particularly relevant in the ambulance setting, where multiple grades of staff with varying levels of education and experience work alongside each other.

If the correct methods for applying a data collection tool or interpretation of results are unclear, then it is likely that significant inter-rater variation will occur. Similar concerns may arise where staff are involved in data collection in areas outside their standard scope of practice. An example of this might be variation in education and experience in electrocardiograph interpretation between ambulance clinicians. Previous studies have noted considerable inter-rater variation in calculating the Glasgow Coma Scale (GCS) score by ambulance clinicians (Feldman et al., 2015). A data collection tool reliant on paramedics determining GCS thresholds might therefore be subject to significant inter-rater variation.

Such concerns may be alleviated to some extent by the provision of adequate training and familiarisation with the proposed data collection tool. This may be conducted face to face or via live or pre-recorded e-learning events. In some cases, it may be appropriate to restrict the staff groups eligible to undertake data collection. Recent examples of this in UK trials include the PARAMEDIC2 and AIRWAYS-2 studies, where only paramedics with the requisite scope of practice were eligible to participate.

Paper or electronic data collection tools?

Methods for the administration of the data collection tool and associated resource requirements are important considerations. Paper-based approaches may be largely immune from technology or infrastructure failure, but are prone to data loss and concern regarding information governance, especially in geographically dispersed services or clinical environments. These concerns must be balanced against the costs of alternative methods such as electronic data capture, which may incur additional costs in the development phase and prove unreliable in the event of software, device or telecommunications failures. The time lag between administration of the tool and data availability to researchers will generally be much shorter where an electronic solution is used. There is some evidence that using apps via a handheld device such as smartphone results in higher response

Chapter 9 — Data collection in observational studies

rates and a reduction in errors, even in geographically challenged or resource-constrained environments (Ahmed et al., 2018).

Ultimately, the data collection tool and approach used will be dependent on the factors highlighted above. Regardless of this, any data collection tool must be as straightforward and usable as possible, considering the practice setting and practitioners involved. Researchers must ensure as far as possible that the application of the tool is standardised. Close attention to the design and pilot phases and associated training requirements are vital in achieving this. Cultural factors such as understanding the purpose of the data collection tool, perception of its usefulness or relevance and overall willingness to participate in research have previously been identified as significant barriers to successful implementation (Rostami et al., 2018). To some extent, these issues may be addressed by appropriate promotion of the programme of work, incentivising participants and adequate training. Nonetheless, the potential for cultural negativity or ambivalence to adversely affect applying a data collection tool, and the associated results should not be ignored.

Data collection tools in paramedic practice

Several data collection tools exist globally in paramedic research relating to areas of practice such as stroke recognition and medication trials (Fothergill et al., 2013; Keeling et al., 2003; Morrison et al., 2009). A UK study comparing prehospital stroke recognition via the Face-Arms-Speech-Time (FAST) test versus the Recognition of Stroke in the Emergency Room (ROSIER) approach (Fothergill et al., 2013) utilised a revised proforma completed by the attending ambulance clinician (Figure 9.1). In this instance, the validated ROSIER procedure was incorporated into a bespoke data collection tool with the addition of a small number of study-specific fields. Training in the application of ROSIER was provided face to face, incorporating procedures for data collection. A total of 312 patients were successfully recruited from the prehospital phase, with a further 32 patients eligible for enrolment but not subsequently assessed via ROSIER.

Figure 9.1 illustrates the ROSIER data collection tool (Fothergill et al., 2013) used by ambulance paramedics. Routine patient information was collected from the patient ambulance report form; this data collection tool was supplemented and used by study paramedics to collect additional information that is not routinely collected.

Another study assessing the potential for out-of-hospital triage of patients with suspected ruptured aortic aneurysm utilised a bespoke app accessible via smartphone. The app's content was based on ten predictive variables identified via retrospective validation using logistic regression analysis (Lewis et al. 2016). Data collection was intended to determine whether a predictive algorithm could be developed rather than altering the care pathway at the point at which the app was accessed. Use of the app in the ambulance environment was feasible in an urban setting by paramedics and other ambulance clinicians at the point of care.

> If BM < 4 mmol/L treat urgently and reassess once blood glucose normal. Please record GCS, BP and BM on the PRF.
>
> **ROSIER ASSESSMENT** Please tick **one** choice for **each** item:
>
> | | | | |
> |---|---|---|---|
> | Has there been loss of consciousness or syncope? | Y (-1) | N (0) | Unable to assess |
> | Has there been seizure activity? | Y (-1) | N (0) | Unable to assess |
> | Is there a **NEW ACUTE** onset (or on awakening from sleep): | | | |
> | 1. Asymmetric facial weakness | Y (+1) | N (0) | Unable to assess |
> | 2. Asymmetric arm weakness | Y (+1) | N (0) | Unable to assess |
> | 3. Asymmetric leg weakness | Y (+1) | N (0) | Unable to assess |
> | 4. Speech disturbance | Y (+1) | N (0) | Unable to assess |
> | 5. Visual field defect | Y (+1) | N (0) | Unable to assess |
> | * **TOTAL SCORE** (-2 to +5): | | | |
>
> A ROSIER score of *ONE* or more suggests a stroke. A score of *ZERO* or less indicates stroke is unlikely but is not completely excluded.
>
> **PROVISIONAL DIAGNOSIS (please tick):**
>
> | | |
> |---|---|
> | | Stroke / TIA |
> | | Non-stroke (specify) |
>
> *Key*: BM = blood glucose; BP = blood presure (mm Hg); GCS = Glasgow Coma Scale; TIA: Transient Ischaemic Attack; PRF = Patient Report Form.

Figure 9.1 The Recognition of Stroke in the Emergency Room (ROSIER) data collection tool.

Source: Reprinted from Fothergill et al., 2013, with permission from the publisher.

Summary

This chapter considers the approach to observational data collection and surveys in quantitative research. Data collection can be both retrospective and prospective in nature. While the former is relatively easy to perform, there are inherent limitations that undermine a study's integrity. The latter approach allows for more control over the data collected and provides the researcher with an opportunity to collect data

Chapter 9 — Data collection in observational studies

that would not usually be available in routine practice. However, prospective research requires an investment in resources to collect these data, and patient follow-up may be challenging. However, if successful, these studies offer a worthy contribution to the evidence base and reflect real-life practice.

The data collection tools used in observational research should be simple in their design. Still, consideration should be given as to who will be using them, what training is required and whether an established tool is available or a bespoke tool is required. These considerations also incur an investment of time or money and need to be factored into a study's design.

Surveys play a valuable role in the early exploration of untapped areas, and can provide a context where other quantitative approaches cannot do so. While surveys have an appeal as they can reach many participants, caution should be exercised as they tend to yield low response rates, and population representation may be specific to particular groups, as those interested in a specific area the survey explores will be more likely to engage than those who are not.

Surveys and data collection tools should be simple in their design. As technology evolves and becomes more accessible, these data collection tools are likely to be found in electronic formats. This reduces the errors associated with paper-based collection tools but raises new data protection and governance issues that researchers will need to be aware of. Patient anonymity is important. While data collection tools can be anonymised, researchers using surveys must be careful not to involuntarily encourage participants to disclose sensitive information that is not required for their research.

Useful resources

- Trauma Audit and Research Network (TARN): www.c4ts.qmul.ac.uk/downloads/procedures-manual-tarn-p13-iss.pdf
- Myocardial Ischaemia National Audit Project (MINAP): www.nicor.org.uk/national-cardiac-audit-programme/heart-attack-audit-minap/
- Out of Hospital Cardiac Arrest Outcomes (OHCAO) registry www.warwick.ac.uk/fac/sci/med/research/ctu/trials/ohcao/overview/projectinformation/

Chapter 10

Data collection in experimental studies

Ruth Fisher and Elicia Austin

> **Purpose of this chapter**
>
> Completion of this chapter will help you to:
> - differentiate between experimental and quasi-experimental study design
> - identify approaches to randomisation in experimental research
> - understand the ethical implications of experimental research
> - recognise how experimental research can be utilised in paramedic evidence-based practice.

Introduction

With much of the historical research into paramedic practice being conducted in hospital and non-comparable settings, reconsideration of the evidence upon which paramedic practice is based has become necessary (Bigham and Welsford, 2015). Experimental research is often described as the most reliable and valid study design in healthcare research, due to the low risk of bias associated with the design strengthening the conclusions that may be drawn. However, it is increasingly recognised that experimental study designs may not always be truly practical in certain healthcare settings (Bärnighausen et al., 2017).

Experimental methodology offers various ways in which knowledge can be generated and theories tested. Experimental research is typically considered to include randomised controlled trials (RCTs) and non-randomised studies (NRS). The unique and unpredictable nature of the prehospital setting can certainly create challenges for researchers in the planning and deployment of experimental studies, which contrasts with the degree of control considered necessary for reliable and valid research.

Purpose of experimental research

Experimental research seeks to test a theory or hypothesis, proving whether it is essentially true or false, and so the positivist ontological belief that a 'single

Chapter 10 — Data collection in experimental studies

tangible reality can be measured' aligns with this type of research (Park et al., 2020). The purpose of experimental research can also be to determine cause-and-effect relationships between different variables, and to show causality the researchers must generate objective knowledge (Bonell et al., 2018). This aligns with the epistemological assumptions in the positivist paradigm, to use quantification and control to generate knowledge which is validated and verified. Following a quantitative methodology allows the research design to create explanation, association or prediction using numerical data. However, for this reason, experimental research can lack context-specific application or considerations with real-life implementation of its results.

A defining feature of all experimental research designs is that they involve the manipulation of an intervention by the researchers, which will often be the independent variable of the study (LoBiondo-Wood and Haber, 2022). For this reason, many experimental studies can be labelled 'interventional' studies, although they can have varying complexities in design. An experimental study design is typically considered to include RCTs, non-randomised controlled trials, cluster, before–after, pre/post, diagnostic and crossover studies (Bootland, 2017; Aggarwal and Ranganathan, 2019).

After the type of experimental design has been considered, the researcher will then seek to collect prospective quantitative data and can do this using a range of different methods. The collected data are then analysed statistically and used to draw conclusions.

Study design

There are several approaches that can be utilised for experimental research, depending on the environment and purposes of the research. Potential methods of data collection include:

- physiological measurements, such as blood pressure, blood tests, and so on
- direct and indirect observation
- questionnaires
- review of records.

However, the key elements of an experimental design lie in the wider study design. True experimental designs have three components: an intervention, randomisation and a control or comparator group. For this reason, an RCT is an example of a true experimental study design.

In applying an RCT study design, researchers will commonly be seeking to establish the effect of one variable on another. The 'independent variable' is what the researchers wish to study as the cause of an effect on the 'dependent variable'. In other words, the independent variable, or 'intervention', is a treatment, drug or process being posited for use as a part of healthcare provision, and the researchers wish to study what effect it causes. The dependent variable in the healthcare context may refer to a medical condition, disease or specific outcome – the effect.

True experimental methods use randomisation to ensure rigour in the research and minimise any potential biases (Hariton and Locascio, 2018). Approaches to randomisation may vary, and notable approaches in paramedic practice have included the provision of pre-prepared, sealed boxes containing the intervention or placebo in the RIGHT-2 trial (Appleton et al., 2019), and the PACKMaN study (Michelet et al., 2023). The random allocation of sealed interventions ensures that neither the patient nor administering paramedic is aware of whether intervention or placebo has been given. This ensures that any genuine effects are captured and can be associated with the cause.

Wherever possible, each group should contain participants with similar demographics who are randomly selected, thus minimising the impact of additional variables not under scrutiny and beyond the control of the researcher. In addition, all other associated care delivered must be the same wherever possible. Wherever there is deviation from the care plan, it should be well documented to enable analysis of any potential impact on the findings of the study.

The use of randomisation within the study design strengthens the rigour of the research, as any differences that occur between the experimental and control groups can be reasonably attributed to the independent variable. Consequently, RCTs are considered nearly the highest level of evidence, second only to systematic reviews and meta-analysis, and a core principle of evidence-based practice (EBP).

Quasi-experimental research

Purpose

Quasi-experimental research (see Box 10.1) may be considered a subtype of experimental research, as there will be an intervention in the design of the study but there will not be either a control group or purposeful randomisation. The approaches taken are frequently similar, but often lack the same rigour and statistical significance of true experimental research. NRS may be considered to fall within this category as they lack true randomisation of participants into experimental and control groups.

Both experimental and quasi-experimental research designs typically involve at least two groups of participants, commonly referred to as an 'experimental' group and a 'control' group. The division of participants can be undertaken using a range of approaches, which is also a key difference between experimental and quasi-experimental designs.

Study design

Quasi-experimental methods are often adopted where the researcher wishes to examine the effect or relationship of interventions but where providing or removing the

Chapter 10 — Data collection in experimental studies

> **Box 10.1**
>
> ### An example of a quasi-experimental design
>
> EXAMPLE: As the paramedic role has developed, the impact and effectiveness of these newly-implemented extended roles should be explored. In 2012 the UK-based NEECaP Trial (Mason et al., 2012) sought to evaluate the impact of paramedics and nurses working as emergency care practitioners (ECP), on different patient pathways and care in various emergency care settings. The intervention in this study was the service employing an ECP to deliver emergency and unscheduled care, this was compared to a control group of services employing usual care providers, who were not ECPs, to deliver care. The authors measured various outcomes for patients such as: time of care episode, likelihood of discharge, investigations, treatment and onward referrals, but the patients who were recruited were not randomised to the intervention or study group. As there was no randomisation, the study can be categorised as quasi-experimental in its design, which also means that any differences in outcomes between the intervention and control services could have been due to characteristics of the services, rather than the intervention itself.

intervention from a current care plan would or could be harmful. In this situation, it is common for experimental and control groups to be assigned based on convenience, grouping those already receiving the intervention as part of their current care plan into the experimental group and subsequently recruiting a control group with similar demographic characteristics. While this approach lacks the rigour of an RCT design, the subsequent inference of a cause-and-effect relationship still carries a degree of reliability and validity in EBP.

Bias

Bias is defined as 'any systematic error in the design, conduct, or analysis of a study' (Althubaiti, 2016). Bias may occur at any stage of the research, in a variety of forms, and can impact the rigour and validity of conclusions drawn, as well as how they are interpreted by a wider audience.

Typically, healthcare studies most commonly experience either selection bias or information bias. Information bias, when referring particularly to experimental research, may more specifically refer to measurement error bias and confirmation bias. Measurement error bias can refer to error that arises out of equipment inaccuracies, the environment in which the experiment is being conducted or errors from self-reporting. Regardless of underlying cause, measurement error bias causes the observed measurement value to differ from the actual value (Althubaiti, 2016). The regular calibration of equipment being used to measure a dependent variable, for example blood pressure monitors, and consistent use of specific equipment can help to minimise potential equipment-based errors.

Selection bias, arising from the way in which participants are selected for inclusion within the study, may be actively addressed in experimental research by the adoption of randomisation in sample selection and allocation of intervention group (Pannucci and Wilkins, 2010). Despite this, experimental designs have the potential to be affected by attrition bias. This can occur between randomisation and follow-up, where participant data may be missing because of loss to follow-up or incomplete data collection. An RCT may struggle in reducing or managing withdrawals and dropouts due to the patients being unable to provide the relevant information (e.g. mortality or severe morbidity), withdrawal from the study because of an adverse occurrence (e.g. side-effects of a drug), withdrawal from the study voluntarily or being lost to follow-up (e.g. move away from the area) (Hewitt et al., 2010). If the withdrawals or data loss from the study disproportionately affect one group of patients (e.g. the intervention group), the attrition bias could impact the results (Phillips et al., 2021).

Confounding, on the other hand, refers to an observed association that has a third, independent and unaccounted-for variable (Pannucci and Wilkins, 2010). An example would be concluding that regular exercise reduces the risk of a myocardial infarction, when all the participants were taking prescribed anticoagulant medication.

Particularly when working with human participants, there needs to be awareness of self-reporting bias (where participants may not accurately recall or record information), and that this may inadvertently contribute to confounding.

Bias is not an inherent component of research but being aware of the potential causes, intentional or accidental, and effects can help to minimise the risk to research validity and rigour.

Quality and reporting

The purpose and design of experimental research mean that confounding factors can often be controlled or reduced through randomisation, restriction and matching, or through tight control of dependent and independent variables. In quasi-experimental designs, where these techniques are not always possible, statistical methods may be used to adjust for confounding effects (Pourhoseingholi et al., 2012), such as multivariable regression. This means that experimental and quasi-experimental designs often have good internal validity – where the analysed results represent the truth in the population studied (Patino and Ferreira, 2018).

When published, experimental designs should adhere to the CONSORT guidelines (Schulz et al., 2010), while quasi-experimental designs should adhere to the TREND guidelines (Des Jarlais et al., 2004). Following a systematic reporting process creates transparency in the research design and processes for the reader, helping them to critically appraise the study's quality. Correctly applying the appropriate guidelines to the study design also helps to reduce reporting errors. However, some reporting errors still occur in published experimental research papers, most commonly in the description of the allocation concealment and implementation of randomisation (McErlean et al,. 2023).

Chapter 10 — Data collection in experimental studies

Ethical considerations

Following ethical controversies identified during World War II, the Declaration of Helsinki served as a reminder for all biomedical researchers of the place of key principles of ethical practice (Jenn, 2006). Biomedical ethical frameworks have developed over the years, with Beauchamp and Childress (2019) defining the most commonly-used framework of 'the four principles approach', also referred to as autonomy, beneficence, non-maleficence and justice (Shea, 2020; Beauchamp and Childress, 2019).

The purpose of embracing an ethical framework within healthcare research is to ensure that the rights of participants are protected throughout the project, including willing participation, not being maliciously harmed, and that the research is both purposeful and beneficial to the healthcare setting. The application of a framework also ensures efficacy and rigour across the research community, as well as honesty and transparency in the work being undertaken.

This is particularly important with experimental and quasi-experimental methods, as they may involve clinical trials of investigational medicinal products (CTIMP), variations on treatment, care or procedures, and access to confidential personal information by named individuals outside the care team. Any research that may affect the participant must consider the potential risks versus benefits, and what potential harm may come to participants if they are given a placebo or comparator treatment rather than the standard drug/treatment. Plans must also be in place to address any adverse events, in line with the International Council for Harmonisation of Technical Requirements for Pharmaceuticals for Human Use (ICH) Good Clinical Practice (GCP) guideline (ICH, 2023).

In the UK, the NHS is the main provider of healthcare and, as such, NHS Research Ethics Committees (REC) are hosted by the Health Research Authority (HRA) Research Ethics Service (RES). In addition, higher education institutions (HEI) will have their own ethical approval processes.

It is important to note that not every project classed as 'research' will require ethical approval from an NHS REC, and it is strongly recommended that researchers consult individual HEI guidelines and the NHS REC Decision Tool in determining which approvals are required. Further details are included in Chapter 16.

Role of experimental research in paramedic research

The concept of evidence-based practice (EBP) within paramedic services remains a point of much consideration amongst practising professionals. Paramedic EBP and guidelines historically evolved from research in other disciplines, such as nursing and medicine, where there was a larger quantity of high-quality research. Intervention-based studies still constitute a small proportion of the out-of-hospital and prehospital research conducted, despite their value in creating valid and reliable research to contribute to EBP (Cavanagh et al., 2023).

As identified by Bigham and Welsford (2015), the environment in which paramedics traditionally work is marked by its unpredictability, with practitioners needing to rely on their knowledge, skills and colleagues in the absence of advanced clinical tests. However, repeated attempts to transfer in-hospital research to the roadside have proved unsuccessful, with subsequent research indicating that there is a need for high-quality, rigorous prehospital research (Bigham and Welsford, 2015).

Rigorous and valid research within healthcare is critical to successful implementation and adoption by both service providers and users. It is key that this relationship is founded on trust that the service provider will act in the best interest of the service user (Tanious and Onghena, 2019). This premise forms the basis of the person-centred approach to care that is emerging at the heart of paramedic practice, following in the footsteps of nursing colleagues. The importance of a person-centred approach to all aspects of patient and service user care has been increasingly emphasised in recent years. While much of the 'person-centredness' of clinical assessment and care may be presumed to be more relevantly addressed through qualitative and non-experimental approaches, the need for experimental research remains ever pertinent in the paramedic profession. As described by Bernard (1957), experimental research in medical fields is necessary to further the understanding of anatomy, physiology, pathophysiology and the efficacy of treatments. As the transferability of some treatment, medication and care has become uncertain, the profession must seek to build a new, applicable evidence base, relevant to the chaotic, unpredictable and low-resource prehospital environment.

The need for strict control within experimental research may be daunting to paramedics, but it is not impossible, as demonstrated by trials such as PIL-FAST (Shaw et al., 2011), ATLANTIC (Montalescot et al., 2014) and PACKMaN (Michelet et al., 2023).

While quasi-experimental methodology may lack the rigour of experimental research, it should not be discarded as it can still contribute to the developing paramedic field. If carefully conducted, quasi-experimental research may have a good degree of internal and external validity.

As the profession continues to grow and expand valid and reliable research upon which an evidence base can be established is necessary. Indeed, recent studies/trials including CRASH-2 (Roberts et al., 2013a) and AIRWAYS-2 (Benger et al., 2018) have signalled the beginning of change for the paramedic scope of practice. However, paramedic practice can only change to best serve those in need of emergency and urgent care if the evidence upon which decisions are made is rigorous.

Limitations of experimental research

If undertaken with a rigorous process, experimental research can have a clear impact on paramedic EBP, given its ability to measure cause and effect. However, experimental research does have limitations, like any other study design. The biggest challenge to overcome may be the time and cost that this type of study often requires.

Chapter 10 — Data collection in experimental studies

RCTs can be very resource-intensive and consequently require large amounts of funding. They may also take long periods of time to reach recruitment numbers and can be at risk of becoming infeasible.

The other potential issue within experimental research may be the lack of long-term follow-up, missing any lasting or extended impact that may affect the patients included (Frieden, 2017). Furthermore, application of the results can sometimes be limited in RCTs. By creating a well-controlled environment in a very specific patient group, this has the potential to lead to a design with unrealistic conditions or a patient group that has been selected based on very narrow eligibility criteria. Consequently, the results of the trial may not be generalisable to patients who differ from the study population, which could lead to low adoption of the treatment being measured (Patino and Ferreira, 2018). With RCTs, it is about weighing up the importance of a controlled design, free from confounding factors (internal validity) and yet maintaining a wide application of the results (external validity).

Summary

The design and delivery of high-quality experimental research within ambulance services rely on the active engagement of paramedics, and their awareness of the factors that contribute to rigour, reliability and validity in a constantly-evolving field.

Experimental research in the prehospital setting comes with many challenges, including the unpredictability of the environment. Paramedics and researchers must actively consider the practical intricacies of any study in the prehospital domain, and the potential biases, ethical considerations and role associated with it.

Chapter 11

Making sense of quantitative data

John Talbot, Hayley Stagg and Anthony Herbland

Purpose of this chapter

Completion of this chapter will help you to:
- identify and differentiate between various types of quantitative data, recognising the importance of selecting the appropriate data types for analysis
- understand measures of central tendency and dispersion, along with summarising datasets using graphical representations to convey information effectively
- grasp the analysis for different epidemiological study designs and the principles of statistical inference, emphasising the ability to draw conclusions about populations from sample data
- examine the diagnostic tests, highlighting the understanding of key metrics like sensitivity and specificity and assessing test performance
- understand the rationale of determining sample size in a research study.

Introduction

In this chapter, we embark on a journey through the complex landscape of numerical information, a realm with a vast array of statistical tests, ratios and numerical values. At the heart of our exploration is a fundamental truth: a lack of proficiency in basic statistical analysis can significantly undermine our ability to critically evaluate research. Statistics, with its promise of clarity and insight, can sometimes become a labyrinth of confusion, where the true significance of data is disguised in biological variability and experimental imprecision (Motulsky, 1995). This chapter aims to demystify the statistical analysis tools and concepts, guiding you through the challenges of quantitative data to uncover the precise and meaningful conclusions that lie beneath the surface.

Chapter 11 — Making sense of quantitative data

The tables, graphs and other visual aids included in this chapter are for illustrative purposes only. They do not contain any real data, unless otherwise stated. Their sole function is to demonstrate key concepts and provide visual examples to support the content of this chapter.

Data types

Datasets are typically derived from a sample of a much larger population of interest. Initially these data can be divided into distinct categories, nominal and ordinal for categorical data, and discrete or continuous for quantitative data. Categorical data may either be unordered (nominal) or ordered (ordinal). Nominal data have distinct categories but no order, for example blood group. A further categorical variable is binary or dichotomous data, for example dead or alive. Ordinal data are mutually exclusive and ordered, for example pain scales such as none–mild–severe.

Quantitative data include discrete and continuous data. In discrete data, the variables can only take whole numbers (integers) and the values cannot be subdivided into smaller parts, for example the number of paramedics working at a complex. Continuous data remove the limitations on the value a variable can take, for example temperature or blood pressure. Continuous data can take many forms which are categorised as normal distribution and non-normal distribution. The normal distribution of data (Gaussian distribution) follows a bell-shaped curve (Figure 11.1). The x-axis refers to the variable of interest (e.g. systolic blood pressure) while the y-axis represents the number of subjects that have a certain value of that variable.

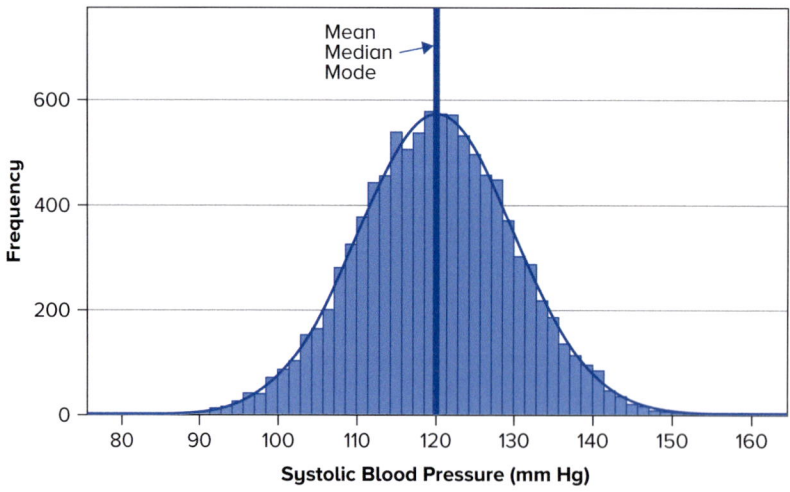

Figure 11.1 Example of a normal distribution for systolic blood pressure with mean of 120 and standard deviation of 10.

Figure 11.2 demonstrates an example of a non-normal distribution, such as survival probability in relation to time until defibrillation.

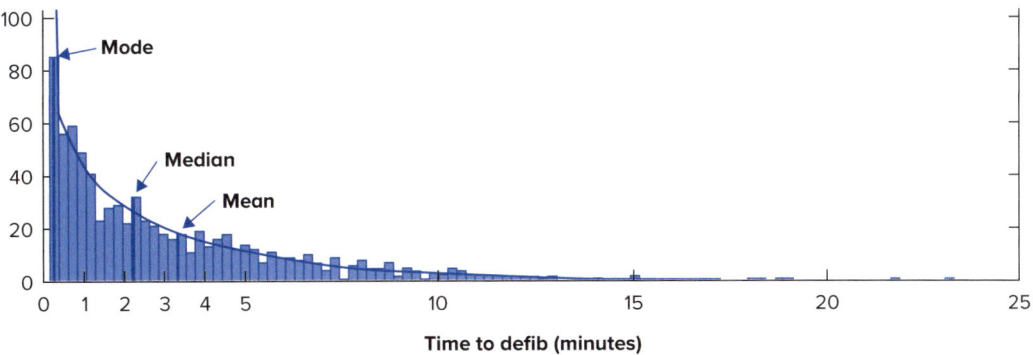

Figure 11.2 Non-normal distribution of survival probability relative to time to defibrillation.

Descriptive statistics

Descriptive statistics vary based on the nature of the variable being analysed. When dealing with nominal variables – categorical data without inherent order or ranking – the analysis, and hence description, primarily focus on determining the frequency and mode of each category. Here, frequency indicates how often a category appears in the dataset, and it is often accompanied by a corresponding percentage to provide clearer context as shown in Table 11.1.

Table 11.1 Reporting the descriptive analysis of nominal variable (i.e. gender).

		Placebo (n = 1238)	Intervention (n = 1249)	Total (n = 2487)
Gender, n (%)	Female	718 (58.0%)	727 (58.2%)	1445 (58.1%)
	Male	520 (42.0%)	522 (41.8%)	1042 (41.9%)

Ordinal variables have categories that are ordered or ranked, but the intervals between these categories are not necessarily uniform. When descriptively analysing ordinal variables, consider the following methods.

- *Frequencies and percentages*: Like nominal variables, you can count the number of occurrences of each category and present them as frequencies and percentages. In Table 11.2, the ordinal age variable is presented with its frequencies and percentages.

Chapter 11 — Making sense of quantitative data

Table 11.2 Reporting the descriptive analysis of ordinal data with frequencies and percentages.

		Placebo (n = 1238)	Intervention (n = 1249)	Total (n = 2487)
Age, n (%)	18–29	112 (9.0%)	136 (10.9%)	248 (10.0%)
	30–39	216 (17.4%)	238 (19.1%)	454 (18.3%)
	40–49	309 (25.0%)	295 (23.6%)	604 (24.3%)
	50–59	320 (25.8%)	305 (24.4%)	625 (25.1%)
	60–69	193 (15.6%)	194 (15.5%)	387 (15.6%)
	≥70	88 (7.1%)	81 (6.5%)	169 (6.8%)

- *Median*: Since ordinal data have a meaningful order, you can determine the middle value when the data are sorted in ascending or descending order. For instance, in their study, Mahta et al. (2021) employed the median to analyse the modified Rankin Scale, a six-point scale ranging from no disability to deceased patients.

Measures of central tendency

Descriptive analysis of continuous variables involves summarising and representing the data in a way that highlights their main characteristics, normally starting with central tendency. The three types of measures of central tendency are as follows:

- The *mean* represents the average calculated by adding all the values and then dividing by the total number of values. Because the mean utilises all the values in the dataset, it can be distorted by outliers, so the mean should only be reported if the distribution is normally distributed as illustrated in Figure 11.1.
- The *median* better represents the average when the data are skewed; not normally being distributed as shown in Figure 11.2. The median effectively splits the data into two separate halves (von Kries et al., 1999). To calculate the median, the values are arrayed in order (lowest to highest) and the middle value taken. If the distribution of the values is normal, then the median and mean will be identical.
- The *mode* represents the most commonly occurring value in a dataset which can also be useful if the data are skewed. It is possible for the mode not to occur if each value only happens the same number of times; moreover, it is also possible to have several modes if different values occur with the same frequency. In health statistics, the mode is rarely reported.

Measures of dispersion

When viewing a dataset, the range describes the 'spread' of results. If the lowest and highest values in the sample are indicated, one must remember that there are only two figures indicated in the range which can give a false impression of the sample distribution.

The standard deviation (SD) is a measure of dispersion around the mean value of a dataset. A low SD indicates that the data points are closely clustered around the mean, while a high SD indicates that the data points are more widely dispersed. For example, we suppose that a set of data for systolic blood pressure has a mean value of 120 and a SD of 10 (Figure 11.1). One standard deviation away from the mean would be a range of values between 110 and 130. This means that approximately 68% of the data points in the dataset fall within this range, while the remaining 32% lie outside this range. Table 11.3 illustrates the reporting of both the mean and the SD within the research article. The SD should only be reported if the dataset is normally distributed. For non-normally distributed datasets, an alternative measure of dispersion is more appropriate.

Table 11.3 Reporting the descriptive analysis of normally distributed data.

	Placebo (n = 1238)	Intervention (n = 1249)	Total (n = 2487)
Mean age ± SD – years	49.6 ± 14.6	48.7 ± 15.0	49.12 ± 14.8

The interquartile range (IQR) are those values that represent the bottom (25th percentile) and top (75th percentile) quarters of the distribution; it is typically reported alongside the median when the data are skewed. Furthermore, the IQR values represent the central 50% of all the values in the dataset. Given the skewness of the continuous age variable, Table 11.4 illustrates that the IQR is used as a dispersion measure.

Table 11.4 Reporting of the descriptive analysis of skewed continuous data.

	Group 1	Group 2
Median age (IQR) – years	33 (24–46.3)	33 (23–45.3)

The range is also used as a measure of data dispersion and is the difference between the maximum and minimum values in a set of data.

Epidemiological studies: assessing risk and outcomes

Epidemiological studies aim to understand outcomes, for example death or disability in a population at risk. Typically, these studies are related to groups rather than individuals and utilise particular statistical tests. For example, in the CRASH-2 trial, the effects of tranexamic acid (TXA) were compared to a placebo on mortality outcomes in bleeding trauma patients. Table 11.5 presents the data extracted and adapted from the original study (Roberts et al., 2013a).

Chapter 11 — Making sense of quantitative data

Table 11.5 Data on mortality outcomes from the CRASH-2 trial comparing tranexamic acid (TXA) to placebo in bleeding trauma patients.

	Event – death	Target – alive	Total
TXA	1463	8597	10,060
Placebo	1613	8454	10,067

Source: Adapted from Table 2 in Roberts et al. (2013a). Reproduced with permission from the National Institute for Health Research.

Absolute risk

Absolute risk (AR) quantifies the probability of a specific event occurring within a defined population at risk. In the context of the CRASH-2 trial, AR measures the likelihood of death. To calculate AR, one divides the number of observed events (i.e. death) by the total population at risk (i.e. TXA group). The AR in the TXA group is determined by the ratio of deaths to the total number of patients in that group:

$$\frac{1463}{10060} = 0.145 \text{ or } 14.5\%$$

Conversely, the AR in the placebo group is:

$$\frac{1613}{10067} = 0.160 \text{ or } 16.0\%$$

By comparing the difference in the risk of death between the two groups, the TXA group exhibits a *1.5 percentage point reduction* in AR compared to the placebo group. Such a difference underscores the potential impact of TXA on reducing mortality in trauma patients.

Relative risk

Relative risk (RR) measures the ratio of the probability of an event occurring in the exposed (or experimental) group relative to a control (or placebo) group. To calculate RR, one divides the event rate in the experimental group by that in the control group. For example, in the context of the CRASH-2 study, the relative risk of death in the TXA group is:

$$\frac{0.145}{0.160} = 0.906$$

This value is typically expressed as a ratio to denominator of 1. In this instance the value of 0.906 is less than 1, indicating that the risk of death is lower in the TXA group relative to the placebo group. For instance, reversing the roles in our calculation to consider the placebo group as the numerator (0.160/0.145) results in an RR of 1.103, indicating a higher risk of death in the placebo group relative to the TXA group. A RR value of 1 means no difference in risk between the two groups.

Therefore, the risk of death is 9.4% (calculated as (1 – 0.906) × 100) lower in the TXA group compared to the placebo group which, one might argue, looks more impressive than the AR reduction of 1.5%

Odds ratio

The odds ratio (OR) is used to compare the odds of an event occurring in one group (exposed group) with the odds of it occurring in another group (non-exposed group). It is calculated by taking the ratio of the odds of the event in each group. The odds are determined by dividing the number of events (e.g. deaths) by the number of non-events (e.g. survivors) in that group.

In the context of the CRASH-2 study the odds of death in the TXA group are:

$$\frac{1463 \text{ deaths}}{8597 \text{ survivors}} = 0.170$$

And for the placebo group, the odds of death are:

$$\frac{1613 \text{ deaths}}{8454 \text{ survivors}} = 0.190$$

The OR is then obtained by dividing the odds in the TXA group by the odds in the placebo group, yielding:

$$OR = \frac{0.170}{0.190} = 0.894$$

This OR value, expressed as a ratio, implies that the odds of death in the TXA group are 89.4% of the odds of death in the placebo group. In practical terms, for every 89 deaths in the TXA group, there are approximately 100 deaths in the placebo group.

It is also important to note that many studies report adjusted odds ratios (aOR). These are calculated using statistical models to control for or adjust potential confounding variables, providing a more precise estimate of the treatment effect or exposure risk by accounting for factors that might skew the analysis. The aOR offers a nuanced understanding of the relationship between exposure (e.g. to TXA) and outcomes (e.g. mortality), enhancing the validity of the research findings.

Hazard ratio

A hazard ratio (HR) quantifies the effect of an intervention on the occurrence of an event over time, crucial in survival analysis. The HR compares the rate of a specified event happening (hazard rate) in a treatment group relative to the hazard rate in the control group. Kaplan–Meier survival curves, as presented in Figure 11.3, illustrate the survival probabilities for patients receiving the new treatment compared to those receiving standard care.

Differences in survival probabilities between patients receiving the new treatment and those receiving standard care are observed over the eight-year period (x-axis). The curve for the 'new treatment' group (upper line, dark blue) consistently lies above the 'standard care' group (lower line, light blue), indicating higher survival rates for patients in the new treatment group throughout the eight years.

Hazard ratios like RR and OR are expressed as a relationship to a denominator of 1. Therefore, for a particular year, if the HR equals 0.5, half as many patients in the 'new

Chapter 11 — Making sense of quantitative data

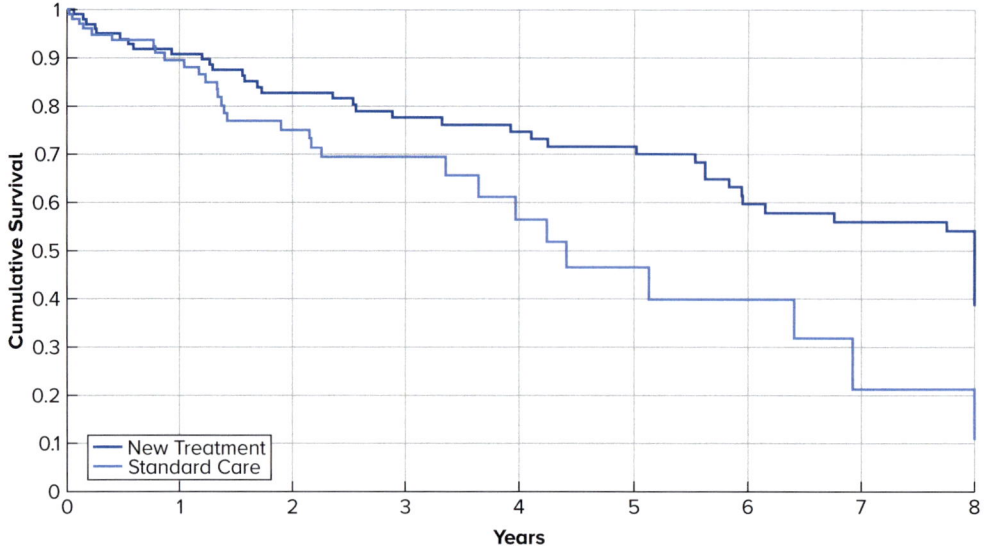

Figure 11.3 Kaplan–Meier survival curves.

treatment' group died compared to the 'standard care' group. If the HR equals 1, the death rates are the same in both groups for a particular year. If the HR equals 2, twice as many patients in the 'new treatment' group died compared to the 'standard care' group for a particular year.

The HR is calculated by dividing the hazard rate of the 'new treatment' group by the 'standard care' group. It may be computed using survival statistical methods. Table 11.6 shows that the HR for the first year is 3.2, meaning that patients receiving standard treatment have a risk of death 3.2 times higher than those on the new treatment. Over an eight-year period, this translates to a notably higher survival probability with the new treatment, with survival rates of 39% for the 'new treatment' group and 11% for the 'standard care' group (Figure 11.3).

Table 11.6 Eight-year mortality hazard rate estimates for each year.

		Hazard ratio	95% confidence interval
New treatment	Year 1	3.2	(1.13–8.97)
	Year 2	3.1	(1.12–7.95)
	Year 3	3	(1.11–6.93)
	Year 4	2.9	(1.10–5.91)
	Year 5	2.8	(1.09–4.89)
	Year 6	2.7	(1.08–3.87)
	Year 7	2.6	(1.07–2.85)
	Year 8	2.5	(1.06–1.83)

Fundamentals of inferential statistics

Confidence intervals

Let us suppose you have an antiarrhythmic drug designed to terminate a specific arrhythmia. In a trial, this medication successfully terminated the arrhythmia in three out of 14 patients, resulting in a success rate of 21.43% for this sample. However, one might question whether this percentage accurately reflects the drug's effectiveness in the wider population. Theoretically, the true success rate in the overall population could range from as low as 0.00001% to as high as 99.999999%, or even beyond these estimates.

This broad range poses a question: how can we ensure that our estimated range accurately includes the true success rate within the entire population? To address this uncertainty, it is important to calculate a confidence interval (CI). This statistical tool helps us define a range that, based on our sample data, is likely to contain the true population proportion. While the exact success rate may vary, using confidence intervals allows us to make informed estimates about the drug's effectiveness on a larger scale, with a specified degree of confidence.

For this reason, the CI is used. It represents a range of values, calculated from statistical techniques, that is likely to contain the true value of a population parameter. Instead of solely relying on significance testing, presenting CIs offers a more comprehensive view of your research findings. Essentially, a CI quantifies the potential error around the observed results, often referred to as the margin of error. A frequently adopted confidence level is 95%, which corresponds to a *p*-value of 0.05. The width of the CI is influenced by the sample size; larger samples typically yield narrower intervals, providing more precise estimates. For example, in a study by Perkins et al. (2015) that investigated whether the LUCAS-2 mechanical CPR improved survival rates from out-of-hospital cardiac arrests, the 30-day survival was lower in the LUCAS-2 group than in the manual CPR group. The adjusted odds ratio was 0.86, with a 95% CI spanning [0.64–1.15]. As this interval includes the value of 1, it indicates no significant difference between the two groups.

Hypothesis testing

Hypothesis testing is a key element of statistical analysis, employed to ascertain whether the evidence from a sample suggests that a particular condition or effect exists in the wider population. It serves as a starting point for a quantitative research investigation or experimentation.

This process revolves around two key hypotheses: the null hypothesis (H_0) and the alternative hypothesis (Ha). While the null hypothesis represents the status quo or a default assumption, the alternative hypothesis is endorsed when the evidence suggests that the null hypothesis is statistically invalid.

For example, suppose you have a coin and you want to test whether it is fair (i.e. whether it has an equal probability of landing heads or tails). You decide to flip the coin 100 times and count how many times it lands heads. The formulation of the hypotheses is as follows.

- *Null hypothesis (H_0)*: The coin is fair. This means the probability P(Heads) = 0.5.
- *Alternative hypothesis (Ha)*: The coin is not fair. This means P(Heads) ≠ 0.5.

In health statistics, it is accepted that the threshold for the significance level (α) is 0.05. This means we are willing to accept a 5% chance of being wrong when rejecting the null hypothesis.

We conducted an experiment by tossing the coin 100 times and, for instance, observed 38 heads. Using a statistical software, we executed a test comparing the observed number of heads with the expected outcome for a fair coin, yielding a specific probability value (*p*-value). The *p*-value is the probability of observing 38 heads in 100 tosses of a fair coin. If this *p*-value is less than our significance level of 0.05, it suggests that our observation would be quite unlikely if the coin were truly fair. In this scenario, our computed *p*-value is 0.021. Since 0.021 is less than 0.05, we reject the null hypothesis and conclude that there is evidence to suggest the coin might not be fair. Let us assume now that the number of observed heads was 55. The computed *p*-value would be 0.368 so we would fail to reject the null hypothesis, suggesting that our observation is not that unusual under the assumption of a fair coin, even if it might seem so.

Parametric versus non-parametric

A lot of common statistical procedures are parametric tests. A parametric test requires the data to follow a specific probability distribution, most commonly the normal distribution, and for the data to be parametric certain assumptions must be true. Other assumptions for running a parametric test are that the variances within each group being compared should be similar and the observations should be independent of each other. Also, the data should be measured at the interval or ratio level. If you use a parametric test when your data do not follow these assumptions, then the results of the analysis are likely to be inaccurate.

Therefore, before you decide which statistical test to do, it is important to check the normal distribution assumptions. The Shapiro–Wilk test, Kolmogorov–Smirnov test and Anderson–Darling test are commonly used to statistically test for normality. A significant *p*-value from these tests indicates deviation from normality.

Non-parametric tests are often known as assumption-free tests because they make fewer assumptions of the data.

Inferential statistics for experimental designs

We are now on to the really thrilling aspects of data analysis. While descriptive statistics focus on individual variables, inferential statistics empower us to answer research questions and draw meaningful conclusions.

As a paramedic, you might pose the following questions.

- Does the administration of epinephrine during out-of-hospital cardiac arrest improve patient survival rates (PARAMEDIC2 trial)?

- Is a supraglottic airway device superior to tracheal intubation as the initial advanced airway management strategy in adults with non-traumatic out-of-hospital cardiac arrest (AIRWAYS-2 trial)?
- What are the effects of tranexamic acid on head injury-related death, disability and adverse events in patients with acute traumatic brain injury (CRASH-3 trial)?

Inferential statistical tests are so called because they allow us to make inferences, conclusions drawn from the data collected, from a sample to the broader target population. Taking the AIRWAYS-2 trial as an example, the study's results indicate that among the general population of adults who experience non-traumatic out-of-hospital cardiac arrests, employing a supraglottic airway device could potentially yield better outcomes, or result in fewer complications, when compared to the use of tracheal intubation.

The goal of inferential statistics is to determine whether there is a significant difference or relationship between two or more variables. Although there are many statistical tests at the researcher's disposal, it is imperative to employ only one particular test for a singular research question. The challenge lies in selecting the most appropriate test. So, how can you confidently choose the correct one? Let us introduce you to our decision-making table specifically for discerning statistical differences (Table 11.7).

Table 11.7 Guide for selecting the appropriate statistical tests for discerning statistical differences.

		Same subject/matched subject design		Different subject design	
		2 conditions	3 or more conditions	2 different groups	3 or more different groups
Non-parametric	Nominal	McNemar test	Fleiss test	Chi-square test	Extended chi-square test
	Ordinal or continuous (non-normal)	Wilcoxon test	Friedman test	Mann–Whitney U test	Kruskal–Wallis test
Parametric	Continuous (normal)	Paired T-test	One-way repeated measure ANOVA	Independent sample T-test or one-way ANOVA	One-way ANOVA

The aim of the decision-making process is to guide you to the appropriate statistical test. To reach the correct test, address the two pivotal questions below in the columns:

- Is the study based on the same subject design or a different subject design?
- Does the study involve two or more than two conditions/groups?

Chapter 11 — Making sense of quantitative data

Subsequently, refine your selection from the row by determining:

- What is the data type of the dependent variable?

To illustrate the process, let us examine how Häikiö et al. (2023) investigated the changes in job satisfaction among Norwegian paramedic students during the SARS-CoV-2 pandemic, specifically between June 2020 (first wave) and March 2021 (third wave). Given that they studied two distinct waves of the pandemic, the research was characterised as employing a 'different subject design' with 'two distinct groups'. The outcome metric was the Job Satisfaction Scale (JSS) score – a continuous variable. This score was sourced from a rigorously validated questionnaire composed of ten items on a Likert scale spanning 1–7, where 1 indicates extreme dissatisfaction and 7 indicates extreme satisfaction. Notably, the scores across both groups adhered to the prerequisites of normality. Consequently, a parametric test was deemed suitable. Referring to Table 11.7, the most appropriate test for this scenario would be the independent T-test or the one-way ANOVA test. In Häikiö et al. (2023), the researchers found, using the independent sample T-test, that the mean value for the combined JSS score was statistically lower in the third wave compared to the first wave ($p = 0.005$).

Correlational analysis

For analysis seeking bivariate correlation or association, the selection process, as illustrated in Table 11.8, is based upon the data type of both variables under consideration.

Table 11.8 Guide for selecting the appropriate statistical tests for statistical correlation or association analysis.

	Data type	Test
Non-parametric	Nominal	Chi-square test for independence
	Ordinal or continuous (non-normal)	Spearman's rank correlation coefficient
Parametric	Continuous (normal)	Pearson's correlation coefficient

In this context, the chi-square test can be used when you want to examine the association between two nominal variables. Take, for instance, the research conducted by Grochowska et al. (2022). One of their primary objectives was to discern any potential association between self-reported burnout (categorised as 'yes' or 'no') among paramedics and nurses. Given that both variables are nominal in nature, the chi-square test for independence emerges as the most fitting analytical method.

Pearson's correlation coefficient is applied when both variables adhere to parametric assumptions, whereas the Spearman's rank correlation coefficient is used when either or both variables do not meet these parametric criteria or are ordinal in nature. When processed by statistical software, both analyses yield a correlation coefficient: 'r' for Pearson's and 'ρ' (rho) for Spearman's. Additionally, the sign denotes the direction of the correlation, indicating whether it is positive or negative. For assessing the intensity of the association, the absolute values of the correlation coefficient can be categorised as follows.

- 0–0.19: Very weak
- 0.2–0.39: Weak
- 0.40–0.59: Moderate
- 0.6–0.79: Strong
- 0.8–1: Very strong.

When interpreting correlation, it is crucial to understand that correlation does not equate to causation. The relationship between two correlated variables might not necessarily be causal. For instance, in a study by Hutchinson et al. (2021) examining the relationship between mental health and three primary lifestyle indicators – sleep, physical activity and alcohol consumption – it was found that alcohol use had a very weak positive association with perceived stress ($r = 0.17$, $p < 0.05$).

Multivariate regression analysis

Linear regression explains the relationship between a dependent variable and one or more independent variables. By using this analytical method, one can quantify the relationship's magnitude, providing precise coefficients for each predictor. Such an approach offers clarity on the expected change in the dependent variable for a unit alteration in a given independent variable, all while assuming other variables remain unchanged. In the study by Keunecke et al. (2019), the dependent variable was paramedic workload, measured using the National Aeronautics and Space Administration Task Load Index (NASA-TLX). This index consists of six subscales, each spanning 10 points. The study highlighted that paramedics assessed the perceived urgency of transports on a scale from 1 (least urgent) to 5 (most urgent). For every increase in urgency level, there was a corresponding 6.9-point surge in the NASA-TLX score ($p < 0.01$). Additionally, transporting patients with potential pathogen transmission elevated the task load by 15.4 points on the NASA-TLX scale ($p < 0.01$).

Another widely-used regression technique is logistic regression, which is particularly applicable when the dependent (or outcome) variable is categorical, often binary in nature. In the study by Eschmann et al. (2010), a multivariable logistic regression model was constructed to examine the impact of crew configuration on the return of spontaneous circulation, a binary dependent variable. The model incorporated several independent variables to account for potential confounders: factors like patient age, gender, date of the event, location of the cardiac arrest, whether CPR was administered by a bystander, the presence of ventricular fibrillation or pulseless ventricular tachycardia, and if the arrest was witnessed. These variables were assimilated in the model to fine-tune the odds ratios among them. The findings

Chapter 11 — Making sense of quantitative data

underscored that the most influential factor was the initial rhythm of VF/VT, which had an odds ratio of 2.58 with a 95% confidence interval of 2.33–2.87 and a significance level of $p < 0.0001$.

Diagnostic tests

Background

Within the realm of paramedic science, as well as in many other fields, a diagnostic test is used to determine the presence or absence of a particular condition or characteristic in an individual or sample. When assessing the effectiveness and accuracy of diagnostic tests, the four outcomes in Table 11.9 are crucial.

Table 11.9 Assessing accuracy of diagnostic tests.

		Condition	
		Present	**Absent**
Test	Positive	True positive (TP) • Test result: positive • Actual condition: present • Description: the test correctly identifies the presence of the condition	False positive (FP) • Test result: positive • Actual condition: absent • Description: the test incorrectly indicates the presence of the condition when it is not there
	Negative	False negative (FN) • Test result: negative • Actual condition: present • Description: the test incorrectly indicates the absence of the condition when it is actually present	True negative (TN) • Test result: negative • Actual condition: absent • Description: the test correctly identifies the absence of the condition

Sensitivity and specificity and their application to clinical practice

Paramedics spend a good deal of their time dealing with undifferentiated patients, often with vague symptoms. So how can one get closer to an accurate diagnosis? Often by employing physical assessment strategies that utilise tests that look for a specific finding that, if elicited, may indicate the presence or absence of the disease in question. Understanding the sensitivity and specificity of tests can be instrumental in making informed decisions in the field.

The sensitivity and specificity of a diagnostic test are useful to describe how well the test performs.

Diagnostic tests

Sensitivity is defined as the proportion of patients *with* the diagnosis who *have* the condition relative to the number of patients *with* the condition.

$$\text{Sensitivity} = \frac{\text{true positive}}{\text{true positive} + \text{false negative}}$$

Specificity is the proportion of patients *without* the diagnosis who do *not have* the condition relative to the number of patients *without* the condition.

$$\text{Specificity} = \frac{\text{true negative}}{\text{false positive} + \text{true negative}}$$

Very few tests offer 100% certainty. Take, for example, the use of Kernig's and Brudzinski's signs in the detection of meningitis; we must consider the:

- *sensitivity* – the extent to which a positive result indicates the presence of meningitis
- *specificity* – the extent to which a negative test result indicates the absence of meningitis.

This is typically derived from a gold standard measure – in the case of Kernig's and Brudzinski's signs, their accuracy in detecting subsequent pleocytosis, the abnormal number of white blood cells in the CSF indicating meningitis.

Nakao et al. (2014) studied the accuracy of these tests and reported the following.

- The sensitivity of Kernig's and Brudzinski's signs was 2%.
- The specificity of Kernig's and Brudzinski's signs was 97% and 98% respectively.

Interpretation of sensitivity and specificity

If you are trying to ensure that a patient does not have a specific condition, such as meningitis, you would use a test with high sensitivity. Why? Because a highly sensitive test excels at correctly spotting those who genuinely have the condition. If this test gives a negative result, it is a strong indication that the patient is probably free from that condition, allowing you to 'rule out' that diagnosis.

Let us illustrate: the Kernig's sign test for meningitis has a low sensitivity of only 2%. If this test comes back negative for a patient, it does not provide much assurance in excluding meningitis as a potential diagnosis. Now, if your aim is to affirm that a patient indeed has a particular condition, you would rely on a test with high specificity. A test with top-notch specificity is adept at rightly pinpointing those without the disease. So a positive result from such a test amplifies the chances that the patient indeed has the condition, allowing you to 'rule in' that diagnosis. For instance, the Kernig's sign test has a specificity of 97% for meningitis. A positive result from this test for a patient can increase confidence in diagnosing meningitis.

In emergency scenarios, the primary objective is often to exclude life-threatening conditions. This prioritises the need for tests with high sensitivity, ensuring that severe conditions do not go undetected. Take, for instance, the findings of Stiell et al. (2003)

Chapter 11 — Making sense of quantitative data

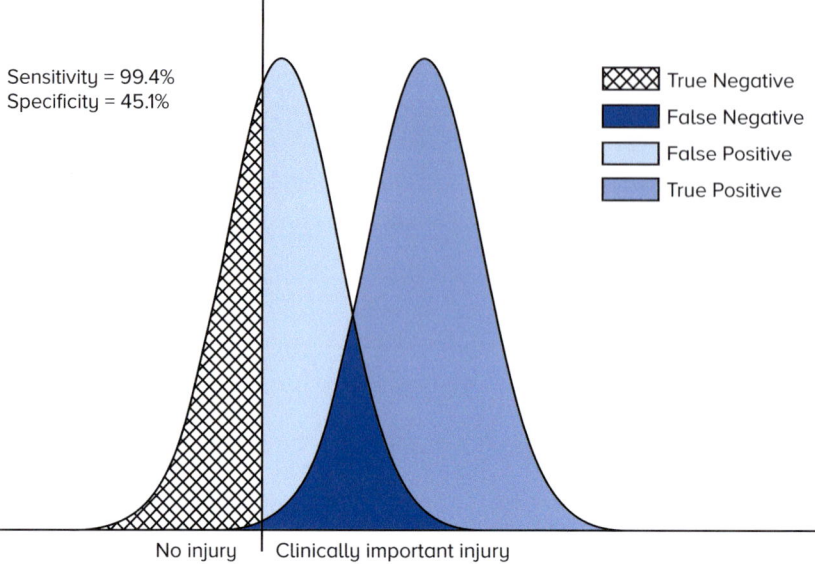

Figure 11.4 CCR probability distribution graph.

who discerned the sensitivity and specificity of the Canadian C-spine rule (CCR) to be 99.38% and 45.09% respectively. As depicted in Figure 11.4, the probability distribution graph for the CCR indicates a notable proportion of false positives. Yet the incidence of false negatives is minuscule. This is paramount for avoiding overlooking patients with clinically significant cervical spine injuries.

Positive and negative predictive values

To distinguish between predictive values and sensitivity/specificity, picture yourself as a paramedic conveying test results to a patient. For instance, if the CCR test yields a positive result, what you would want to convey is the likelihood of the patient genuinely having a clinically significant injury. Essentially, you'd be addressing the question: 'Given this result, how concerned should you be?'.

The *positive predictive value* (PPV) is the proportion of patients with a positive test result who truly have the condition:

$$PPV = \frac{\text{true positive}}{\text{true positive} + \text{false positive}}$$

The *negative predictive value* (NPV) is the proportion of patients with a negative test result who truly do not have the condition:

$$NPV = \frac{\text{true negative}}{\text{false negative} + \text{true negative}}$$

Revisiting the research by Stiell et al. (2003), the positive predictive value stands at 3.87%. This indicates that if a patient tests positive, there's a 3.87% probability that they truly have a clinically significant injury. Conversely, the negative predictive value is 99.97%, signifying that if a patient tests negative, there's a staggering 99.97% likelihood that they don't have any clinically significant injury.

Sample size calculations

Trials, clinical or otherwise, require participants to ensure that results are robust and generalisable. The key question here is: how many participants, often termed the 'sample', are needed for the study? However, it is essential to differentiate between trials and observational studies. In trials, the participants receive a specific treatment or intervention, where they are intentionally assigned to specific conditions to determine the effect of the intervention. In contrast, observational studies do not involve any active intervention by the researcher. Hence, observational studies often do not require a sample size estimation because they aim to describe and analyse existing data or conditions without manipulating any variables and the participants are not typically selected from a predefined target population.

An appropriate sample size ensures that the study can reliably detect a difference if one actually exists. The ability of a test to detect an effect is known as the statistical power of a test. All statistical tests can produce incorrect results, which are categorised into two types of error. A type I error occurs when the test says there is an effect when there is not, that is, diagnosing a patient with a disease when they do not have it. A type I error has a probability of α. Typically, the significance level (α) is set at 0.05 or 5%. A type II error therefore is when the test says there is no effect when there is, that is, saying a patient does not have the disease when they do. A type II error has a probability of β. The statistical power of a test is simply $1 - \beta$.

Cohen (1988) recommends that the statistical power of a test should be at least 80%. For example, in Ostadal et al. (2023), the sample size was determined to detect clearly clinically significant 50% reduction in death from any cause at 30 days, with 80% power at $\alpha = 0.05$. The calculation indicated an enrolment of 120 subjects (60 individuals in each arm). The purpose of this study was to determine the effectiveness or otherwise of extracorporeal membrane oxygenation (ECMO) when used on patients in cardiogenic shock, either immediately or delayed following a more conservative supportive approach. The trial used a multicentre approach, that is, several similar care facilities were used, which, as well as adding numbers to the sample, increases the external validity of the study (the extent to which the trial results can be extrapolated to a wider population).

Note: you can estimate the power of a test after you have conducted your experiment by using the number of data points in your data, the estimated effect size based on collected data and the probability level at which you will accept the effect as being statistically significant (commonly known as the α-level and in most cases, this is set to 0.05).

Chapter 11 — Making sense of quantitative data

Summary

In this chapter we explored the essentials of quantitative data analysis, laying a solid foundation for understanding and applying statistical methods in research. We began by identifying and differentiating various types of quantitative data, underscoring the significance of selecting the correct data types to ensure accurate analysis. Through an exploration of measures of central tendency and dispersion, readers have gained the ability to summarise datasets effectively. We have also navigated through the analytical approaches applicable to different epidemiological study designs. A section dedicated to the fundamentals of inferential statistics guides readers from the initial steps of hypothesis testing through the careful selection of appropriate statistical tests. The chapter concludes by mentioning regression analysis, giving readers the knowledge necessary to make well-supported conclusions about populations based on sample data. The chapter further discusses diagnostic tests, focusing on understanding key metrics such as sensitivity and specificity, which are essential for assessing test performance accurately.

Finally, we tackled the aspect of determining sample size in research studies, explaining the rationale behind sample size calculation and its impact on the validity of research findings.

This comprehensive journey through quantitative data analysis prepares readers with the knowledge and skills to interpret, and potentially apply, statistical data in their research activities, encouraging a deeper appreciation for the role of quantitative analysis in advancing paramedic research.

Useful resources

- Brown RB and Saunders M (2008). *Dealing with Statistics: What You Need to Know*. Buckingham: Open University Press.
- Campbell MJ (2021). *Statistics at Square One*, 12th edn. Chichester: John Wiley & Sons.
- Field AP and Iles J (2024). *Discovering Statistics Using IBM SPSS Statistics*, 6th edn. London: Sage.
- Field AP, Miles J and Field Z (2012). *Discovering Statistics Using R*. London: Sage.

Chapter 12

Qualitative research design

Georgina Murphy-Jones and Joel Symonds

> **Purpose of this chapter**
>
> Completion of this chapter will help you to:
> - understand the value and role of qualitative research
> - recognise different theoretical approaches in qualitative research
> - describe key characteristics of different qualitative approaches
> - consider key factors within different qualitative approaches to help you decide which approach gives you the best 'fit' to answer your research questions.

Introduction

The cornerstone of a successful study is determining the most appropriate methodology to answer the research problem or question posed. Methodological design is the framework that sculpts the study. While qualitative designs have processes to follow, these are not rigid protocols that order and restrict, but are more akin to guidelines that offer flexibility, creativity and support to the inductive nature of a qualitative study.

The methodological design and research objectives drive the choice of research methods, with which to collect and analyse data. Qualitative methods such as focus groups, interviewing and thematic analysis feature across varying methodologies; they are the foundations of the design that influence not just the selection but how they are adopted and applied.

If methodology guides the choice of research methods, what guides the initial choice of methodology? Primarily, consideration as to what the research aims to achieve, after which more pragmatic factors emerge: the researcher's experience, access to methodological expertise, time and resource availability. The theoretical assumptions of the researcher also influence methodological choice, a more challenging consideration for the philosophically naïve. The work of Crotty (1998) is

Chapter 12 — Qualitative research design

a valuable guide in helping navigate the researcher's worldview and their standpoint on the nature of social realities and knowledge. Critical to producing high-quality research is concordance between methods, methodology, theoretical perspective and epistemology (Crotty, 1998), in addition to integrating rigour-enhancing processes and rationalising choices made.

The numerous qualitative methodologies on offer provide an abundance of opportunities to explore issues from clinical practice and can be tailored to paramedic practice in settings as diverse as primary care, education, military environments and ambulance services. This chapter outlines the leading qualitative methodological designs, their associated methods, advantages of use and the challenges to deliberate. Designing a study requires numerous decisions. Qualitative methodologies offer pliable structure and enable innovative practice and rigorous enquiry for paramedics.

Generic qualitative research

What is it?

Generic qualitative research keeps company with methodologies that are considered to be the giants of qualitative enquiry: grounded theory, ethnography and phenomenology. Its relative infancy, debated definition, challenges in judging credibility and absence of a ready-made framework may cause novice researchers some trepidation. However, being a creative, flexible and pragmatic methodology makes it an attractive choice for researchers.

It is not feasible to neatly categorise generic qualitative research. Merriam and Tisdell (2009) recognised the challenges in labelling such an approach, opting for 'basic qualitative study'. Caelli et al. (2003) defined it by what it is not: 'that which is not guided by an explicit or established set of philosophical assumptions in the form of one of the known qualitative methodologies'. Interpretative description, suggested by Thorne et al. (1997), has been rivalled by Sandelowski's (2000, 2010) basic qualitative description, sharing principles but differing in the extent of interpretation.

Using the term 'basic' in naming such an open methodology is perhaps misleading, as it is not an easy option of pick and mix. A generic qualitative study may claim no specific methodological standpoint, or it may combine numerous methodologies or approaches (Caelli et al., 2003). Alternatively, Kahlke (2014) offers an approach that adapts and deviates from the purpose or rules of only a singular methodology. With careful reasoning and justification, the extraction, merging or transformation of methodologies, processes or techniques can create a unique enquiry.

When is it best used?

The function of generic qualitative research varies depending on the influencing approach. Sandelowski (2000) seeks the unearthing of the 'who', 'what' or 'where' of events or experiences; more interpretative approaches add 'how' and 'why' (Chamberlain, 2000; Thorne, 2008). While more traditional methodologies may appeal, caution should be exercised when the methodology does not seem the right fit to answer the research question. If the study goal is not thick description, high-level interpretation or theory development (Sullivan-Bolyai et al., 2005) then generic qualitative research may be the right approach.

More pragmatic considerations can drive this design choice, particularly for clinical researchers who do not want to engage in lengthy, theoretically complex studies. For health researchers, a generic qualitative research approach is favoured for its ability to produce straight, factual answers that are directly applicable to clinical problems and can be rapidly applied to practice (Colorafi and Evans, 2016; Kelly, 2010; Sandelowski, 2000).

Appropriate sampling strategies

Almost any sampling strategy can be employed, the decision being guided by the phenomenon, the research question and strategic aims. Purposive sampling aims to recruit participants with relevant experience of the phenomenon and a willingness to provide detailed information. Both Sandelowski (2000) and Thorne (2008) underline the benefits of theoretical sampling, driven by emerging concepts and the use of maximum variation sampling, to achieve diversity and a broad understanding. Sample size is often determined by the achievement of data saturation, originating from theoretical saturation in grounded theory (Glaser and Strauss, 1967), although the concept of, and need for, saturation has been challenged (Braun and Clarke, 2021b). As with the sampling approach, sample size is determined by that which is required to meet the study objectives.

Most common data collection methods

The mainstay of data collection is through observation or interview, both individual and group, but any data source is feasible. Again, the decision is based on appropriateness of the tool to gather the type and depth of data required to answer study objectives. In paramedic practice, pragmatic concerns also feature in these decisions, such as availability of researchers or participants, impediment of health conditions or acceptability of the method. A range of supplementary data sources may strengthen findings and the overall enquiry (Thorne et al., 1997), for example the addition of documentary analysis.

Management of data

The degree of data interpretation fluctuates depending on which generic qualitative approach is of influence. Basic qualitative description takes a less explanatory approach, avoiding abstract inferences. Adopting a content analysis strategy and *in vivo* coding, the researcher stays close to the data, presenting facts and their meanings in a descriptive summary (Sandelowski, 2010).

Moving beyond description and seeking meaningful analytic interpretations, Thorne et al. (1997) avoid content analysis, considering such preplanned strategies as inhibitory to inductive analysis. Instead, Thorne (2008) advocates for a 'borrowing technique', selecting analytic guidance from other methodologies, but warns against plucking these out and using them uncritically. The analysis process is outlined once study objectives and analysis goals are determined; most importantly, choices must be justified and clearly communicated to the reader.

Strategies to enhance rigour

Rigour-enhancing techniques may be adopted, adapted and combined from varying approaches. Universal strategies such as Lincoln and Guba's (1985) trustworthiness criteria can be applied (Bradshaw et al., 2017) or strategies customised to the study design. Interpretive description may be enriched via Thorne's (2008) criteria to aid credibility, integrity and analytic logic, while Caelli et al.'s (2003) four principles focus on philosophical assumptions and congruence of methodology and methods. When considering epistemological assumptions, Avis (2003) has argued that adhering to a particular methodological theory is not necessary to justify knowledge claims. Instead, theoretical choices used to generate evidence should be justified and this is of critical importance for researchers creating their own design.

From planning to dissemination, researchers must clearly demonstrate that their unique methodological design has produced credible evidence and trustworthy knowledge claims.

Significant challenges in this type of research

In the absence of a specific framework, the challenge when adapting or extracting procedures from other methodologies is to avoid misjudged amalgamation, critiqued as methodological slurring (Kahlke, 2014). Influential approaches must be acknowledged, while clearly demonstrating how the study is distinct from more established methodologies. Acknowledgement of this 'non-traditional' methodology can be problematic when seeking publication, especially in journals with a clinical focus, where capacity for explanation of research methodology is limited. An example of a generic qualitative study is given in Box 12.1.

> **Box 12.1**
>
> ### An example of a generic qualitative study
>
> A generic qualitative research study (Murphy-Jones and Timmons, 2016): Aiming to explore paramedics' end-of-life care decision making, this study used a pragmatic self-designed methodology, influenced by phenomenological and interpretative approaches. A purposive snowball strategy sought paramedics who were unaware of the researcher's background and views. Six participants were interviewed in their workplace setting, using a semi-structured approach and photo elicitation to clarify the patient context and prompt discussion. Data were collected by text message, although this was limited in breadth and depth. Notes on researcher influence were documented in a reflective diary, alongside decisions relating to the thematic data analysis method adopted. This supported a reflexive approach and awareness of the impact of the researcher's 'insider position' on study rigour.

Source: Murphy-Jones and Timmons (2016).

Phenomenology

What is it?

Phenomenology may be defined as the study of individual human experience; it seeks to describe both *what* was experienced and also *how* it was experienced (Teherani et al., 2015). The concept has deep-seated philosophical bases (Neubauer et al., 2019) and has been broadly categorised as 'descriptive' and 'hermeneutic'.

The descriptive phenomenological approach argues that experiences and their essence are anchored firmly to how our consciousness interprets them; phenomenology practitioners must abandon their presuppositions or past knowledge when examining these experiences, a practice known as 'bracketing' (Tuffour, 2017). It is the researcher's role to report and describe the subject's lived experience.

In stark contrast to this, hermeneutic phenomenology embraces the interpretation and 'lens' of the researcher's involvement, arguing that the suspension of personal opinion is impossible, and that deeper meaning arises from the human interpretation of human experience (Tuffour, 2017).

When is it best used?

Phenomenology is exceptionally useful in healthcare research, particularly when seeking to understand the experiences of patients, practitioners and others within healthcare contexts. It is particularly valuable when considering the psychological, emotional and social facets of illness and health, in addition to biological and physical aspects.

Appropriate sampling strategies

Phenomenology focuses on the exploration of experiences, so recruitment and sampling must focus on finding subjects who have had the experience in question. Like many other qualitative methodologies, phenomenological study samples tend to be smaller than quantitative approaches, and it is not uncommon to find sample sizes ranging from one to ten people (Starks and Brown Trinidad, 2007). Initially, this small sample size may seem a point of contention and source of peer challenge from those more familiar with quantitative research. However, it must be remembered that through interview, focus groups or observation, hundreds of data points may emerge which inform thematic analysis.

Most common data collection methods

The collection of phenomenological data is universally geared towards facilitating the understanding of another's lived experience. Common methods include the use of focus groups and direct participant observation, though others have used participant diaries to the same end (Morrell-Scott, 2018). Most predominant, however, is the participant interview, considered to be the discipline's mainstay (Kvale and Brinkmann, 2009). Researchers should approach the design of interviews with an open mind, to ensure that the reflexive nature of these events is productive (Kallio et al., 2016).

Chapter 12 — Qualitative research design

Management of data

Phenomenology immediately produces an inherent challenge in the management of data. How does one begin to codify, quantify and ultimately analyse the inherently abstract and qualitative nature of human experience? A systematic process for this may include the categorising of statements into clusters of similar meaning, allowing common themes to emerge and to be examined (Creswell, 2016). Analysis of these is predominantly a writing exercise, as the analyst composes a story via which the reader may feel that they too have experienced the studied phenomena.

Strategies to enhance rigour

A common phenomenological practice is the use of a semi-structured interview format, where question sets are prescripted, with additional flexibility for the interviewer to go 'off script' to explore or expand on interesting discussion points.

This combination of structured and free-flowing interview allows participants to share their experience and stories with the interviewer while maintaining rigour and data validity. Without this, researchers may find themselves at the mercy of an enthusiastic but unguided research participant who, while saying a lot, fails to produce any relevant data for analysis.

Phenomenological researchers must remain permanently aware of their own perspective and pre-existing thoughts and beliefs. A range of practices exist to minimise the impact and influence of these, including the 'bracketing' of prejudices (where said prejudices are recognised and deliberately set aside during analysis) (Ahern, 1999). It should be noted that, despite appropriate bracketing, it may be difficult for researchers to set aside their own presuppositions and prejudices. Alternative practices include regular consultation with research colleagues or the maintenance of a research journal in which analysts record their thoughts and responses to emerging themes and data (Cutcliffe, 2003). Such journalling may greatly inform the analyst's understanding of the phenomenological themes and concepts.

Significant challenges in this type of research

Being rooted in complex and historical philosophical bases, phenomenology is potentially one of the less accessible research methodologies to relatively inexperienced researchers. Determining a philosophical foundation for one's phenomenological project is an essential aspect of planning and process, requiring an early decision with regard to which philosophical tenets will be carried forth throughout the project (Pringle et al., 2011). Ethically, care must be taken to ensure the participants are not subjected to introspection and examination of their thoughts and feelings (or reliving traumatic events) in such a manner that they may suffer emotional harm; researchers should ensure that they are prepared for such outcomes. An example of a paramedic-led and focused phenomenological study was the work on paramedics' experiences during the PARAMEDIC2 trial by Charlton et al. (2019).

Action research

What is it?

Action research is a process in which research and project work occur concurrently to solve a problem or investigate an issue within a sphere of practice. It occurs when researchers systematically analyse and reflect on processes and roles in which they are themselves involved. Since many healthcare professionals already practise self-reflection, it is argued that action research is not itself a methodology, but rather a research style focusing on the study of one's own practice or practice environment (Meyer, 2000). How, then, do we find a clear definition of action research? Is it, arguably, simply a more-structured form of reflective practice?

Action research differs from typical reflective practice due to its systematic approach, careful planning and critical analysis. Carr and Kemiss (2003) refer to a 'democratic impulse' as a feature of action research; the drive for research to be completed arising from those parties involved in the research question itself. This embodies the concept that action research can empower and authorise 'grass roots' or operational practitioners to implement change by identifying and exploring processes within their own practice.

When is it best used?

Action research is often driven by a requirement to make a change or gain a deeper understanding within one's own practice. It is particularly well suited to situations on the peripheries of traditional research structures. An increased focus on globalism, attitudinal changes around 'developing' and 'developed' countries and increased professional fluidity amongst specialisms (Reason and Bradbury-Huang, 2007) mean that action research encourages participation from practitioners of varied backgrounds, in environments that are not typically considered 'academic'.

Such approaches to non-'siloed' practice boundaries and recognition of the overlap between clinical disciplines and professional cultures make action research an exciting process for examining and improving practice environments, cultures, norms and social constructs.

Appropriate sampling strategies

Predominantly, in healthcare, action research is delivered by researchers within their own teams, although external researchers may embed themselves within an existing team. Action research differs from other approaches as it begins with the identification of a tangible problem within an existing context. It then studies the associated people and surrounding concepts, rather than identifying a group of subjects to be recruited specifically to the project (Mills and Fitzgerald, 2008).

Most common data collection methods

Action researchers must maintain a concept of responsiveness and flexibility in collecting their data, which is reflected in the broad range of data-gathering methods

Chapter 12 — Qualitative research design

that may be used. Researchers might consider using observation, questionnaires, surveys, interviews or individual case studies. It can be helpful to maintain a diary or personal research log throughout the process to ensure you have a record of when, how and why you have changed or added to the data-gathering processes in place. A structured system of ongoing re-examination is discussed below.

Management of data

The action research process involves a cyclical process of data planning, gathering, observation and reflection that drives each subsequent step and focus of the project. As conclusions develop, they allow researchers to refocus or realign their attention and research question as time goes on – action researchers must be flexible and responsive to these developments (Taylor and Francis, 2013). This has been described as a participatory research cycle (Kemiss and McTaggart, 2005), a spiralling series of planning, observing, reflecting and then replanning which will probably be familiar to many healthcare professionals as they continue to expand their practice.

Strategies to enhance rigour

Action research prompts an important question. If the research is simply the study of what we already do or the recording of an experimental new element of practice, how can academic rigour be maintained and results defended? Numerous systems of academic research have emerged, although they predominantly have one theme in common, that of systematic and cyclical project management. Taylor and Francis (2013) advocate a repeating cycle of problem identification, diagnosis, planning, intervention and action evaluation, while others describe the same process in the form of flowcharts or spirals (McNiff and Whitehead, 2010).

Common to all of these is a planned and published process by which action researchers can demonstrate a premeditated structure to their research practice that evaluates, adapts and builds upon outcomes, discoveries and learning. By engaging with practitioners as co-investigators, action researchers can gain deeper understanding and analysis of complex issues within specific contexts and environments. The process has attracted criticism due to its 'grass roots' approach, arguing that action research is relevant only to the context and environment within which it occurs and, as such, has limited generalisability and applicability (Taylor and Francis, 2013).

Significant challenges in this type of research

Due to its collaborative nature, it can be attractive and extremely useful to incorporate patients into action research, bearing in mind that appropriate consent and ethical consideration are essential. Furthermore, due to the contextual nature of action research conclusions, any publications must ensure that environmental, contextual, social and professional surroundings relating to the research setting are fully understood by the reader. While one of the strengths of this process is to allow detailed analysis of events within their own context, it is essential that this context is well understood by external parties when reading at a later date.

Ethnography

What is it?

Ethnography is a holistic form of study. Researcher observation of everyday behaviour is supplemented with participants' voices and wide-ranging sources, to describe the meaning of human activity. Commonly equated to 'doing observation', ethnography can be misrepresented as a method; it is a methodology but beyond a study design it is also the product, the process of creating written, visual or auditory output.

Notorious for its anthropological roots, early ethnographers travelled long distances to study what were known at that time as 'primitive societies'. Gaining scientific foundations in the early 20th century, the concept of fieldwork as a distinct feature of ethnographic theory is attributed to Bronislaw Malinowski (Rabinow, 1985). This 'classic ethnography' has evolved to be more localised, studying communities, including the researcher's own, nearer to home. The ethnographer's aim is to 'get inside' how groups of people see the world, the socially acquired, collective knowledge of members allowing a culturally immersed researcher to describe the overall picture that may not be seen by those inside the community (Angrosino, 2007; Maanen, 1979).

Criticism of ethnography's relevance, value, practice contribution and epistemological claims is well documented (Hammersley, 1992). The evolutionary response has been the development of differing types — critical, feminist, focused, organisational and autobiographical ethnography. These acknowledge constructs such as emancipation, power, change and transformation (Draper, 2015; Tedlock, 2000) and in keeping with contemporary practices, 'digital spaces' of habitation have led to online ethnography or 'netnography' (Hallett and Barber, 2014).

When is it best used?

Ethnographic study is beneficial in its own right, but also has a complementary role, enriching wider evidence and providing a deeper understanding of a subject. It can support study design, define research problems, establish what is acceptable to a community and how people understand potential research tools (Angrosino, 2007). Another benefit of including ethnography in a multi-method approach is the ability to examine the differences between what people say they do and their actual actions and activities.

Ethnography can provide detailed narratives about the cultural context of health and illness, how they are characterised and experienced by society and individuals. Furthermore, the nature of clinicians' professional and interprofessional relationships, patient interactions and management of care can be examined (Reeves et al., 2008). For patients with cognitive or expressive impairments or difficulty communicating thoughts verbally, an ethnographic design can provide a unique insight (Ottrey et al., 2019).

Chapter 12 — Qualitative research design

Appropriate sampling strategies

A primary consideration is the study's setting, which may lead to or arise from the research problem. Hammersley and Atkinson (1995) recommend assessing suitability of sites by 'casing the joint', but choice may be driven by pragmatic reasons or be reliant on permissible access. Not all of the setting may be relevant; there may be a focus on specific aspects, for example triage within an urgent care centre. Sampling progresses within the setting; what data to collect, from whom, when and how? Beyond categorisation and representation of people, Hammersley and Atkinson (1995) identify additional sampling dimensions including variation of time, resulting in fluctuating patterns of activity and the contexts within which people act.

To facilitate successful recruitment, researcher entry into the setting is important; first impressions, researcher presentation, building rapport all help with acceptance. Selection and recruitment can be purposive, strategic, opportunistic or fortuitous but not all areas of the setting will be accessible, not all people welcoming and negotiation with gatekeepers a continuing process (Hammersley and Atkinson, 1995).

Most common data collection methods

The researcher's role in ethnography is central, absorbing and recording interactions, appearance, conversations, relationships, behaviours and actions. Data collection is unstructured, the researcher taking nothing for granted and collecting details of the informal and unplanned: 'The ethnographer becomes like a little child, to whom everything in the world is new' (Angrosino, 2007). Most commonly, adopting the role of a participant observer requires striking a balance between forming socially involved relationships with participants and holding back to enable space for critical, analytical thought (Hammersley and Atkinson, 1995). Interviews, of varying structure, provide understanding about the motivation, experience and significance of observed behaviours but any source of information, for example photos, documents and videos, are valid to gain additional insight.

Management of data

The results of ethnographic analysis can be description, explanation or theory. The development of each uses an analytic approach akin to Glaser and Strauss' (1967) grounded theory, comparing categories as analysis evolves, guiding further sampling and data collection (Hammersley and Atkinson, 1995). Adopting a thematic approach allows the researcher to discern patterns and relationships in the data, but reflexivity is important in interpretation. The important factor is what is perceived as meaningful through the researcher's lens, as opposed to the extent to which meaning is true to the participants.

Multiple methods exist for the presentation of data. Computer-aided analysis programs or pictorials, such as a hierarchical tree, matrix or typology, aid the emergence of connections (Angrosino, 2007; Hammersley and Atkinson, 1995). Situational and contextual data must also be incorporated into analysis, giving meaning to witnessed behaviours and participant accounts. Detailed descriptions when reporting findings are essential, enhancing rigour and fully illustrating the study setting. Textual output is not the only form of ethnographic narrative as film, music, pictures and plays offer added benefits, performances with participants giving richness to the sharing of findings (Goldstein et al., 2014).

Strategies to enhance rigour

Prolonged time in the field is a defining ethnographic feature, greatly increasing rigour, and is required to understand language, cultural codes and meaning of behaviour (von Koskull, 2020). Extended time to capture the voices of those who usually go unheard leads to diversity in how a phenomenon is viewed and deeper levels of accuracy and authenticity. Given the time and active role the researcher occupies within the setting, a reflexive attitude is indispensable – questioning and accounting for their potential impact on participant selection and responses, data interpretation and presentation. Acknowledging their background, characteristics, cultural beliefs and existing standpoints allows readers to judge their influence on the study.

There will always be a degree of behaviour modification once people know they are being observed. Angrosino (2007) suggests that such bias is minimised as people are not being asked to act differently, and subjective observations are cross-checked with information from other data sources. This concept of triangulation enables inferences to be checked against data from other collection techniques, different phases of fieldwork or from participants in other areas of the setting (Hammersley and Atkinson, 1995). A combination of methods enables interpretations about a concept to be checked from multiple sources, thus enhancing rigour. Participant observation may allow the witnessing of practices that remain concealed to other forms of investigation.

Significant challenges in this type of research

Being immersed in a community is beneficial to gain a deep understanding, but may place burdensome demands on the researcher including entering unknown situations, exposure to uncomfortable experiences or a range of emotions, from hostility to reliance. The well-being of both researcher and participants is an important consideration.

There are significant ethical issues that, while applicable to all research, are particularly relevant due to participant observation. Concerns regarding informed consent, the nature of private spaces and information, harm and exploitation have been raised and the difficulties in gaining ethical approval for an emergent design that cannot be fully defined in advance (Roberts et al., 2013b; Hammersley and Atkinson, 1995). Depending on the research topic, utilising ethnography within prehospital care may create additional challenges due to the unpredictability and mobility of ambulance service work. For example, studying a particular condition or patient group may not be logistically possible. Opting to study interactions in more static environments where paramedics work, such as primary care or police custody, may be more successful options.

Case study

What is it?

The definition of the term 'case study' is widely debated. The phrase is used to describe a research method, meaning the technical approach used, and a methodology, meaning the factors surrounding the researcher's analysis and conclusions (Harrison et al., 2017). Primarily, the aim of a case study is to explore the complexities of a situation within its real-life context.

Differing approaches to case study have led authors to promote their own definitions of the term and practice. These vary but common themes (Harrison et al., 2017) refer to:

- *singularity*: a clearly defined subject
- *context*: the clinical, practical, political, social or geographical factors surrounding the subject and their mutual influence
- *nature*: the subject's specific features and relationship to the study
- *description*: a design that discusses and explores the subject themes.

This complexity and potential ambiguity could dissuade researchers from employing case study as a methodology, considering these factors as weaknesses in academic rigour. However, it is this flexibility that allows case studies to have a deeply practical application, allowing in-depth study of real-world situations by closely engaged researchers. This close relationship of researcher and subject, and the inherent subjectivity that arises from such a relationship, is both acknowledged and welcomed within the literature. It must, however, remain in the forefront of researchers' minds, accounting for this need for reflexivity in both study design and subsequent analysis.

When is it best used?

Case studies are particularly useful when attempting to understand a complex situation with many involved parties or moving parts. Contrary to other forms of research which may take place in an artificial or controlled environment, case studies often take place '*in situ*'. Rather than attempting to separate the data from their context or environment, case studies embrace all aspects to provide an in-depth and extensive analysis of a phenomenon within the context in which it is encountered. They are of particular utility when a research question is posed as 'how?' or 'why?' and can allow researchers to explore, describe and explain complex situations (Yin, 2014).

Appropriate sampling strategies

While case studies provide enormous capacity to explore complex situations and presentations, it is essential to ensure that the *right* cases are selected to study. It can be particularly valuable to focus on cases which are already known to be unusual or extreme, as these situations are more likely to yield a high volume of useful data and information (Flyvbjerg, 2006).

An extreme example of this would be choosing to study the dynamic working relationship between transport staff and ambulance personnel at railway-related suicides; hypothetically, it might be easier to conduct this research in central London (with its large population and wide-reaching railway network) rather than in rural Scotland, since the incidence in the former is likely to be far greater. However, consideration would need to be given to the potential impact of this context, recognising that attitudes and social norms may be specific and unique to such a busy metropolitan area. The design may therefore include interviews with personnel in both locations, in the interests of uncovering common themes and 'universal truths' despite their differing contexts.

Most common data collection methods

Case studies allow researchers to gain insight and data from an enormous range of sources, including existing documentation, observations of participants and events, archive material and interviews. Quantitative data may also be gathered and used to support, contextualise and solidify case study findings and hypotheses (Baxter and Jack, 2008).

Management of data

Case study research has, historically, been criticised for its lack of data credibility and veracity, often being accused of only being useful for 'storytelling' (Krusenvik, 2016). As discussed above, the convergence of multiple data sources of both a qualitative and quantitative nature to inform contextual considerations and discussion can be seen as one of the greatest elements of data credibility and rigour within case study research. However, the risk exists of enormous collections of data developing to such an extent that researchers become overwhelmed and unable to manage the data in a meaningful way. An organised database in which to collect, collate and codify received data is an essential aspect of this work.

Strategies to enhance rigour

Baxter and Jack (2008) recommend clearly specifying the case's limits, advocating for an approach that specifically considers what the case is not. Suggested boundaries to define a case may include time and place, type of activity, or definition and context (Baxter and Jack, 2008). However, the ability to uncover new elements and concepts within a subject can be the methodology's strongest advantage, so research design must allow for discoveries to be made and for terms to flex in response (Cypress, 2017).

In attempting to understand, define and thus manage the potential weaknesses of case study research, many authors have adopted varying philosophical tenets when conceptualising case study research:

- *Realist* – postpositivism (Yin, 2014). Researcher bias is inevitable and must be recognised. The bias may be minimised through use of multiple cases, meticulous design, and process.
- *Pragmatic constructivist* (Merriam and Tisdell, 2015). Cases are selected to provide holistic and thematic understanding, allowing concepts to be defined and sorted. Bias is reduced through rigorous data collection, triangulation and continual analysis.
- *Relativist* – constructivist/interpretivist (Stake, 2006). Information is contextual and subjective; using interviews and observations, it falls to the researcher to interpret and illustrate individuals' experience.

Significant challenges in this type of research

Case-study research, while open-ended and expansive in its capacity to explore complex phenomena, also faces a risk whereby parameters are insufficiently defined, leading to accusations of insufficient investigative rigour. As a case's complexity and nuances become more known, poorly-prepared researchers may find themselves rapidly overwhelmed by a seemingly unending source of contradictory and complex findings. Promoters of case-study research cite its ability to understand complex and interacting factors and associated processes within a wider social context (Baxter and Jack, 2008). However, debate around case study use regularly levels the accusation that the study of a specific subject within a specific context cannot then be extrapolated to make generalised conclusions about a broader environment, or necessarily applied to other contexts and situations.

Grounded theory

What is it?

Grounded theory (GT) has been on a journey of transformative growth since its inception by Glaser and Strauss (1967) as a means of generating theory. Three leading variations exist: classic or 'Glaserian' GT was advanced by Strauss and Corbin (1990), their 'Straussarian' GT later evolving into constructivist GT (Charmaz, 2014). Alongside this journey of procedural change has been ontological and epistemological progression, each variation prompting continued debate between their authors and in wider methodological literature.

Classic GT was designed to challenge the dominance of quantitative verification of theory in sociology (Glaser and Strauss, 1967), offering a systematic and structured constant comparative method to analyse data and generate theory. It is renowned for these procedures, but integral to this methodological approach are concurrent data collection and analysis; theoretical sampling; saturation and sensitivity; memo writing; *in vivo* coding; and the interconnection of categories to form a core that is central to the theoretical framework (Glaser and Strauss, 1967).

These elements have persisted throughout methodological progression, but movement has occurred in the underlying philosophy, use of literature and coding procedures (Kenny and Fourie, 2015). The many approaches and variations of GT create perplexity. Essentially, there is one GT, a methodology with fundamental techniques at its foundation that has taken many directions (Bertero, 2012). Although it is an adaptable methodology, it is important to ensure there is clarity and well-defined use of the chosen variation.

When is it best used?

Grounded theory has a fundamental practicality, underlined by the philosophical assumptions of Strauss and Corbin's (1990) variation. The process of GT does not produce descriptive findings but knowledge of practical use, described by Glaser and Holton (2004) as theory that has implications. By definition, GT is best adopted where there is a lack of existing theory; the types produced frequently focus on a behavioural concept or phenomenon, for example trust, caring, coping (Morse, 2001). As such, this methodology lends itself to studying healthcare and answering problems from clinical practice. Adopting an interpretative approach of GT enables the creation of theory with patients, their perspective contributing to the understanding of key processes in healthcare (Charmaz, 2014; Foley and Timonen, 2014).

Appropriate sampling strategies

There is limited preparation when formulating the sampling strategy. A couple of participants are purposively selected, based on the researcher's existing knowledge of the phenomenon or problem to be addressed. Remaining sampling, recruitment and sample size are controlled and driven by the emerging theory using theoretical sampling, a defining feature of GT.

Glaser and Strauss (1967) suggest that participant selection is based on theoretical purpose and relevance, selecting groups who will generate as many properties of the category as possible. These decisions are based on data collected and analysis undertaken; once categories are formed, sampling is simultaneous as the study unfolds. Having identified gaps in the theory, the researcher is directed by these towards subsequent sources and styles of data collection (Glaser and Holton, 2004). The aim is to saturate and refine categories, enabling relationships to be drawn between them and continuing until no new properties emerge (Charmaz, 2014).

Most common data collection methods

Choice of collection methods is summed up neatly by the advice that 'all is data' (Glaser and Holton, 2004); while there are favoured methods, any type of data can be used to generate theory. Glaser and Strauss (1967) advocated for variety and the use of complementary quantitative and qualitative data sources as a means of verification. However, qualitative data are preferred for providing an abundance of detail and lines of enquiry for mapping, discovering and building strands of the theory. Selection and combination of methods are determined by the evolving theory and understanding of formed categories. Interviews are common, with Corbin and Strauss (2015) revealing a preference for unstructured interviews to provide the richest source for theory development.

Management of data

While each GT approach advocates different analytical processes, all share the constant comparison process and use of theoretical sensitivity to give data meaning and develop theory. It is important to appreciate the significance of the entwining of both obtaining and evaluating data: 'Data collection and analysis procedures are explicit and the pacing of these procedures is, at once, simultaneous, sequential, subsequent, scheduled and serendipitous' (Glaser and Holton, 2004). By this process the theory is grounded in the data.

The constant comparison process begins by comparing incidents found in data with each other, seeking similarities and differences. This process generates the properties of a category, after which coding and comparison continue, contrasting individual incidents with properties of categories. Ultimately, the comparison of categories and their integration around a core category give structure to final theory development (Glaser and Strauss, 1967).

Straussarian GT offers a more detailed structure to analysis, the questioning of data and additional coding procedures (Corbin and Strauss, 2015; Strauss and Corbin, 1990). Conversely, Charmaz's (2014) constructivist GT has more flexible guidelines and a simplified two-stage coding process, based on interactions and shared experiences.

The final requirement for any GT analysis is memo writing. The systematic writing of theoretical memos moves data to a conceptual level, defining categories and theorising connections between them and, in so doing, mapping the theory development (Glaser and Holton, 2004).

Strategies to enhance rigour

Credibility is supported by using multiple data sources, researcher collaboration in analysis and participant recognition and validation of the theory produced. Glaser (2002) believed researcher impact could be mitigated by close adherence to methodology, eschewing literature and constant data comparison. Likewise, Strauss and Corbin (1990) advise observance of their procedures, designed to provide rigour and disperse bias, with the oscillation of data collection and analysis verifying emerging theory. Accepting that researchers bring presuppositions and that theory is formed through researcher/participant interactions, incorporating reflexivity into GT increases transparency and enhances rigour (Hall and Callery, 2001). Charmaz's (2014) constructionist approach maintains that reflexivity is critical, offering a questioning framework to aid self-examination of influential standpoints and appraisal of analysis.

Significant challenges in this type of research

Researchers need to fully understand the basic principles and variations and how to adapt processes, without creating a jumbled and confusing study design. Given study strategy is driven by the emergent theory, design specifics cannot be predetermined, making ethical approval challenging. Explanation will be required about initial sampling, location and recruitment, and how this could progress using a theoretical sampling strategy.

Summary

Practitioners engaging with qualitative research for the first time may have conflicting thoughts and opinions about its methodologies. At first glance, the concept can appear vague and poorly defined – how does a researcher defend their findings when so many qualitative outcomes can appear subjective and dependent on environment, subjects and context? However, with an understanding of the strengths and challenges inherent within each methodology, researchers can select a qualitative approach that allows them to study, understand and report upon situations of enormous subtlety and complexity. A qualitative approach lends itself exceptionally well to the humanistic aspects of healthcare, considering both the practitioner's and patient's perspective. Qualitative methodologies offer paramedic researchers a conduit to profound and rigorous study.

Chapter 13

Qualitative data collection

Mike Brady and Enrico Dippenaar

> **Purpose of this chapter**
>
> Completion of this chapter will help you to:
> - understand the three main tools used to capture qualitative data
> - recognise the five major methods of qualitative data collection
> - identify the key strengths and weaknesses of different methods of data collection
> - understand the common challenges with data collection
> - outline the ethical considerations when using different methods of data collection.

Introduction

Throughout the chapter, you will be signposted to various sources, published works and useful tools to help you through your journey of qualitative data collection. Put simply, you will have the dos and don'ts of data collection with useful examples from research practice written by those who have had the opportunity to learn along the way.

As paramedicine progresses both clinically and academically, with more paramedics researching in a range of settings, it is important to understand the role of qualitative research in this advancement. Although there are still some researchers caught up in the paradigm wars of qualitative versus quantitative and what is 'good' science versus 'bad', it is accepted generally that the aims of qualitative research are distinct from quantitative, and that its utility in healthcare remains valid. Such is the case in paramedic-led qualitative research.

Ensuring that qualitative data are collected properly and with suitable rigour is part of accepted validity. High-standard data collection is equally important to the validity of the researcher themselves and their profession, thus forming part of expectations set out by registering bodies, such as the Health and Care Professions Council. Ensuring

Chapter 13 — Qualitative data collection

all paramedic researchers from novice to expert have access to reputable sources of information, instructional references, advice and support is key to ensuring adequate data collection. Whether you, as the reader, are working in phenomenology, ethnography or grounded theory, this chapter sets out to support you through the process of collecting these data.

Tools for data collection

Researchers capture qualitative data in several ways, primarily through written records, audio or visual recordings. These tools allow for the capture and recording of information for later analysis. The type of data to be captured depends on the needs of the researcher, who may use these tools individually or in combination:

- *Written records*: Researchers may make field notes or keep journals during the process of data collection, or information can be sourced from books, notebooks, diaries, documents, websites, blogs or social media.
- *Audio recordings*: Researchers may record vocal, musical, noise or other specific sounds of people talking, singing, acoustic or nature sounds, ambient or background noise.
- *Visual recordings*: Researchers may record video, pictures or images of people, nature, artwork, paintings, drawings or digital media.

Useful tips

Whichever data capture tool you use, be sure to protect it:

- Use two recording devices at the same time.
- Use one visual recorder and one audio recorder at the same time.
- Save documents in two different, but secure, locations.

Should one method fail, break, or get lost (it does happen), you have an immediate back-up option. Most importantly, you would have not squandered your participants' time, energy, and contribution.

Data collection methods

Interviews and focus groups

Interviews are a form of facilitated conversation. They are an important method of data capture, and involve the administration of specific questions or a conversation focused on a specific topic with selected individuals or groups. Interviews are quite different from questionnaires, as they involve social interaction and reaction to social interactions.

The purpose of undertaking interviews is to collect meaningful data that might not otherwise be captured or understood in as much depth by other methods. Interviews help researchers to better explain, understand and explore participants' reactions, attitudes, opinions, behaviours and lived experience of a specific subject.

Types of interviews include the following:

- *Structured interview*: A structured (or standardised) interview involves interview questions being asked in a very specific manner. The aim is for all participants to be given the exact same set of questions, in the exact same order, within the exact same context and for there to be no difference. This ensures that answers to such interviews can be aggregated reliably. Participants can respond in their own words, but the topics within their answers are pre-decided and limited. Structured interviews are usually most useful when researching areas in which the literature is well-established.

- *Semi-structured interview*: A semi-structured interview involves developing a range of questions that can be put to participants, and from which a conversation can develop between interviewer and interviewee. Boasting the benefits of both structured and semi-structured processes, these interviews allow the researcher to spontaneously respond and explore topics which arise throughout. Semi-structured interviews can often feel less intimidating for the participant and more conversational in nature, which may be of benefit, depending on the nature of the research and those involved.

- *Narrative interview*: Narrative interviewing is a method of data collection whereby a story is generated through the interview process – a listening approach rather than a questioning one. The emphasis of narrative interviewing is less on a range of questions, but rather focuses on an opening question that allows and invites the participant to narrate their experience – to tell the story. This method is useful for exploring transformations and transitions in people's lives. The key advantage of narrative interviewing is the control and ownership the participant holds through telling their story. They can confirm their sense of identity and their perspective of reason, blame and praise.

- *Episodic interview*: Episodic narrative interview is a qualitative method that can be useful for researchers who are new to narrative research and are developing their interview control techniques. It integrates elements from several qualitative approaches, and has a clear focus on a particular time or episode in someone's life, but is still an open-ended approach that allows an understanding of the participants' experiences to be told and owned by them. This method can help researchers understand how sense is made of people's experience and can be used to compare different times in people's lives and the meanings associated with those times (Mueller, 2019).

An alternative to interviewing individuals is to interview groups of people. This type of interview is commonly known as a group interview or group discussion.

Focus group research typically applies the same qualitative method as interviews, but to a group of participants. The group usually have experiences, conditions or an attribute that is of interest to the researcher. Unlike interviews, the thoughts and perspectives being explored by the researcher are often elicited solely through group discussion, comparison and interaction between participants from which the researcher discovers how individuals understand and perceive subjects.

Chapter 13 — Qualitative data collection

The subject questions of focus groups can be determined from previous quantitative research to form a mixed-methodological study. Quantitative research is limited in its ability to tell the lived experiences of individuals or groups in as much depth as qualitative, but has a role to play in generating focus group questions. The same is true in reverse, in that qualitative research can generate theories and hypotheses that require quantitative methods to address them.

There are different types of focus groups that can be utilised. There will be times when a particular type of focus group will be most beneficial to the type of research being undertaken, and other times when the sample group available dictates the type of focus group that can be conducted.

Types of focus groups include the following:

- *Single*: A single focus group is the most typical form, and involves a group of participants and an individual facilitator, or a team of facilitators undertaking the same research with different participant groups.

- *Two-way*: A two-way focus group exercise involves using two separate groups of participants. One group discusses a topic and the other observes the first group's discussion. This focus group method is usually conducted with the use of video conferencing software. The observation group analyses the discussion group's interactions, opinions and conclusions. This observation and analysis will often lead to further discussion being generated, comparisons being made between groups or opinions, and different conclusions being drawn through different perspectives.

- *Dual-moderator*: Dual-moderator focus groups involve two moderators working collaboratively throughout the session. Each moderator will have a different role, which usually involves supporting the other and ensuring the session runs smoothly and that all subjects are covered. This type of focus group can be particularly helpful to novice researchers in mentorship.

- *Duelling-moderator*: Just as it sounds, a duelling-moderator focus group involves two moderators who take opposite sides on purpose. This disagreement or different approach taken to a topic helps the group to think critically and achieve more in-depth discussion through the promotion of respectfully delivered contrary views.

- *Respondent-moderator*: A respondent-moderator focus group involves the recruitment of some of the group participants. Recruits take up the temporary role of moderator themselves. It is thought that having one of the participants lead the discussion in this way will impact on the dynamics of the group by influencing participants' answers, and increasing the chances of varied and more honest responses. Caution should be exercised when adopting this method. Ensuring that the normal group hierarchy (rank, seniority, the loudest) is considered and understood is important in ensuring that the group does not transition into a normal business-type meeting with normal levels of engagement and prepared response.

- *Mini*: A mini focus group is usually undertaken because there are a limited amount of participants able or wanting to be involved in the research. Mini focus groups can be undertaken with minority or hard-to-reach groups, or where numbers can be naturally small. Between two and six participants can still make for a meaningful discussion with valid findings.

- *Remote (online, telephone)*: Remote focus groups use the same methods as other focus groups, but are carried out using remote methods, such as video conferencing software or phone conference platforms. Remote focus groups can often increase access and availability of those with additional needs or disabilities that limit travel. However, they can also marginalise those with limited technological skills, internet access and up-to-date hardware (phones, laptops). The remote focus group can often create very different group dynamics where body language and eye-to-eye contact cannot be seen by the moderator or other participants. Remote focus groups should be used with caution when undertaking research about sensitive and possibly upsetting subjects. Often, remote focus groups limit the face-to-face support participants may need when affected by sensitive subjects such as child abuse, rape and death.

Focus groups as a method can present the researcher with different ethical challenges and considerations from one-to-one interviews with participants. Focus group control, ground rules and confidentiality are all key aspects to consider.

The challenges associated with focus groups lie in their unpredictability. One can plan for sensitive subjects to be discussed in one-to-one interviews in a way that steers or prepares both interviewer and interviewee, but due to the free-flowing dialogue of focus groups, it is unpredictable what sensitive subjects people may raise throughout and how this may affect others. Similarly, this unpredictability can lead to patient or colleague identifiable information being shared inadvertently, which can sometimes lead to conflict within the group or the facilitator needing to interrupt and reaffirm ground rules.

A balance should be struck between outlining clear expectations of focus group behaviour and topics for discussion, while also not wanting to dominate or dictate the discussion, which can sometimes inhibit free-flowing conversation. Focus groups need to have clear objectives, involve the correct group of people, create a supportive atmosphere, and not turn into a group of professionals complaining.

Useful Tips

- Be relaxed. If you are not relaxed, your participants will not be relaxed; and will not share.
- Be mindful of power struggles in large groups and how such dynamics can affect some participants' willingness to contribute. Hear from everyone.
- Try to avoid long-winded complicated questions.
- Try to avoid jargon, insider talk, acronyms, or abbreviations.

Chapter 13 — Qualitative data collection

- Assume you know nothing. Allow yourself to be led by the answers, not vice versa.
- Never ask leading questions or guide the answers to suit your preconceived ideas.

Qualitative questionnaires

Many people think of a questionnaire as a quantitative approach; however, a qualitative questionnaire is a valid method of qualitative data capture, and can be a useful tool in reaching more participants than would be possible in focus groups or interviews, in a relatively short timeframe. There may be quantitative elements to such questionnaires, such as age, occupation, gender, which can be captured descriptively (Box 13.1).

Box 13.1

An example of a survey collecting qualitative and quantitative data

Lazarus J, Iyer R. Fothergill R. (2019). Paramedic attitudes and experiences of enrolling patients into the PARAMEDIC2 adrenaline trial: a qualitative survey within the London Ambulance Service. *British Medical Journal*, 9(11). DOI: 10.1136/bmjopen-2018-025588.

This study surveyed paramedics using qualitative questionnaires with open and closed questions. The aim of the study was to gather the views and experiences of paramedics who participated in a large-scale randomised controlled drug trial and to identify barriers to recruitment. It found a strong appetite for involvement in prehospital research among paramedics and an understanding of the importance of research that prevailed over the complexities of the trial. This is an important finding demonstrating that potentially ethically controversial research can be undertaken successfully by paramedics in the prehospital environment.

Qualitative questionnaires tend to use open-ended questions to elicit written responses which can then be analysed. They aim to collect opinions, experiences and narratives of participants, and can be an accessible way to reach groups with various needs, such as those who may be deaf and those with verbal communication difficulties, as they are able to write their response.

Like all methods of data capture, the design is crucial. Poor design can often be the downfall of a research project. Qualitative questionnaires look for in-depth responses to topics, and ensuring the participant understands what is being asked in a way that does not lead them or influence their response is integral to gaining valid data. Qualitative questionnaires can be used as a preparatory tool for more intimate methods such as interviews or focus groups. If designed in a way that biases the responses or confuses participants, an entire research programme can be affected.

When designing a questionnaire, it is important to ask yourself as a researcher: *Are these questions really needed?* An eager novice researcher or student may fall into the trap of overcomplicating a questionnaire, and run the risk of wasting participants' time – a serious ethical concern.

There might be an urge to add questions without fully evaluating their ability to contribute to answering the research question. There may be a tendency to add questions to which the answers are 'nice to know' and are interesting, but not required to meet the research objectives. Adding such questions can often confuse the analysis, waste participant time, add cost and reduce participant uptake and completion rates. Avoid this temptation.

Qualitative questionnaire design

Table 13.1 compares weak to strong questions. Tips for developing strong questions for your qualitative questionnaire include the following:

- Questions should not be closed and should invite elaboration (avoid Yes or No answers).
- Questions should be no more than a single sentence.
- Including the research topic in a question will help the participant focus their answer.
- Use words that express the type of response you want to measure – the quality of the subject (discover, understand, experience, perceptions, feelings, views, opinions).
- Avoid questions which increase ambiguity (compare, contrast, cause, measure, relate).

Useful Tips

Strengths

- Inexpensive
- Scalable
- Can facilitate participant anonymity
- Standardised approach to questioning
- Quick results.

Limitations

- Participants may skip questions
- Participants may not complete the entire survey
- May be accessibility issues for those with additional needs
- Lack of personal approach
- May be unsuitable for very sensitive subjects.

Chapter 13 — Qualitative data collection

Table 13.1 Developing questions for a qualitative questionnaire.

Weak question example	Strong question example
Is the atmosphere good in your favourite restaurant? **Explanation:** Avoid having questions that can be answered 'yes' or 'no'.	Thinking about the atmosphere, what do you like most about your favourite restaurant? **Explanation:** Encourage a response based on the quality of the subject that has more richness and depth.
How much time in a week do you spend watching documentaries? **Explanation:** Avoid quantitative based questions that give you a defined (often estimated) answer. It actually tells you very little.	Why do you prefer watching documentaries over other types of television? **Explanation:** Encourage a response that tells you more about 'why' rather than 'how much'. 'Why' responses might lead to more questions and a richer understanding.
What is the meaning of happiness? **Explanation:** Avoid asking very broad questions that are unlikely to give you focused specific responses.	Describe what makes you most happy. **Explanation:** This question allows multiple answers, from which themes can be identified. It allows expression and personalisation of an answer as opposed to a dictionary definition of an emotion.

Observations

Observational data collection in the context of qualitative research refers to the study of people and/or things by observing in a systematic and meaningful way. The purpose of human observation is focused on capturing behaviours and interactions, from either individuals or groups. Depending on the research goal, attention can be placed on the individual, intragroup or intergroup dynamics. In paramedic research, this translates to watching and listening to how people behave and interact within certain environments and settings. Observation is thus a method of exploring complex human phenomena from the outside in, and from the observer's viewpoint (Box 13.2).

Box 13.2

An example of an observational study

Johnson M, O'Hara R, Hirst E, et al. (2017). Multiple triangulation and collaborative research using qualitative methods to explore decision making in pre-hospital emergency care. *BMC Medical Research Methodology*, 17(11): 1-11. DOI: 10.1186/s12874-017-0290-z.

This study used multiple qualitative methods to investigate decision-making in pre-hospital emergency care. A key component was the direct observation of paramedics' day-to-day working practices.

Types of observations include the following:

- *Direct vs indirect*: A direct observation takes place in the present as events occur. It is an active process whereby the researcher has access to the participant either in person or via communication media. Indirect observation may deduce or infer conclusions based on events in the past. It is a passive process whereby the researcher examines previously recorded material. In modern times it has become easier to conduct both direct and indirect observation as audio and video recording equipment has become more readily available, allowing researchers to actively observe in the present and passively review recorded material at a later stage. Research can be conducted using pre-recorded material such as TV programmes (Shapiro, 2019).

- *Structured vs unstructured*: A structured observation is meticulously planned to look for and document specific behaviours and interactions that are predetermined by the researcher. This approach is directed, systematic and focuses around gathering information that would assist the researcher in gaining understanding of a specific phenomenon. Unstructured observation is the opposite, where there is no predefined plan for specific observation. A structured approach usually includes some checklist components that allow the researcher to focus on a given phenomenon without being distracted by other factors. An unstructured approach provides a broader and more exploratory view of all factors that may affect the phenomenon being studied. This could further lead to incidental findings that may enrich understanding.

- *Overt vs covert*: In overtly conducted observations, all intentions are declared to the participants at the beginning of the study. They are informed about the purpose of the observation and what data will be collected in the process. Participants need to be aware of and consent to the observations taking place, including information about incidental findings that may be captured based on their behaviours and interactions. Covert observations take place where participants are unaware that they are being observed. In some cases, there are a mix of observation strategies, as participants may consent to being observed but do not know when the observational data capture will take place. Following the ethical principle of autonomy, it is generally expected that participants consent to and know when they are being observed, following an open and overt process. The use of covert observation is problematic from a legal and ethical standpoint as it violates personal privacy. Although covert observation has been used historically, the modern protections of individual rights preclude such methods in most instances.

Using a qualitative observational data collection design is challenging but extremely rewarding. Some of the key challenges relate to phenomena known as observer bias and the Hawthorne effect:

- *Observer bias*: Observation by design allows for an external viewpoint to be formed based on participant behaviours and interactions. However, this introduces the perspective and interpretation of the observer into the phenomenon being observed. Interactions by the observer in the process of observation or past personal experiences can thus affect or influence the data being collected and the outcome of the inquiry. Structured observation tries to alleviate potential observer biases by fixing the data points to be collected and using the observer merely as the mechanism for data capture. Unstructured observations are thus more susceptible to such biases, as the observer is free to capture any data that is believed to be relevant. Data collected during direct observation are mostly on information available at the time of occurrence, and thus it is the perspective of the observer that is relied upon for accuracy of events and immediate interpretation. The use of indirect observation in combination allows for behaviours and interactions to be evaluated not only by the primary observer but secondary observers, who may formulate different viewpoints of the phenomenon being studied. It is not only advantageous for multiple researchers to review recorded observations in formulating a more robust understanding of the phenomenon observed, but also allows researchers to reflect on their inherent biases and the impact thereof on their findings.

- *Hawthorne effect*: The Hawthorne effect was first formulated by Landsberger in the 1950s when he reviewed and analysed the interviews conducted during the 1920s at the Western Electric's Hawthorne plant in Illinois, USA (Given, 2008). The purpose of the research was to investigate what factors would maximise workers' effectiveness. It was found, as is now associated with the term, that when individuals are aware of being observed, they react, modify or change their behaviours and interactions. The change in behaviours and interactions may be a conscious decision or a subconscious reaction to the observation. This may substantially affect the authenticity of the data being captured and whether it is a true reflection of observed reality and thus the phenomenon being studied.

This form of data collection is not commonly used within paramedic research studies due to its seemingly complex and intrusive nature. Researchers have found innovative ways to navigate these challenges by allowing less-intrusive and more indirect observation to take place as audio and video capture devices become smaller and less noticeable by participants. This helps mitigate the Hawthorne effect and allows more natural participant behaviours and interactions to emerge. While modern innovations make it more feasible to conduct observations, researchers should remain aware of the concepts that underpin this design and appreciate the potential influence observers have on a studied phenomenon.

Useful tips

- Observations can be seen as intrusive, so it is important to make participants comfortable with the process.
- Ensure everyone understands the process and communicates their expectations before and after the observation.

- Things will happen that you have not planned for, so be pragmatic and flexible with your approach.
- Participants will ask you not to record certain behaviours or events, so ensure this is discussed beforehand and keep true to the documentation structure you agreed.
- It has been shown that participants quickly forget they are being recorded when using small or inconspicuous camera systems, like body-worn types.
- Do not be afraid to get involved when a participant requests your assistance, especially to aid in clinical treatment; this may help your immersion into the phenomena you are studying.

Documentary research and the use of documents in research

Documents are key to research, not solely as a tool for researchers themselves but as a source of rich, often in-depth, personal data from individuals and societies throughout history that can be analysed. As diaries, letters, notepads, wills, shopping lists, death and birth certificates and other documentary evidence can be highly valuable qualitative tools.

Documents themselves can also be highly useful for the researcher, as a planning tool but also as a reflective one. Field notes, research diaries and illustrations of conversations are all key in helping the researcher be effective, and hold a place in the research governance process also.

Types of documentary evidence include the following:

- newspapers and magazines
- maps
- organisational documents
- posters
- diaries and blogs
- official certificates
- adverts
- health records
- notepads
- online messaging transcripts
- books.

The analysis of such documents needs to be systematic. Documents need to be examined and the content interpreted to be able to identify and understand the meaning, social context and purpose of the communication, to ultimately inform the

Chapter 13 — Qualitative data collection

researcher's question. Documentary evidence allows one to view a snapshot in time from the perspective of a particular individual, group or society.

Documentary research will often involve thematic or content analysis. Content analysis is a technique used to make valid inferences by interpreting and coding documentary material. It is possible to convert qualitative data into quantitative data for further interpretation although it is not always necessary to do so.

Content analysis can be used to reveal patterns in communications, determine what the priorities were at a particular time, identify intentions and focus of communication, and understand trends and describe responses.

- How many times was a deity mentioned in a document? *Belief systems*.
- How many times was the word 'evaluation' used in a group of emails? *Organisational culture*.
- Was the male pronoun used more than the female in the documents? *Societal norms*.

By coding this information, qualitative documentary evidence can be used in a quantitative manner and further inferences can be determined, especially from a statistical perspective.

Documentary evidence should, where possible, be used with other methods, as context can be challenging to understand. Context describes the circumstances that create the event or setting, idea or statement. Context provides clarity and meaning to wider events and describes the interrelated conditions in which something exists, occurs, is said or recorded to documents.

Think about the following in terms of context.

- A man walks into a bank with a gun. What are your thoughts? Robber, hostage taker?
- A man walks into a bank with a gun but is wearing police uniform. What are your thoughts? Security guard, routine patrol? The police uniform provides context for the gun in the bank and changed our situational view.

A documentary researcher is always required to understand the context in which something has been recorded while also understanding that they will never fully experience that context.

Useful tips

- Understand the context involved. This will change the analysis.
- Generally content analysis is less obtrusive and invasive research, and therefore may raise fewer ethical concerns. This may be of use for projects with shorter timelines.

- Ensure you consider the reliability and validity of the evidence sources and advertise their strengths. This will reduce the possibility of your analysis being dubbed as being subjective and of poor scientific rigour.

Physical and digital materials

Apart from the traditional and direct methods of data collection, there are indirect approaches that may seem unconventional at first, but should be considered when undertaking healthcare research. These include physical and digital materials created by people through which to express themselves, their thoughts, experiences and feelings. These materials are rich in qualitative data and capture vast amounts of information that is commonly used in conjunction with direct methods. The extraction, interpretation and understanding of such information can be a complex task and is mostly dependent on perspective, usually that of the researcher(s) analysing the materials.

Any physical or digital material created by an individual or group can be considered under this form of data collection; however, photography, video/film, voice/music/noise, art, social media and computer software are the most common.

- *Photography*: The phrase 'a picture is worth a thousand words' comes to mind when looking at photographs that depict people and/or situations. Photographs create context that supports meaningful investigation. Participants are often asked to take photographs (Box 13.3) and depict their view of the world or to capture an image that could later be used as a memory reference point that could elicit thoughts and feelings from a particular time. The modern 'selfie' can also be used as a rich source of information about self-expression and perception. Photographs of historical events or places are often used to help understand human developments or behaviours over time.

- *Video/film*: In modern society there are many devices that fit in our pockets that can take high-quality videos at any time. Just as photographs capture the world around us, video can further expand that world to include motion and audio. Videoing ourselves, our surroundings or participants provides key insights to actual events that can be analysed at a later stage. Participants can use video to record visual diaries or researchers can record the actions of participants during events, such as simulations or clinical practice. Using video to make a film not only allows investigators to capture information, it also provides an opportunity to disseminate key messages to a wider audience.

- *Voice/music/noise*: The ability to speak and communicate information between people is one of the greatest tools we as humans have in understanding ourselves and our environment. It is becoming easier for participants to use their voice to make audio recordings, rather than writing down their thoughts and feelings. Music is an expression of self, and usually has a message or feeling it wants to convey. We can often follow the life journey of musicians as they express themselves through their work. Similarly, the same approach can be used to elicit information from participants through the creation of music using their voices and/or instruments. Music or other noises can also be used as triggers or distractors to elicit responses from participants in various settings.

- *Art*: Art is one of the oldest forms of expression, from plays and performances to paintings and sculptures. Art provides a rich source of information in terms of content and context. It can be used as a medium to explore complex and sometimes abstract phenomena. There are various ways in which participants could be asked to create works of art to bridge their thoughts and feelings into manifestations of physical expression. People, especially children, may find it easier to play-act, draw pictures or sculpt a set of behaviours or circumstances that represent real-world interactions and experiences.

- *Social media*: In the modern digital era, social media has become part and parcel of daily living, providing a unique means of communication and expression. Large amounts of metadata are captured every day that describe, for example, our human behaviours, preferences and social norms. A range of social media platforms can be used to capture and convey, in real time, information about a person's views and opinions. The use of hashtags or similar identifiers attached to posts has become a common method to collate information within this vast space. Although social media information is viewed in the public domain, its use within research comes with a sense of caution as this method of data capture is further explored and understood.

- *Computer software*: Computer software relies on data points drawn from user input to produce outputs in the form of analyses, predictions or modelling. Researchers can use software to capture and transform almost any information into a digital data format. These digital data can then be used to further inform researchers in their investigations and potentially speed up data capture, processing and analysis.

Using alternative means to capture information gives researchers an opportunity to explore qualitative inquiry from a different perspective, often uncovering deeper and sometimes hidden meaning. There are many subconscious elements associated with our behaviours, experiences and thoughts that could be explored using such indirect data capture tools and methods. Healthcare researchers can benefit greatly from these bold approaches to help them understand complex phenomena beyond face value.

> **Box 13.3**
>
> ### An example of a study using photo-elicitation
>
> Houston J, Rae J, Brewster L. (2020). A photo-elicitation study of paramedics' perceptions of mental illness. *Irish Journal of Paramedicine*, 5(1): 1–17. DOI: 10.32378/ijp.v5i1.225
>
> This study used photographs during interviews to extend the conversation about paramedic perceptions of mental illness, through social and personal meaning. The meaning and emotions elicited supplemented the verbal inquiry.

Useful tips

- The interpretation of information from indirect sources is key to the generation of credible data and should thus be done by at least two or more people.
- It would be impossible and unnecessary to extract every bit of detail from photographs, videos and art, so set reasonable parameters.
- Involve your participants in the process of data capture and do not be afraid to give them tasks to complete and plenty of time.
- Capturing digital materials can be a daunting task and take up a lot of storage. Ensure you keep separated back-ups to avoid losing your information.
- The methods of data capture described here often come with some form of copyright protections or intellectual property rights, so ensure you understand your responsibilities and consult with an expert(s) before starting to collect data.
- Content available within the public domain does not necessarily translate to free use by researchers, so ensure you respect ethical procedures and conduct when collating such materials.

Summary

This chapter has provided a comprehensive overview of qualitative data collection methods in the context of paramedicine research. We have explored three main tools and five major methods used to capture qualitative data, enabling you to select the most appropriate approach to answer your research question.

We have looked at strengths and weaknesses inherent to different data collection methods, and discussed common challenges encountered during data collection, providing practical strategies for overcoming them and empowering you to navigate potential obstacles with confidence and resilience.

As you reflect on the wealth of knowledge and insights gained from this chapter, remember that qualitative data collection is both an art and a science, requiring creativity, methodological rigour and ethical responsibility. Whether you are embarking on your first research project or refining your skills as an experienced researcher, the principles and guidelines presented here will serve as a valuable resource in your journey towards conducting meaningful and impactful qualitative research in paramedicine.

Chapter 14

Making sense of qualitative data

Ursula Rolfe and Alison Porter

> **Purpose of this chapter**
>
> Completion of this chapter will help you to:
> - understand the complexities surrounding qualitative data analysis
> - become familiar with the characteristics of content analysis, framework analysis, thematic analysis, grounded theory method, discourse analysis and conversation analysis
> - consider some of the challenges that you will encounter in qualitative analysis and how to navigate these
> - consider how to manage and present qualitative data.

Introduction

Qualitative research method is like a submarine that patiently waits to be used as a powerful instrument of investigation. It silently waits to be submerged into the ocean, its favourite and natural habitat. Above sea level it is noisy, hot or cold and one is considered as just another species of existence. Below sea level it is quiet, swift and beautiful. Qualitative researchers abandon the noisy outside world to enter the quiet and sacred realms of their data. The researcher submerges themselves in the deep waters to reach the answers.

Jimenez, 2023

Previous chapters have guided you through collecting qualitative data. Now that you have your data, the next step is to analyse them. But what are you trying to do through the process of analysis?

First, you are simply reducing your thousands of words of text, hundreds of pages of material or other data to something which is manageable, and that your reader is going to be able to assimilate. Second, you are selecting what is important or significant within that data – think of this as telling a story or choosing a path through a landscape to find a destination. What is important or significant is a matter of judgement, and will vary according to the questions you are asking and the context for the research. Third, you are going through a process of interpretation. Qualitative data can be likened to user behaviour records and customer feedback. Data may yield direct reporting of facts, direct statement of perceptions or opinions, and implicit messages. The researcher has to take all this information and transform it using analysis and interpretation into something with significance and meaning.

Approaches to analysis of qualitative data have developed and diversified enormously over the last few decades, but the characterisation of qualitative data as 'an attractive nuisance' by Matthew Miles (1979) remains true. It is attractive because it is very rich and full of possibilities, but a nuisance because of the difficulty of finding analytic paths through it. You are not seeking to uncover a single absolute truth but instead to build a plausible and meaningful narrative which is rooted in the data.

Analysis of qualitative data can be thought of as a mix of art and science. There is no single formula about what to do, but rather guidelines for approaches which range in how structured or flexible they are. Whatever approach you take, there will be a large element of subjectivity and individuality – this is accepted as part of the qualitative research process. Since qualitative analysis is all about making choices – what you include, what you leave out, what you emphasise, what dead ends of reasoning you abandon – two different researchers or different research teams could start with the same dataset but may not end with the same conclusions. This is not something to worry about, but it is something to acknowledge and think about in reflexive terms – what assumptions and expectations are you bringing to the analysis because of who you are, and because of your background and experience?

Your approach to analysis is something you need to think about when you are designing your study, not once you have your data. You will need to decide on the goals of your analysis; what you consider appropriate information or data; and how best to capture, understand and convey these data. These considerations are part of a continuous process that begins when you first consider what research you will undertake, and will continue throughout your data collection, analysis and write-up phases.

The study design will inform the nature of the analysis, which in turn will have implications for how you plan your data collection. In this chapter, we give some pointers about qualitative data analysis and introduce you to a range of approaches, but we strongly recommend that before embarking on a qualitative analysis project, you read up on methods in more detail, and we have suggested some key texts for you to look at.

Making choices – what is your starting point?

One of the first big choices you need to make when designing your study is how inductive you want to be in your approach. Do you want to be mostly driven by exploring what is in the data (inductive) or by the specific questions which you bring to the data to test them (deductive)? It is not necessarily a case of either/or but a continuum, and you need to choose where to position yourself on it. This will in turn help to shape your research objectives and plan for data collection, as well as your plan for analysis.

The other decision you need to make at the start is about how you want to use theory. We are not talking here about high-level theories of knowledge, but about theories which explain and support our understanding of a particular phenomenon. 'Mid-range theory' can give you a lens through which to examine your topic and help to focus your analysis, and can support comparison across settings and across studies, to produce transferable knowledge and develop a wider body of evidence. If you choose to use theory to inform your analysis, it will help to guide you through the process, as in the example in Box 14.1.

> **Box 14.1**
>
> ### An example of an ethnographic study using mid-range theory
>
> *Example:* Using computer decision support systems in NHS emergency and urgent care: ethnographic study using normalisation process theory
>
> Pope et al. (2013) were interested in what is needed for people to successfully bring new information technology into use – specifically, software to support decision making by call handlers in urgent and emergency care settings. They drew on normalisation process theory (NPT), which explains these changes in terms of four mechanisms, including 'coherence' (people collectively recognising that an innovation is meaningful and desirable) and 'reflexive monitoring' (the continuing process of reviewing the innovation and making adjustments). The study team spent 500 hours observing how call handlers and clinical supervisors used the software in three different settings – an ambulance call centre, a GP out-of-hours service, and a single point of access service for urgent and emergency care – and made notes of what they saw and heard. They also carried out 61 formal interviews with people using the software, recording those interviews so they could produce a full transcript. The researchers found that using NPT to inform their analysis helped them to understand the similarities across the three settings, and to produce insights which could also be relevant to other settings.

Somewhere between the inductive and deductive approaches to analysis is the abductive approach (Box 14.2), which is informed by existing theory, but in what Timmermans and Tavory (2012) call an 'agnostic' way. Researchers compare the data with existing theory, but look for surprises within it: things which are novel or puzzling, and can help to advance, refine or challenge the theory.

The choices you make will influence the approach you take to analysis. Sometimes a researcher will shift their position as they go through analysis – commonly, starting with a more deductive position and then realising that there is a lot of significant material in the data which does not relate to the questions they are using, and

Chapter 14 — Making sense of qualitative data

> **Box 14.2**
>
> ### An example of a study using an abductive approach to analysing feedback to paramedics
>
> Wilson et al. (2022a) interviewed 24 EMS professionals about their perceptions of current provision of prehospital feedback and their views on how feedback impacts patient care, patient safety and staff well-being, and how feedback might be improved. From their reading of the background literature, they found two theories they wanted to explore in relation to the literature: clinical performance feedback intervention theory (CP-FIT) which outlines the mechanisms by which feedback works within healthcare and considers what makes it effective; and theory around feedback-seeking behaviour (FSB), which explores what motivates people to seek feedback. Wilson and colleagues took an abductive approach to analysis, drawing on these theories in their interpretation of the data to develop a single model setting out how prehospital clinicians are highly motivated to get feedback to improve patient outcomes and for their own professional development.

adjusting the analysis to take account of this. Conversely, the researcher may start with a very inductive approach, but during the course of analysis realise that there is an existing theory which they want to use to help them interrogate the data. It is important to be wary of mission creep – producing answers to a different question may not meet the purpose of the study or the expectations of the funders – and to be cautious of findings which may be superficially interesting but not actually significant. Be particularly careful not to be distracted by the glittering diamanté in your data – things which are catchy or funny, but ultimately don't mean much.

Dealing with Data

Types of data have been largely covered in Chapters 12 and 13. Your data type will inform your approach to analysis. For example, if you have collected data via observation of conversations, this lends itself more to discourse or narrative analysis.

There are two broad approaches to dealing with data:

- Tagging or labelling data
- Grouping tagged or labelled data.

Tagging is the process of selecting bits and pieces of information that satisfy your curiosity and help support the aim of your research study (Baptiste, 2001). You will need to decide what to count as important and what to reject. Labelling (assigning some distinguishing mark to selective data) is part of tagging. These labels may naturally follow the data itself, for example images, numbers, symbols, words or phrases (Baptiste, 2001). Once you have tagged and labelled your data, you need to consider if there are similar features in a group of categories, also known as themes, constructs, concepts or variables. Remember that your categories can overlap. Your choice of theory will also inform how you decide on these categories.

This phase is a messy one as you may change your mind about labels and categories. Remember to go back to the question of whether you are tagging inductively or deductively, and most importantly, how will you demonstrate trustworthiness in dealing with your data (Denzin and Lincoln, 2000)?

Approaches to qualitative analysis

Finding the meaning and making sense of your data is the main purpose of qualitative data analysis. Miles and Huberman (1994: 10) said that "the strengths of qualitative data rests on the competence with which their analysis is carried out".

Carl May (2003) set out a useful breakdown of the different types of work involved in qualitative analysis, showing how it starts with simple process of classification, coding the data and putting it in order, which may lead to a set of categories or taxonomy. This can then support what he calls analytic work, which involves looking at relationships between different themes in the data, and their relative significance, which may lead to a map or model. Finally comes interpretative work, which seeks explanation for what's going on, and develops plausible claims which may be presented as hypotheses, propositions or theories. The balance of these three different types of work will vary between qualitative studies, according to the aims and research questions, and the analytical approach taken.

There are many approaches to qualitative analysis. We will be considering the following: content analysis, framework analysis, thematic analysis, grounded theory method, conversation analysis and discourse analysis.

Content analysis

Content analysis is used to identify patterns in the text by grouping content into words, concepts and themes, and is a popular method created by journalists and later adopted by social scientists (Curtis and Curtis, 2011). It sits at the more deductive end of the analysis spectrum, best suited to looking for answers to particular questions. It is a useful approach for quantifying how often words, phrases or concepts appear in the text, and to highlight associations, for example whether one type of participant is more likely to express concerns about a particular issue than another.

When conducting content analysis (example in Box 14.3), follow considerations suggested by Grbich (2013): researchers should ensure that they have enough documents and determine the aspects of the documents to be analysed; establish the sampling approach when selecting documents; decide on the level of analysis to be done and how the codes will be generated; consider the relationships between concepts, codes and contexts; record the number of times categories appear; and ascertain the reliability of the coding scheme.

Chapter 14 — Making sense of qualitative data

> **Box 14.3**
>
> ### An example of a study using content analysis
>
> *Example:* Paramedic identification of patients with end-of-life care needs
>
> Eaton-Williams et al. (2020) wanted to examine the timely identification by ambulance paramedics of patients with potential end-of-life care (EoLC) needs. They had some specific questions: do paramedics think they are currently identifying patients within the last year of their life for subsequent referral to their primary care provider for EoLC needs assessment? What are current levels of awareness and utilisation of the Gold Standards Framework Proactive Identification Guidance (GSF PIG) amongst paramedics? What are paramedics' attitudes towards using the GSF PIG in their clinical practice?
>
> The research team recruited registered paramedics from nine English NHS ambulance service trusts to complete an online questionnaire, which included questions about paramedics' attitudes, inviting free-text responses in a box for 'any other comments'. The researchers used content analysis to categorise responses, and to count the number of comments in each category. 587 free-text responses were submitted by participants. The researchers grouped these into categories, of which the most commonly mentioned were: further EoLC clinical education (n = 139); provision of responsive EoLC referral pathways, accessible at all hours (n = 97); and the unique opportunity provided by the ambulance clinical setting (n = 95). These responses helped Eaton-Williams and colleagues to interpret and build on other findings from their survey.
>
> They concluded that predominantly, ambulance paramedics believed that EoLC was a role both appropriate to and achievable within their clinical environment, but that paramedics faced barriers to delivering it. Identification of EoLC patients within ambulance-based clinical practice would be facilitated by the provision of formal EoLC education and the establishment of dedicated, accessible and responsive referral pathways.

Framework analysis

This is an approach that has been used since the 1980s, especially in large-scale social policy research (Ritchie and Lewis, 2003). The process often starts with transcribing data from audio recordings. This is also a great opportunity for you as the researcher to become more immersed in your data. After becoming familiar with the interview using audio recordings, making reflective notes while listening to the recordings is the second stage.

The defining feature of framework analysis is the matrix output: cases, columns (codes) and 'cells' of summarised data, providing a structure into which the researcher can systematically reduce the data, to analyse it by case and by code. The 'case' is usually a participant interviewee, but it can be adapted to groups or organisations. The view of each participant is connected to other aspects within the matrix so that the context of one participant is not lost. As with most qualitative analysis methods, constant comparing and contrasting of data is vital.

Framework analysis provides the ability to compare data across cases as well as looking at individual cases with ease (Gale et al., 2013). However, it can be time-consuming and resource-intensive. It often includes a multidisciplinary research element, and critical to its success is the use of an experienced qualitative research lead (Box 14.4).

Box 14.4

An example of a study using framework analysis

Example: The research paramedic experience (RESPARE) study: a qualitative study exploring experiences of research paramedics working in the United Kingdom

McClelland et al. (2023) were interested in exploring the experience of people who work, or have worked, as research paramedics. The authors gathered data from interviews and focus groups with 18 research paramedics from across England. Volunteers were recruited via ambulance research leads and social media. Online focus groups allowed participants to discuss their roles with peers who may be geographically distant. Semi-structured interviews expanded on the focus group findings. Data were recorded, transcribed verbatim and analysed using framework analysis. Eighteen paramedics representing eight English NHS ambulance trusts participated in three focus groups and five interviews lasting around one hour, in November and December 2021.

Six key themes were identified: starting as a research paramedic; barriers and facilitators to working as a research paramedic; research careers; opportunities; the community (support and networking); and the value of a clinical identity. McClelland et al. (2023) concluded that many research paramedics had similar experiences in terms of starting their career by delivering research for large studies, then built on this experience and the networks they created to develop their own research. There are common organisational and financial barriers to working as a research paramedic. Career progression in research beyond the research paramedic role is not well defined, but often involves building links outside the ambulance service.

Thematic analysis

Thematic analysis is a very widely-used approach when working with qualitative data (see example in Box 14.5). It is a structured approach to developing themes from the data. It starts with coding the data, identifying repeated content which may be

Chapter 14 — Making sense of qualitative data

semantic (on the surface, what people say) or latent (implicit, what you interpret from what people say or how they express themselves). Codes are then used to build up themes.

Braun and Clarke (2021a) made the useful distinction between themes as buckets (where you bring together all the codes relating to a particular topic) and themes as stories (where the researcher interprets the codes to weave them together into a narrative). Both types of themes are valid and may be used to a greater or lesser extent in each study. Braun and Clarke (2021a) also place great importance on being reflexive in thematic analysis, arguing that the researcher(s) should constantly be checking and reviewing their assumptions, and considering how their own position (role in relation to the topic, past experience) may influence their interpretation.

Box 14.5

An example of a study using thematic analysis

Example: Emergency ambulance call-takers' experiences in managing out-of-hospital cardiac arrest

Perera et al. (2023) were interested in what it was like for call-handlers in an ambulance control centre to deal with calls where a patient had experienced an out-of-hospital cardiac arrest. They interviewed ten call-handlers in a service in Western Australia about how they perceived the interaction with the caller in these circumstances. Interviews lasted 30 minutes to 2 hours and were loosely structured to allow the respondent to take the conversation in the direction they wanted.

When analysing the transcripts, the research team followed the six stages set out by Braun and Clarke (2021b): 1. familiarising themselves with the data; 2. generating initial codes; 3. searching for themes; 4. reviewing themes; 5. defining and naming themes; 6. producing the report. The team developed four themes from the data. The first was the time-critical nature of the call, which meant that the call-taker was aware of working in a situation of urgency and pressure; the second was the call-taking process, where the respondents emphasised the value of the software they used to help them identify a cardiac arrest and offer an appropriate response; the third was caller management, by which call-takers adapted their response to suit the range of emotional presentations (including anger and panic) which callers may have; and the final theme was protecting the self, where the call-takers discussed the emotional impacts of dealing with such calls.

Grounded theory method

Grounded theory approaches to analysis sit at the most inductive end of the analytical spectrum. Originally developed in the 1960s by Glaser and Strauss (1967), grounded theory method (GTM) seeks to develop theory inductively from the data – so the theory is grounded in the data. This original model of GTM asks the researcher to approach the data with an open mind, without bringing any pre-existing theoretical constructs. Data collection and analysis proceed in parallel: the researcher analyses each data item as it is gathered, looking for patterns and concepts, then seeking further data which may challenge or refute emerging ideas. This process stops at the point of 'data saturation' – when collecting and analysing data brings no new insight. Subsequently, other methodologists have proposed evolved versions of GTM, which acknowledge the impossibility of washing the researcher's mind of pre-existing theories, and challenge Glaser and Strauss's idea that theory is there to be 'discovered' in the data, like fossils in rock.

Grounded theory method is slow, laborious, intellectually demanding and a poor fit with research regulatory systems which expect tight plans at the outset, which means it is rarely delivered in its true form. However, GTM remains influential on qualitative analysis methodology in its emphasis on interpretation and insight throughout the analytical process (Box 14.6).

> **Box 14.6**
>
> ### An example of a study using grounded theory
>
> *Example:* Paramedics' perceptions of the care they provide to people who self-harm: a qualitative study using evolved grounded theory methodology
>
> Rees et al. (2018) aimed to understand more about how paramedics feel about providing care to people engaged in self-harm (SH), a complex situation which makes up about 5% of calls in the UK but which is not well understood. The study used evolved grounded theory methodology – a development of the original grounded theory approach which incorporates the constructivist ideas of Charmaz (2006) who considers the meaning in the data to be constructed by the researcher, rather than pre-existing as a truth. This puts the reflexivity of the lead author centre stage: Rees brought 28 years' experience as a paramedic to the analysis, including caring for many people who had engaged in acts of SH, and witnessing some deaths following acts of SH.
>
> Rees and colleagues developed a grounded theory to describe *wicked complexity in paramedics' care for people who self-harm*, centred on the basic social process of decision-making in the context of risk. This process is influenced by three categories of factors: usual factors, such as tiredness and frequent callers, common to routine paramedic work; heightened factors including lack of support and pathways which are found to a greater degree in work with people who SH; and factors specific to SH such as assessing suicide risk.

Chapter 14 — Making sense of qualitative data

Conversation analysis

Conversation analysis is an approach which examines how people communicate (see example in Box 14.7). It uses naturally-occurring data, such as conversation between a clinician and patient, rather than, for example, an interview conducted as part of the study. A researcher doing conversation analysis may be interested in how people communicate or how decision-making takes place. They will draw on ideas from the fields of sociology and linguistics about how people use language, including the role of utterances and the conventional sequence in conversation. Recordings of conversations are transcribed in a very high level of detail for conversation analysis, with special notation used to identify things such as sighs, pauses and emphasis.

Conversation analysis may tell you interesting things about how power works in decision making, or about how people understand or misunderstand each other.

Box 14.7

An example of a study using conversation analysis

Example: 'Primary care sensitive' situations that result in an ambulance attendance: a conversation analytic study of UK emergency '999' call recordings

Booker et al. (2018) were interested in why ambulance services despatched ambulances to deal with situations which could be dealt with by primary care – 'primary care sensitive' situations. They decided to examine in detail the conversations which took place during the 999 calls, to understand what might be the challenges to identifying an appropriate triage response. In total, recordings of 48 conversations were analysed, selected after Booker – himself a GP – had spent many hours riding out on shifts to identify primary care sensitive incidents.

In their analysis of the ways in which the call-handler and the caller (patient or friend/relative) communicated, the researchers identified the many ways in which the highly scripted triage process didn't always fit with the way in which the caller expressed themselves. Their description of the problem may not have fitted the codes in the triage system. Callers may not have had full understanding of what the problem was or how urgent it was – in two-thirds of the calls, it was not the patient doing the talking but someone speaking on their behalf, which may have added extra challenges. The way in which some of the set questions were phrased seemed tricky for some callers, and the ambulance service and the caller may have different perceptions of the 'purpose' of particular questions. The findings contribute to the understanding of how risk is negotiated and managed in triage decisions, and how call-handlers use unscripted talk to get through blocks in the triage process.

Discourse analysis

This approach is used to obtain an understanding of political, cultural and power dynamics that exist in specific situations. The main focus is on how people express themselves in different social contexts (see example in Box 14.8). The ability of discourse analysis to deal with dialogue, texts and language makes it popular with those in sociology, psychology, media studies and health sciences – especially when wanting to explore social patterns and practices (Liamputtong and Serry, 2013). This approach is all about dealing with talk and text, and can be closely linked to conversation analysis.

> **Box 14.8**
>
> ### An example of a study using discourse analysis
>
> *Example:* Evidence from the scene: paramedic perspectives on involvement in out-of-hospital research
>
> Burges Watson et al. (2011) sought to understand paramedics' perceptions of involvement in research and the barriers and facilitators to their involvement, in the UK and USA. The study used semi-structured focus groups with 58 UK paramedics and interviews with 30 US firefighter-paramedics. The researchers focused on out-of-hospital research (trials of prehospital treatment for stroke) where paramedics identify potential study subjects or obtain consent and administer study treatment in the field. Data were analysed using a thematic and discourse approach. The study's participants use 'discourses' (their version of the world) to interpret and present descriptions of that world. The researchers aimed to gain a richer understanding of the cultures and customs encoded in the participants' speech. Preliminary analyses were presented in various ways back to paramedics and other researchers to check and challenge the interpretations made.
>
> Three key themes were identified as significant facilitators and barriers to paramedic involvement in research: 'patient benefit', 'professional identity and responsibility' and 'time'. Paramedics showed willingness and capacity to engage in research but also some reticence due to the perceived sacrifice of autonomy and challenge to their identity. Paramedics work in a time-sensitive environment and were concerned that research should not increase the time taken in the field.

How to do analysis – the technical bit

You can analyse your data manually or with the help of computer-aided qualitative data analysis software (CAQDAS). Manual approaches can involve using paper and handwritten margin notes, highlighter pen, Post-it notes and filing cards. Drawing mind maps to indicate developing grouping of themes and ideas can certainly help the process, but it takes some work to learn how to use it effectively.

Chapter 14 — Making sense of qualitative data

There are a variety of CAQDAS programs, including NVivo, ATLAS.ti, Provalis Research Text Analytics Software, Quirkos, MAXQDA, Dedoose, Raven's Eye, Qiqqa, webQDA, HyperRESEARCH, Transana, F4analyse, Annotations and Datagrav, which generally need to be bought or used under licence. Programs generally help you to classify, sort and arrange information contained in textual data; examine the relationships in the data; search the data in a structured way; and map and present findings. However, they do not do the work of analysis for you.

Paulus et al. (2014) provide a useful list of questions that may guide a researcher when selecting a CAQDAS system:

- What features will support my analytical approach?
- Does the system allow me to annotate, link, search, code and visualise data?
- How does the software assist in data management?
- What are the benefits and constraints of the software package?

Once you have decided whether you want to use a CAQDAS or do it manually, or even a combination of both, you need to connect and organise your data. This will initially feel quite overwhelming. Make sure your data are accessible and in one place — the key is to be consistent and keep pressing 'save'! If you have decided on a manual approach, the best starting point is inputting your data into a spreadsheet. Remember that how and where you store these data will also be aligned to the requirements of the organisation you work for.

Once you have your data organised in one place —on your spreadsheet, CAQDAS or a feedback repository such as Dovetail or EnjoyHQ — you need to start sorting your data depending on the analysis approach (see section on analysis approach) you have decided to use in your study. Once you have coded or sorted your data in alignment with your analysis approach, you will start to find some meaningful insights — this is where your research journey becomes more exciting and fulfilling, especially as you discover insights and themes that provide an interesting perspective and theory linked to the aims of your research study.

Who is doing the analysis?

Qualitative analysis may be a solo activity or it may be carried out by a team (see example in Box 14.9). Working in a team has several advantages: sharing out the labour; sense checking each other's work; and getting alternative angles on interpretation, as different members of the analysis team bring their own background, experience and values. However, team working needs careful handling, and is not always easy to achieve. An analysis team may combine researchers with methodological skills, members of the wider study team with particular clinical insights or knowledge of relevant organisational issues, and patient and public involvement (PPI) partners who may be bringing lived experience of healthcare (see Chapter 17).

> **Box 14.9**
>
> ### An example of a team approach to qualitative analysis
>
> *Example:* The ERA study of electronic records in ambulances
>
> Porter et al. (2020) studied how electronic health records can be most effectively implemented in a prehospital context to support a safe and effective shift from acute to community-based care, and how their potential benefits can be maximised. Part of this study involved gathering a large qualitative dataset from four case study ambulance services, consisting of transcripts, observation notes and documentation.
>
> The analysis was carried out by a team bringing together university-based researchers, four site researchers who had collected the data while embedded in the ambulance services, and two PPI partners. Each participant read a sample of texts before meeting to discuss ideas and themes and develop an analytical framework. Each text was then coded by a minimum of two researchers and developed into an initial analysis. The research team invited partners from the study sites to a workshop event to discuss this initial analysis and seek feedback and check interpretation with those involved in using electronic health records, before the final report was published.

Verifying and presenting qualitative data

A large part of presenting qualitative data is considering their validity and being able to verify your findings. Analysis of qualitative data is arguably more subjective than the processes associated with quantitative data analysis (Burnard et al., 2008).

There are two key ways of verifying your data. The first is participant validation – returning to the study participants (see example in Box 14.10) and asking them to validate analyses. The second is peer review (or peer debrief, also referred to as inter-rater reliability) whereby another qualitative researcher analyses the data independently (Mays and Pope, 1995; Barbour, 2001).

Long and Johnson (2000) suggest that participant validation involves returning your data to the participants of your study and asking them to carefully read through their interview transcripts and/or data analysis for them to validate, or refute, your interpretation of the data. While this can arguably help to refine theme and theory development, the process is hugely time-consuming and, if it does not occur relatively soon after data collection and analysis, participants may have changed their perceptions and views because of temporal effects and potential changes in their situation, health and perhaps even as a result of participation in the study.

Barbour (2001) and Cutcliffe and McKenna (1999) add that peer review involves at least one other suitably-experienced researcher independently reviewing and

Chapter 14 — Making sense of qualitative data

exploring interview transcripts, data analysis and emerging themes. It has been argued that this process may help to guard against the potential for lone-researcher bias and to provide additional insights into theme and theory development.

There are two ways to consider writing and presenting your qualitative research. You can begin by simply reporting your key findings by using verbatim quotes to support these findings. This is supported by linking a separate discussion section where your findings are discussed in relation to existing research The other approach is where you combine your discussion and your findings (using verbatim quotes to illustrate points) into one integrated section.

The keys to quality reporting of qualitative research results are clarity, organisation, completeness, accuracy and conciseness in communicating the results to your reader.

Box 14.10

An example of verifying qualitative data

Example: Paramedic performance when managing patients experiencing mental health issues – exploring paramedics' presentation of self

Rolfe et al. (2020) aimed to explore how paramedics perform in practice when managing patients experiencing mental health issues. Methods included qualitative observation over 240 hours and interviews involving 21 paramedics and 20 patients with mental health issues. The authors began by describing the complexity of paramedic work in the prehospital environment, moving to a focused phase analysing the range of problems paramedics faced while managing patients experiencing mental health issues. The final phase of analysis was selective, exploring how paramedics managed particular cases in more detail. Goffman's concept of presentation of self was used as a theoretical framework, to help understand the behaviours of paramedics and their coping strategies as a performance. To support credibility of the data, several paramedic participants of the study scrutinised the initial observation notes and later some of the analysis. Advisers drawn from the ambulance trust, and working on education and policy development for the professional body (the College of Paramedics), were also asked to review the data and its interpretations. They provided feedback and comments which were integrated into the analysis and results. The first author kept extensive reflexive accounts about her experiences of participant observations and had regular meetings with experienced supervisors to discuss these experiences and to critique the emerging analysis.

The findings of this study revealed that paramedics 'perform' on two stages: front stage and backstage. Their coping mechanisms, in the metaphorical sense, include props such as uniform and scripts filled with humour, stereotyping and nostalgia to aid in their management of this specialist patient group. Rolfe et al. (2020) concluded that paramedics feel frustrated and unsupported when dealing with patients experiencing mental health issues.

Johnson et al. (2020) recommend using a standardised framework such as Standards for Reporting Qualitative Research (SRQR). This framework provides detailed explanations of what should be reported in each of 21 sections of a qualitative research manuscript. While the SRQR does not explicitly mention a conceptual framework, the descriptions and table footnote clarification for the introduction and problem statement reflect the essential elements and focus of a conceptual framework. An alternative reporting checklist is the 32-item Consolidated Criteria for Reporting Qualitative Research (COREQ) (Tong et al., 2007). COREQ has also been frequently used in reviews on qualitative studies to assess the quality of the included studies in the absence of a checklist specifically developed for this purpose.

Summary

Analysis is about distilling complex narratives into digestible insights. This process involves three key steps: condensing the data to manageable proportions, discerning what is significant amidst the noise and unravelling the underlying meanings embedded within.

Qualitative data offer richness and depth but demand patience and skill to navigate. There is no one definitive path; rather, it is a journey of exploration guided by methodological frameworks yet framed by individual perspectives.

This chapter provides an initial roadmap for qualitative analysis, offering insights into different approaches and methodologies. However, it is not a substitute for deeper exploration and understanding.

Ultimately, qualitative analysis is a transformative process, empowering researchers to uncover hidden truths, challenge assumptions and drive meaningful change in their practice. It is a continuous process, evolving from study design through to data interpretation and write-up. While this chapter offers insights into qualitative analysis, further reading and exploration of methodological texts are encouraged to refine your analytical toolkit.

Useful resources

- Braun V and Clarke V (2021). *Thematic Analysis: A Practical Guide*. London: Sage.
- Grbich C (2013). *Qualitative Data Analysis: An Introduction*, 2nd edn. New York: Sage.
- Mills J and Birks M (2014). *Qualitative Methodology: A Practical Guide*. London: Sage.
- Pope C and Mays N (eds) (2020). *Qualitative Research in Health Care*, 4th edn. Oxford: Wiley Blackwell .

Chapter 15

Mixed methods research design

Gregory A. Whitley and Scott Munro

> **Purpose of this chapter**
>
> Completion of this chapter will help you to:
> - understand what constitutes mixed methods research
> - describe the different types of mixed methods research
> - understand the strengths and limitations of mixed methods research
> - understand the philosophical and theoretical challenges of mixed methods research
> - understand how to apply mixed methods to paramedic research.

Introduction

Evidence-based practice (EBP) involves the 'conscientious, explicit and judicious use of current best evidence' (Sackett et al., 1996). EBP has been accepted as the 'gold standard' for prehospital healthcare development and improvement and is achieved through the integration of best evidence, individual clinical expertise and patient preferences/values (Swanson et al., 2010).

Evidence informing the treatment and management of patients in the prehospital environment has primarily favoured quantitative methods (McManamny et al., 2014), including experimental and observational studies. However, the volume of qualitative research has been steadily increasing in recent years (Pope and Mays, 2009).

Individual quantitative studies such as randomised controlled trials (RCTs) aim to determine the effectiveness of interventions (Law and Pascoe, 2013). Their goal is to determine causation, where conclusions are drawn based on appropriate numbers of patients. With appropriate sample selection, the results should be generalisable. A disadvantage of individual quantitative research is the objective nature of the findings, which provides a limited understanding of context (Creswell, 2014).

Chapter 15 — Mixed methods research design

Prehospital healthcare research often involves people. This makes qualitative methods useful to understand lay and professional views, attitudes, beliefs, behavioural intentions (Pope and Mays, 1995), experiences and cultures (Al-Busaidi, 2008). A limitation of individual qualitative research is the subjective nature of the findings (Creswell, 2014), which can be difficult to demonstrate with rigour (Cypress, 2017).

Considering the inherent disadvantages of individual quantitative and qualitative research, coupled with increasing healthcare complexity (Plsek and Greenhalgh, 2001), mixed methods research may provide a helpful solution. This is particularly useful in the prehospital setting due to the unpredictable environment (Abelsson and Lindwall, 2012), where mixed methods are an ideal solution to the difficulty faced when attempting to fully understand complex problems.

What is mixed methods research?

Although there is no formally-established or universally-agreed definition of mixed methods research (Johnson et al., 2007), it is considered essential to contain quantitative (numerical) *and* qualitative (non-numerical) data within one overall study. The collective strength of combining both types of data provides a better understanding of the research problem than can be achieved with either form of data alone (Creswell, 2014).

The *integration* of quantitative and qualitative data from two or more studies is considered essential to mixed methods research (O'Cathain et al., 2010; Creswell, 2014). Integration can be achieved at the design, methods, interpretation and reporting levels. This is achieved via connecting, building, transforming (Fetters et al., 2013), following a thread, triangulation (O'Cathain et al., 2010) or using a joint display (Guetterman et al., 2015), amongst other techniques. See Table 15.1 for a description of these methods. Without integration, a study involving quantitative and qualitative data has been termed 'multi-methods' (Creswell, 2014).

The aim of mixed methods research is to create depth and breadth of understanding (Johnson et al., 2007) that is considered more than, or beyond, the sum of its parts (Teddlie and Tashakkori, 2009). Such conclusions are termed 'meta-inferences', defined as:

> a conclusion generated by integrating the inferences obtained from the qualitative and quantitative strands of a mixed methods study.
> (adapted from Teddlie and Tashakkori, 2009)

Types of mixed methods research

The three basic types of mixed methods design, described by Creswell (2014), are sequential explanatory, sequential exploratory and convergent. More advanced designs include the embedded (or intervention) design, where qualitative research is incorporated into quantitative experimental research, for example a process evaluation within an RCT, to better understand the patient's experience of the

Table 15.1 Methods of integration.

Level	Method	Description
Design	Sequential explanatory	Data are inherently integrated in these designs as they are *explained* (sequential explanatory), *tested* (sequential exploratory) or *merged* (convergent).
	Sequential exploratory	
	Convergent	
Methods	Connecting	When the findings from one study inform the sampling of the other.
	Building	When the findings from one study inform the data collection approach of the other.
	Following a thread	When a question or theme from one study is followed across to the other study to elicit deeper understanding.
Interpretation and reporting	Triangulation	Assessing the level of agreement, complementarity[a] and contradiction between both sets of findings.
	Data transformation	Transforming one type of data into the other, followed by combining the data.
	Joint display	Visually bringing together quantitative and qualitative findings into a figure or table to facilitate the generation of meta-inferences.[b]

Source: Adapted from Fetters et al. (2013).
[a] Quantitative and qualitative data may address different aspects of a phenomenon and therefore may not be able to confirm or refute each other. Instead, they may offer complementary information which can help build a more comprehensive understanding of the problem.
[b] 'a conclusion generated by integrating the inferences obtained from the qualitative and quantitative strands of a mixed methods study' (adapted from Teddlie and Tashakkori, 2009).

intervention or of the trial itself (O'Cathain et al., 2013), including examination of how the intervention is working and how, if it is successful, it may be sustained or spread (Moore et al., 2015).

Sequential design

The sequential design is the most popular mixed methods approach in prehospital research (McManamny et al., 2014). It can either be explanatory, in which quantitative findings are *explained* using qualitative methods (commonly notated as QUAN(qual)), or exploratory, in which qualitative findings are used to generate hypotheses that are *tested* using quantitative methods (commonly notated as QUAL(quan))

Chapter 15 — Mixed methods research design

a) Sequential explanatory design

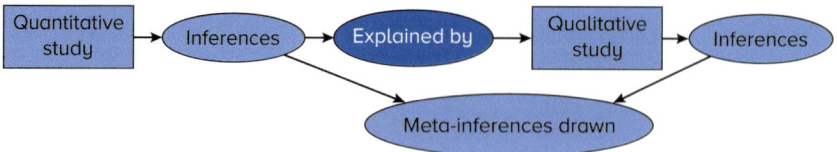

b) Sequential exploratory design

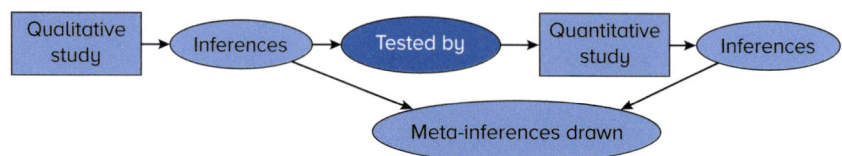

Figure 15.1 Procedures for mixed methods sequential designs.
Source: Used with permission from Whitley et al. (2020b).

(Schoonenboom and Johnson, 2017). Figure 15.1 illustrates the procedures for both types of sequential design.

The sequential explanatory design (see Figure 15.1a) is often utilised by researchers who have a background in quantitative research (Creswell, 2014), due to the familiarity of the initial statistical phase. The conclusions, or 'inferences', generated from the initial quantitative study are observational in nature and offer little depth of understanding or explanation, hence the need for a second qualitative phase to *explain* the findings.

The sequential exploratory design is often used when little is known about a topic, for example perhaps due to an understudied population (Creswell, 2014). The hypotheses and theories generated from the initial qualitative work can then be *tested* quantitatively (see Figure 15.1b).

One of the major drawbacks of sequential designs is the time taken to perform the overall study; they must be performed sequentially, as the findings from the initial study are needed to inform the second study. However, this drawback is also a benefit; integration occurs when the initial study informs the second study in the form of 'connecting' (when the findings from one study inform the sampling of the other) and 'building' (when the findings from one study inform the data collection approach of the other) (Fetters et al., 2013), explained in Table 15.1.

To demonstrate how a mixed methods sequential design can be adopted effectively within a prehospital research project, a prehospital pain management study in children is described below.

Types of mixed methods research

Prehospital pain management study in children

Prehospital pain management in children is an extremely complex phenomenon; the illness or injury must be considered along with the child's perception of pain (influenced by many factors), the ambulance clinician's ability to assess and manage the pain, the role of the parents and the theory of pain (Whitley et al., 2019). Pain management for children attended by the ambulance service is considered poor (Samuel et al., 2015). Before improvements can be made, the problem must be fully understood. It was unlikely that individual quantitative or qualitative studies would create findings of sufficient depth and breadth to fully understand the problem, therefore a mixed methods approach was adopted.

The study aimed to understand which children were likely to achieve effective pain management (defined as the abolition or reduction of pain ≥2 out of 10) and to explore potential reasons for any disparity. A sequential explanatory design was adopted (Figure 15.1a) and predictors of effective pain management were identified using electronic data from completed clinical records; this formed the initial quantitative study (Whitley et al., 2020a).

A qualitative study was then used to explain the predictors of effective pain management (see Figure 15.2 for the diagram of procedures).

Figure 15.2 shows that the mixed methods study was informed by a systematic mixed studies review (Whitley et al., 2021a); previously identified predictors of effective pain management in children were included in the cross-sectional study and previously-identified barriers and facilitators were explored further during the generic qualitative study. The objectives of the qualitative study were to (a) explain the identified predictors of effective pain management (completing the mixed methods

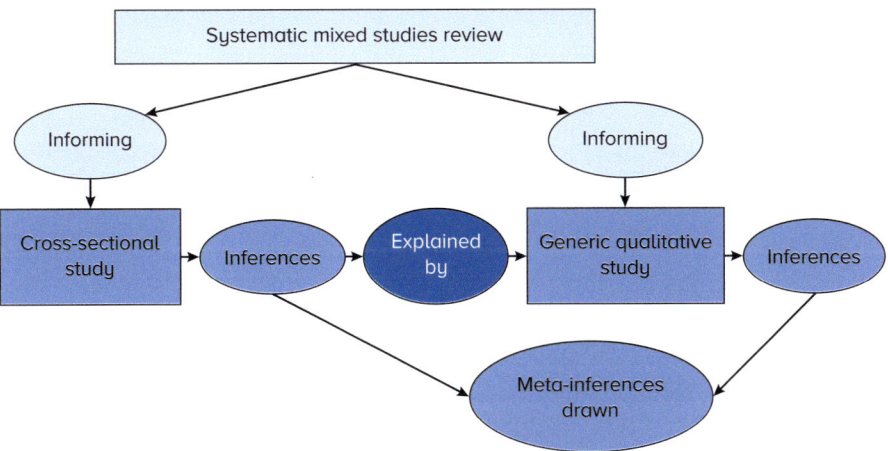

Figure 15.2 Procedures for the Prehospital Pain Management in Children study.
Source: Used with permission from Whitley et al. (2020b).

Chapter 15 — Mixed methods research design

sequential explanatory study), (b) identify barriers and facilitators and (c) explore ways to improve pain management. The qualitative study was therefore used for more than explanatory purposes. Considering participants were already in a face-to-face interview with their mind focused on the specific topic of prehospital child pain management, it was a pragmatic choice to seek more than explanation, but to also explore barriers, facilitators and potential improvements.

One of the key benefits of using a mixed methods approach was that it allowed the study to 'follow a thread' (O'Cathain et al., 2010) to help explain findings that could not be explained comprehensively using qualitative techniques. For example, the quantitative study found that children living in more deprived areas were less likely to achieve effective pain management (Whitley et al., 2020a). When asked at interview, participants gave a broad variety of reasons for this finding, none of which fully explained the difference. The study then 'followed this thread' back to the quantitative data and performed further statistical analyses. It was found that clinicians spent significantly more time on scene when attending children who lived in more affluent areas (Whitley et al., 2021b). This would have allowed more time for analgesics to take effect and more time for children's fear and anxiety levels to reduce. These quantitative insights allowed the strengthening of some of the qualitative explanations, helping to develop a more comprehensive explanation for the disparity (Whitley et al., 2021b). Without the mixed methods approach, this depth of knowledge may not have been gained.

A method of separate publication was chosen for pragmatic reasons and the cross-sectional study was published first (Whitley et al., 2020a), followed by the first 'explanatory' phase of the qualitative study, including the integration (Whitley et al., 2021b).

Convergent design

The convergent design (Figure 15.3) involves the separate and often simultaneous collection and analysis of quantitative and qualitative data (Creswell, 2014) (commonly notated as QUAL + QUAN or QUAN + QUAL). The separate findings are then merged through techniques such as triangulation, which is the 'process of studying a problem using different methods to gain a more complete picture' (O'Cathain et al., 2010) by assessing the level of agreement, complementarity and contradiction between both sets of findings. Triangulation may identify contradictions in the data; this is not a failure of the research but an important part of the process, as discrepancy may lead to a better understanding of the research question (O'Cathain et al., 2010).

Meta-inferences produced from triangulation techniques may be illustrated within a joint display, providing visual structure and facilitating the process of integration (Guetterman et al., 2015). Another method of merging data is through transformation, when qualitative data are transformed into quantitative form, or vice versa (Fetters et al., 2013).

A major benefit of the convergent design is that quantitative and qualitative data can be collected at the same time, reducing the time taken compared to sequential

Types of mixed methods research

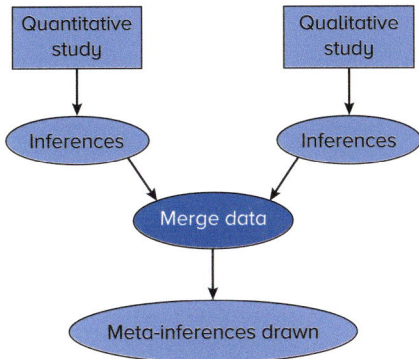

Figure 15.3 Procedures for the mixed methods convergent design.
Source: Used with permission from Whitley et al. (2020b).

designs (Creswell, 2014). However, the process of analysis is arguably more challenging, especially when performing data transformation (Fetters et al., 2013).

To demonstrate how a mixed methods convergent design can be used effectively, a prehospital stroke care study is described below.

Prehospital stroke care study

Stroke is a leading cause of death and disability across the globe (Johnson et al., 2019; Gorelick, 2019). Emergency medical services (EMS) play a vital role in the recognition, management and transportation of stroke patients to hospital (Munro et al., 2018). Prior to 2019, the UK national clinical practice guidelines, set out by the Joint Royal Colleges Liaison Committee (JRCALC), recommended that EMS staff consider recording a prehospital 12-lead electrocardiogram (PHECG) for stroke patients, providing this did not cause significant delay (Joint Royal Colleges Ambulance Liaison Committee, Association of Ambulance Chief Executives, 2013, 2016). This recommendation was based on expert opinion rather than robust evidence. A systematic review (Munro et al., 2018) found no studies undertaken in the prehospital environment investigating the use of 12-lead ECGs in acute stroke patients at the time. To address the gaps highlighted in the systematic review, an overarching research question was articulated: 'What is the use and impact of PHECGs in acute stroke patients?'.

To answer this question, a mixed methods study within a critical realist paradigm (Bhaskar, 1975, 2009, 2014), comprising both quantitative and qualitative studies, was designed. The research questions for these studies are stated below:

- Study 1 research question: *In acute stroke patients presenting to the ambulance service, is PHECG associated with functional outcome (as measured by modified Rankin Scale) and hospital processes of care?*
- Study 2 research question: *What are the views, practice, attitudes towards and perceived value of recording a PHECG in acute stroke patients from the stakeholder groups involved in their care?*

Chapter 15 — Mixed methods research design

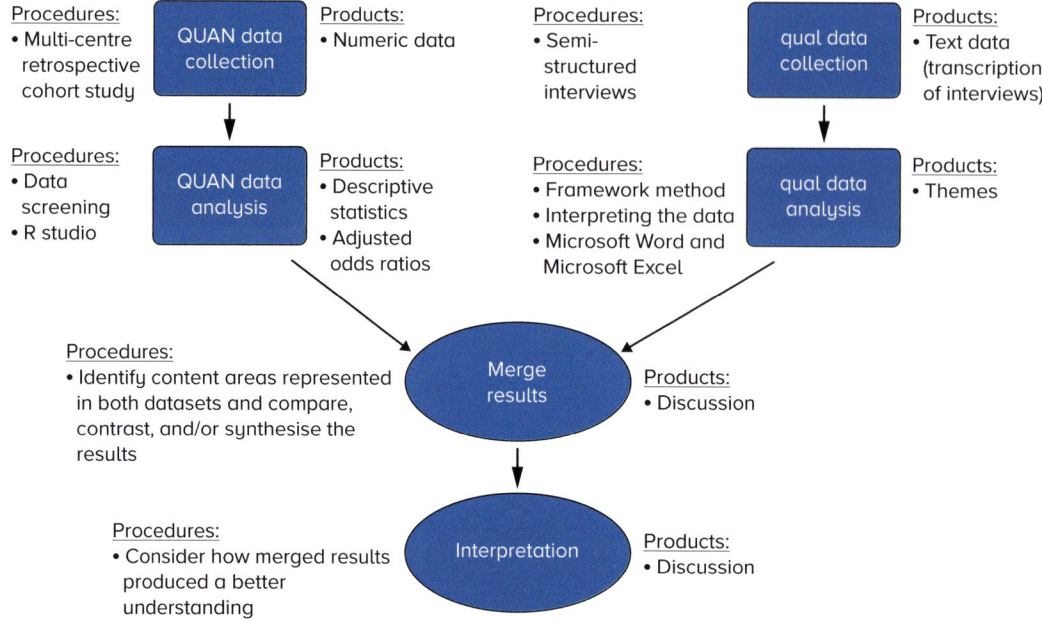

Figure 15.4 Procedures for the prehospital stroke care study.
Source: Used with permission from Whitley et al. (2020b).

The convergent design (Figure 15.3) was used, incorporating a quantitative linked retrospective cohort study (Study 1) and a cross-sectional qualitative interview study (Study 2). See Figure 15.4 for the diagram of procedures.

The justification for using a mixed methods design was to develop a more comprehensive understanding of the use and impact of the PHECG in acute stroke patients, which could not be achieved by adopting one method alone (Bryman, 2006). The phenomenon of recording PHECG for stroke patients was too complex to be fully captured by quantitative enquiry alone, and a qualitative exploration was needed to provide additional detail and understanding.

Study 1 was a multicentre retrospective cohort study, which linked data collected from the participating EMS trusts' patient clinical records (PCRs) with routinely collected data from three hospitals with hyperacute stroke units. Ordinal and logistic regression analyses were used to investigate the association between patients who received a PHECG and functional outcome at discharge from hospital (measured using the modified Rankin Scale), hospital mortality rate, prehospital interval time, rate of thrombolysis and door-to-scan and door-to-needle times.

While the quantitative methods of Study 1 could address 'what', 'who' and 'when' questions (Crabtree and Miller, 1999; Silverman, 2000), they were not able to adequately answer 'how' or 'why' questions which help give a more complete picture of the process of EMS stroke care (Denzin and Lincoln, 2000; Silverman, 2000).

Study 2 was a cross-sectional qualitative interview study, exploring the views, practice, attitudes towards and perceived value of EMS undertaking PHECGs from the stakeholders involved in acute stroke care. The PHECG decision-making process of paramedics was explored using the cognitive continuum theory (Hamm, 1988; Standing, 2008). A purposeful sample of 14 paramedics, two emergency department nurses, three stroke nurses and three stroke physicians were recruited. Data were collected via semi-structured interviews. Themes were generated using the framework analysis method (Ritchie and Lewis, 2003).

Both studies were undertaken concurrently, and the results were merged and integrated during analysis. Common concepts across both quantitative and qualitative sets of findings were identified using triangulation techniques (O'Cathain et al., 2010). Merging both sets of results created a deeper understanding of the use and impact of PHECGs for acute stroke patients in the prehospital setting; this was presented as a narrative discussion. The findings from study 2 helped to contextualise and complement the findings from study 1, providing a deeper, different and augmented understanding of the phenomenon, aiding in the generating of recommendations for future practice and research.

Embedded design

The embedded design is where a smaller qualitative study is conducted within a larger quantitative study, or vice versa. It is often used in clinical trials in the form of a process evaluation. Historically, clinical trials were conducted without regard for patient or clinician experience. The difference in outcome measure between groups was considered the most important aspect of the trial. Yet as we discussed earlier, patient values are a core component of EBP. Not only is understanding patient experience important from an EBP perspective, but it is also important from an implementation perspective. An intervention may be effective in terms of outcome measure but if it is uncomfortable, painful or impractical, for example, and patients are subsequently less likely to use the intervention as intended, then it is less likely to normalise into routine clinical practice.

Interventions to improve patient outcomes are becoming increasingly complex. While clinical trials are the gold standard to evaluate the effectiveness of interventions, understanding the implementation *process* is of equal importance (Oakley et al., 2006). Interviews, focus groups and questionnaires are often used to collect data as part of a clinical trial process evaluation, particularly for complex interventions. Such qualitative data help to understand the implementation process and fundamentally what the barriers and facilitators to implementation are.

An example of a qualitative process evaluation embedded in a clinical trial is the Paramedic Acute Stroke Treatment Assessment (PASTA) study (Price et al., 2019). This study evaluated whether an enhanced care pathway delivered by paramedics increased the number of acute ischaemic stroke patients who received intravenous thrombolysis (Price et al., 2020). The team sought patient experiences and professional (ambulance and hospital) views regarding the acceptability and feasibility of the new pathway in the clinical setting. Interviews were proposed for enrolled patients and interviews or focus groups were proposed for paramedics who did and did not complete the trial training. It was felt important to understand the experiences of paramedics who did not complete the trial training to gain insights into barriers to pathway implementation. Focus groups were also proposed for the hospital staff to gain in-hospital views. The experiences of the paramedics who participated in the study were captured and revealed benefits to the process not captured elsewhere (Lally et al., 2020).

Whether the PASTA pathway is deemed effective or not, the insights gained from the process evaluation were extremely useful to the study team and facilitated normalisation into clinical practice as PASTA was recommended in the 2021 JRCALC stroke update.

Strengths of mixed methods research

Findings from mixed methods studies are considered more than the sum of their parts (Teddlie and Tashakkori, 2009). Integrating statistical analysis with a rich understanding of concepts generated through qualitative methods provides a better understanding of the research problem (Creswell, 2014) than performing two separate studies in isolation. This allows for a deeper understanding of complex clinical problems from well-designed and conducted mixed methods studies than can be achieved with conventional quantitative or qualitative approaches alone. Minimising the inherent limitations of individual quantitative and qualitative studies and harnessing their strengths is a clear benefit of conducting mixed methods research.

Mixed methods research enables researchers to ask exploratory and confirmatory questions at the same time, thus generating and verifying theories within the same study (Teddlie and Tashakkori, 2009) through the process of 'following a thread' (O'Cathain et al., 2010). This unique ability allows questions to be addressed in a rapid iterative fashion. From the personal experiences of the authors, mixed methods research allows more questions to be answered than can be achieved with a single research method. Study designs that rely exclusively on a quantitative or qualitative approach often lead to more questions, which take time to answer as new studies must be set up to answer them.

Limitations of mixed methods research

A limitation of mixed methods research is the increased time taken to complete the overall study, particularly with sequential designs (Hansen et al., 2016). This must be considered early in the development phase because data collection, analysis and interpretation of two or more individual studies take a significant amount of time. This limitation may be offset, to some degree, through the benefit of answering exploratory and confirmatory questions within the same study. Individual researchers may not have the skill set to undertake a mixed methods study and therefore additional researchers may be required to assist with the project (Hansen et al., 2016). Not only will quantitative and qualitative knowledge and skills be required, but an understanding of integration will also be needed.

Due to the recent history of mixed methods research, the quality, validity and reliability of the meta-inferences generated can be difficult to judge (Teddlie and Tashakkori, 2009). It has been argued that design quality and interpretive rigour should be assessed to determine inference quality, as set out by Teddlie and Tashakkori (2009) within their 'integrative framework for inference quality'. The Good Reporting of a Mixed Methods Study (GRAMMS) criteria have also been proposed as a mixed methods reporting guideline (O'Cathain et al., 2008).

Another limitation is the publication process; many journals limit the word count, making it difficult to publish a full mixed methods study within the word limit without losing necessary detail. A pragmatic approach is to either append data as a supplementary file or publish the studies separately, although care must be taken not to lose the depth of integration. O'Cathain et al. (2007) argued that separate publication of studies within a mixed methods approach *may* produce findings that are 'the sum of its parts' rather than 'more than the sum of its parts', potentially negating the inherent strength of performing mixed methods research. An example of utilising the separate publication model was described earlier in the 'Prehospital pain management in children study' section (Whitley et al. 2020a, 2021b). Detailed explanation of the level of integration achieved and comprehensive discussion of the meta-inferences are required if a model of separate publication is to be adopted as the dissemination strategy.

Philosophical and theoretical challenges of mixed methods research

Philosophy is an extremely broad subject that is considered to have three main divisions: metaphysics (nature of existence), epistemology (nature of knowledge) and axiology (nature of value) (Figure 15.5). One of the branches of metaphysics is ontology, the study of 'being and reality'. When someone has a set of beliefs about the study of 'being and reality' (ontology) and the nature of knowledge (epistemology), they are said to have a paradigm.

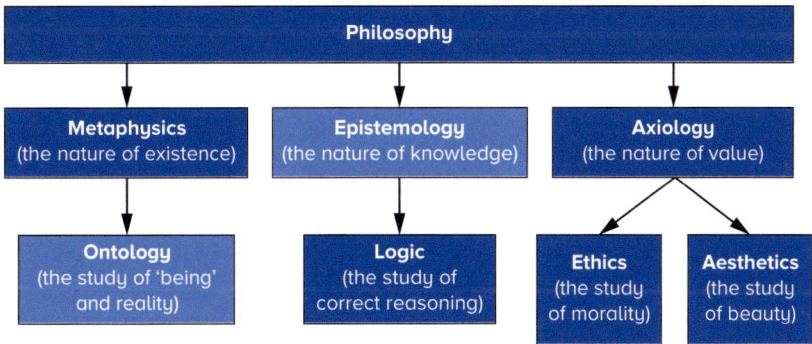

Figure 15.5 Philosophical branches and divisions.

A paradigm, also called a 'worldview' or 'lens', is a way in which researchers view and conduct research. Quantitative and qualitative research studies are conducted with different paradigms; quantitative research is often conducted within a positivist/postpositivist paradigm and qualitative research is often conducted within a constructivist/interpretivist paradigm (Guba and Lincoln, 1994). These paradigms have different beliefs about reality (ontology) and knowledge (epistemology).

Paradigms have been discussed in Chapter 5, so we will not go into any detail here, but it is important to consider the implications of these different paradigms. If quantitative and qualitative research are conducted within different paradigms, how can they be combined without violating their underpinning philosophical assumptions?

Tashakkori and Teddlie (2010) proposed several conceptual stances that aimed to address the contemporary issue described above. One solution was to adopt an a-paradigmatic stance. This argued the irrelevance of paradigms within 'real-world' settings such as applied research. Another solution was the substantive theory stance, which argued again that a paradigm was less important, but a relevant theory should be adopted to support the research. Multiple paradigms could be used within mixed methods research, specifically a paradigm for each type of mixed methods design, for example postpositivism for the sequential explanatory approach or constructivism for the sequential exploratory approach (Creswell et al., 2003). The dialectic stance is one that argues multiple paradigms can be used within a single study type to provide greater understanding of the phenomenon of interest. Finally, a single paradigm stance was proposed, where one paradigm could suit all mixed methodologies, for example pragmatism.

Summary

Mixed methods is a useful design to help researchers understand complex clinical problems in the prehospital setting. Researchers should be aware of the strengths and limitations before embarking on a mixed methods project. We have provided methodological guidance along with examples of how mixed methods research has been used in the prehospital setting. We hope this chapter provides useful information for clinicians and early-career academics who wish to undertake mixed methods research.

Useful resources

- Creswell JW (2014). *A Concise Introduction to Mixed Methods Research*. London: Sage.

- McManamny T et al., (2014). Mixed methods and its application in prehospital research: a systematic review. *Journal of Mixed Methods Research*, 9: 214–231.

- Teddlie C and Tashakkori A (2009). *Foundations of Mixed Methods Research: Integrating Quantitative and Qualitative Approaches in the Social and Behavioral Sciences*. London: Sage.

SECTION 3

Chapter 16

Ethics and governance in research

Georgette Eaton and Helen Pocock

> **Purpose of this chapter**
>
> Completion of this chapter will help you to:
> - understand ethical principles in research
> - describe ethical behaviours in research
> - outline the role of ethics and governance in paramedic research
> - identify what research ethics and governance approval processes apply when doing paramedic research in the UK.

Introduction

What history teaches us here is very clear. Having a code of ethical practice for experimentation on humans, even if ratified by laws is no insurance against atrocity... Their existence is one thing; our adherence to them is quite another.
(Gaw, 2009)

Also known as moral philosophy, ethics is concerned with how individuals (as moral agents) ought to act, and how they can best conduct themselves to achieve a 'good life'. This is the main crux of the problem when considering ethics: one person's idea of a good life may be different from that of another person. Rather than offering a prescriptive outline of how one should live, ethics instead offers a system of principles that enable individuals to make decisions about how they may achieve a good life (Eaton, 2024b).

What is ethical behaviour in research?

Debates about ethical behaviour in research are typically accompanied by well-documented cases of ethical transgressions in research. The problem with such notoriety is the implication that ethical concerns are only prevalent in certain methodologies (such as disguised/covert observation), whereas some methodologies (such as questionnaires) are considered as immune from ethical problems – which no methodology can claim.

Chapter 16 — Ethics and governance in research

Most researchers will justify their behaviour based on one of the following stances.

Anything goes

Under a libertarian view (which seeks to maximise autonomy and freedom of choice), researchers would argue for flexibility in ethical decision making. Anyone in any setting may be studied, provided the work has a scientific purpose, does not harm participants and does not damage the discipline under which the study falls.

Consequentialist ethics versus deontology

Consequentialist ethics judges the consequences of an act to determine whether the act is right or wrong, and deontology considers an act as good (or bad) in and of itself (Eaton, 2024b). The tension between these stances underpins many approaches to research. Generally, deontological behaviours prevail, where transparency is advocated since deceiving research participants is ethically wrong. But consequentialist ethical arguments are often considered in social research. For example, covert ethnography (or lurking) may be thought to harm the reputation of the profession, as well as the authorising institutions, so implicating other researchers and the wider profession. But in some cases, this is the best and only method of investigation if natural behaviours are to be observed. It is perhaps a combination of the two ethical behaviours that would enable a widely morally permissible approach.

Consequentialism: ethical transgression is inescapable

Behavioural approaches here would be concerned that all research elements are ethically questionable. Gans (1962) is perhaps the best-known proponent of this, arguing that 'If the researcher is completely honest with people about his activities, they will try to hide actions and attitudes they consider undesirable, and so will be dishonest. Consequently, the researcher must be dishonest to get honest data'.

Consequentialism: situation ethics

Also considered as 'principled relativism', this argument is represented in two ways:

- *No choice*: this approach suggests that, on occasion, there is no choice but dishonesty to investigate the issues of interest.
- *The end justifies the means*: this approach suggests that, unless there is some breaking of ethical rules, we will never understand certain phenomena (Brotsky and Giles, 2007).

Deontology: universalism

A universalist behavioural stance holds that any infringement of any ethical principles is wrong in a moral sense and damaging to research.

What is the role of ethics in research?

The investment of so much time and energy in ensuring that research is ethical is not due to a belief that researchers will deliberately inflict harm on their participants.

Rather, it is to protect participants from thoughtless or careless acts or omissions by researchers that may cause harm (Beecher, 1966). There are, however, some examples from history that serve as a stark warning of how human rights can be abused in the name of research.

A long-running and infamous example is the Tuskegee syphilis study initiated in 1932 in Alabama, USA. This publicly-funded study invited African American men, a severely socially-disadvantaged group at the time, to receive special treatment for 'bad blood'. Participants were not told that their illness was syphilis and were not given the known treatment, penicillin. Diagnostic spinal taps were conducted and placebo medication administered under the guise of 'treatments'. The real aim of this research was to study the course of untreated syphilis (Brandt, 1978). This study flouted many ethical values: participants did not grant informed consent, they could not leave the study, were denied a beneficial treatment, subjected to unnecessary harms and bore the entire research burden on behalf of wider society.

In response to the Tuskegee study, a national commission was established. Over the course of three years, leading experts in the fields of medicine, ethics, law, religion and industry met and discussed the ethical aspects of human research. The resulting Belmont report, published in 1978, described three fundamental principles that should guide the design and conduct of research (Rice, 2008).

First, that respect for persons should be demonstrated; this assumes that every individual has the right to self-determination. Additionally, those with diminished autonomy should be afforded additional safeguards to protect against exploitation. Second, that beneficence (doing good to others) should be inherent in research; this is ensured by maximising the benefits and minimising the harm to individuals. Third, that justice should be applied, whereby the risks of research are fairly distributed across the population likely to benefit from the research. Researchers cannot, for example, enrol children in a medicine trial where that medicine is only for adults.

These considerations are very similar to the principles of biomedical ethics which underpin modern healthcare: autonomy, beneficence, non-maleficence (do no harm) and justice (Beauchamp and Childress, 2019). Both sets of principles arose from the move from paternalistic healthcare, where doctor knows best, to one of shared decision-making where the power differential is diminished, and doctor and patient are equal partners.

Legislating ethical practice

Ethical standards in research

The development of international standards for ethics in research, in response to ethical transgressions of the past, is one of the most significant moments in the history of clinical research. These standards, outlined below, have all contributed to the UK Policy Framework for Health and Social Care Research, which provides a comprehensible summary of the principles of good clinical practice in the management of health and social care research (Health Research Authority, 2023a).

Chapter 16 — Ethics and governance in research

Nuremberg Code (1947)

Stemming from the Nuremberg trials of Nazi doctors in 1947, this code emerged from the ten principles that formed the Court's judgement to protect future individuals from harm during experimental and non-experimental research (Shuster, 1997). Two main principles that emerged from this trial were the importance of informed consent and the right of participants to withdraw.

Declaration of Helsinki (1964)

Originally outlined in 1964 and revised in 2013 and 2024, the Declaration of Helsinki (World Medical Association, 2024) has become the benchmark for ethical consideration for researchers conducting research involving human subjects. The principles set out by the Declaration were transposed into UK law by the Medicines for Human Use (Clinical Trials) Regulations 2004 amended in 2006 and adopted by the Good Clinical Practice Directive (Commission Directive 2005/28/EC).

International Conference on Harmonisation (ICH) Good Clinical Practice E6(R3)

The first version of the ICH E6 Good Clinical Practice (GCP) Guideline was finalised in 1996, describing the responsibilities and expectations of all participants in the conduct of clinical trials. The Harmonised Guideline was amended in 2016, and again in 2025, to encourage implementation of more efficient and flexible approaches to clinical conduct, design, oversight, recording and reporting, while continuing to ensure human subject protection and reliability of trial results.

Human Tissue Act 2004

This Act regulates activities concerning the removal, storage, use and disposal of human tissue – defined as material that has come from a human body and consists of, or includes, human cells. Consent is the fundamental principle of the legislation and different consent requirements apply when dealing with tissue from the deceased and the living (outlined in the Act as Scheduled Purposes).

Medicines for Human Use (Clinical Trials) (Amendment) (EU Exit) Regulations 2019

Updated from the previous Medicines for Human Use (Clinical Trials) Regulations 2004 to reflect the UK's departure from the European Union, this legislation is the principal piece of legislation that sets the legal standard for clinical trials involving human participants. This legislation has particular emphasis on registration of clinical trials, publication of clinical trials and General Data Protection Regulation (GDPR).

Clinical Trials Regulation

In the EU, the conduct of clinical trials was originally governed by the Clinical Trials Directive (2001), which was updated in January 2022 to the Clinical Trials Regulation (Regulation (EU) No 536/2014). The goal of the Clinical Trials Regulation builds on the original Clinical Trials Directive to create consistent rules for conducting clinical trials to ensure that trials have increased transparency in their construct, conduct and reporting.

Professional guidelines

While the ethical standards listed above focus on clinical trials, this is only one paradigm in the research sphere. Statements of professional principles are provided by a range of professional organisations, regulators and research associations:

- The British Educational Research Association's *Ethical Guidelines for Educational Research: Fourth Edition* (2018)
- The British Psychological Society's *Code of Ethics and Conduct* (2021)
- The British Sociological Association's *Statement of Ethical Practice* (2017)
- The Economic and Social Research Council's *Framework for Research Ethics* (2022)
- The General Medical Council's *Good Practice in Research and Consent to Research* (2013)
- The Medical Research Council's *MRC Ethics Guide: Good Research Practice: Principles and Guidelines* (2014)
- The Medical Research Council's *MRC Ethics Guide: Involving Children in Research: MRC and ESRC Joint Guidance* (2021).

Common themes in ethical standards

Ethics should not be an afterthought. Rather, it should be inherent in the design of a research project. An ethical research project should fulfil the seven requirements in Box 16.1.

> **Box 16.1**
>
> **Seven requirements of ethical research**
>
> 1. Social or scientific value
> 2. Scientific validity
> 3. Fair subject selection
> 4. Favourable risk–benefit ratio
> 5. Independent review
> 6. Informed consent
> 7. Respect for participants.

Source: Emmanuel et al. (2000).

1. Social or scientific value

Researchers must ask themselves if their project has the potential to improve the lot of humanity. If it does not contribute in any way then it lacks social or scientific value and scarce resources (research participants, time energy and funding) should be directed elsewhere.

2. Scientific validity

A state of genuine equipoise must exist, meaning there is currently insufficient good evidence supporting the intervention under investigation. Researchers must demonstrate rigour in their methods and enrol sufficient participants to give the study the power to detect meaningful differences in outcome.

3. Fair subject selection

Study participants should be restricted to those members of society who might benefit from the outcome of the research. For example, it would be unethical to recruit children to a trial where the intervention is only for adults. Additionally, the research burden should be fairly distributed across society. No group should be singled out for recruitment merely for convenience (as was the case in the Tuskegee study).

4. Favourable risk–benefit ratio

Harms should be minimised and benefits maximised. For example, if the study requires a blood sample, it is better to take this at a time when routine blood sampling is happening than subject the patient to venepuncture twice. If risks and benefits to the individual are balanced, then benefits to society may also be taken into consideration.

5. Independent review

This reassures society of the ethical acceptability of a project. Projects cannot be deemed acceptable simply by designing according to a set of 'rules'; ethics is not fixed and absolute. A project's merits should be judged against the moral compass of society. This happens through review provided by a group of individuals not involved in the research so as to exclude bias.

6. Informed consent

There are three elements of informed consent:

- *Information*: individuals must be provided with clear, accurate information about the research and the risks/benefits to themselves. Careful thought must be given to how information is provided. Interviews have revealed that most participants struggle to understand the information they were given, with many being unclear as to whether they might receive a placebo (Corrigan, 2003).
- *Competence*: this is decision-specific; for instance, a 13-year-old may be competent to consent to a study involving food preferences, but perhaps not to a study involving vaccination against a sexually transmitted infection (Slowther et al., 2006).
- *Voluntariness*: the decision to take part should be made freely and without coercion. Researchers should carefully consider the effect of offering payment, or the impact of the relationship between the healthcare professional/researcher and the participant/patient on decision making.

Provision must also be made for situations where an individual does not have the capacity to grant consent. Alternatives include deferred consent, whereby consent is granted after the intervention, and proxy consent, whereby a personal consultee may declare that they consider the person would not object to taking part. Where participants have the capacity to agree to treatment but cannot give informed consent, assent may be sought at the time of treatment and informed consent sought later (Armstrong et al., 2017). Permission for employing such models of consent is considered by specialist ethics committees.

7. Respect for participants

Respect must be demonstrated throughout the research process, from invitation to participate to sharing of study results. The right to privacy is a tenet that is held especially dear in the 21st century. Information and data collected from participants need to be handled correctly and stored safely to protect their confidentiality and right to privacy (Health Research Authority, 2020a). In quantitative research, it is relatively easy to report findings in a way that protects participants' identities, as data are rarely presented on an individual basis. However, this is less easy in qualitative research. Pseudonyms are often used to anonymise people and places, although this can add complexity to follow-up and secondary data analysis, and individuals may still identify themselves. Safeguards concerning confidentiality must be guaranteed as far as possible while honestly and accurately reporting the research, regardless of methodology.

Transparency must be demonstrated throughout, for example at the outset, the possible harms to which the participant may be exposed and, during the study, any new information that comes to light about the condition of interest. Hiding such information, as in the Tuskegee study, has the effect that power is retained by the researcher, leaving participants powerless (Higgs, 2006).

Demonstrating ethical intent: ethical approval processes

Within the UK, there are ethical approval processes that paramedic researchers need to follow to ensure their research will be undertaken ethically, with legislative and professional principles addressed. More detail is given on this process by Renshaw (2019), and a brief overview of the ethical approvals process is outlined below.

Is my study research?

The Health Research Authority (HRA) has created an online decision tool entitled 'Is my study research?' to help prospective researchers decide whether their study meets the definition of research as described by the UK Policy Framework for Health and Social Care Research (Health Research Authority, 2023b). Most often, projects that are not classed as research do not require Health Research Authority or NHS Research Ethics Committee (REC) approval.

Integrated Research Application System (IRAS)

The IRAS is a single-system online platform used to streamline the application process for research approvals within health and social care research (www.myresearchproject.org.uk/). Completing an IRAS application form is one of the steps in applying for both HRA and NHS REC approval (Health Research Authority, 2018a).

Chapter 16 — Ethics and governance in research

Health Research Authority

The HRA approval service provides an expert assessment of research governance and legal compliance for research applications within the NHS in England and Wales (Health Research Authority, 2018b, 2023a). If the project does match the criteria for HRA approval, then applicants will need to contact the Online Booking Service to book an appointment with a REC and submit their IRAS application on the same day (Health Research Authority, 2022a). Research that does not meet the criteria for HRA approval but does involve a research tissue bank or a research database or is taking place in a non-NHS setting may require approval from the NHS REC and/or Confidentiality Advisory Group (CAG) (Health Research Authority, 2020a).

NHS Research Ethics Committee

Research Ethics Committees (RECs) examine research applications to determine whether the research is considered to be ethical, based upon the information provided (Health Research Authority, 2020b). Once paramedics have submitted the IRAS form and have contacted the Online Booking Service, they will attend a REC meeting (Health Research Authority, 2022a). The four possible outcomes are:

- a favourable opinion to proceed
- a favourable opinion to proceed, but with conditions
- a provisional opinion
- an unfavourable opinion which does not give permission.

Applicants who receive a favourable opinion to commence with their research record the HRA and REC approvals within their research.

Confidentiality Advisory Group

For research or non-research (such as evaluation or audit) that requires access to confidential patient information without consent, consideration must be given to whether an application should be submitted to the CAG in England and Wales (Health Research Authority, 2020a). Research applications are required to submit via IRAS, whereas non-research applications use a Section 251 form. There are 11 precedent set categories that describe commonly arising requests, and applications that fall into one of these categories will be processed within that pathway.

Health and medical research exempted from ethics review

In the UK, there are four types of research that are exempt from ethics review by NHS RECs (Health Research Authority, 2020b):

- Previously collected, non-identifiable, tissue samples.
- Healthcare market research conducted by professional market researchers, if it complies with the guidelines of the British Healthcare Business Intelligence Association.

- Research involving NHS staff acting in professional roles. This decision was based on legal advice that any ethics issues that arise (such as those surrounding consent or risks) are already covered by employment law (Health Research Authority, 2020b).
- Audit and service evaluation.

However, it is recognised that research falling into these areas may require approval by the CAG, and a confirmation of exemption should be obtained by researchers if there is uncertainty (Scott et al., 2020).

Capacity and capability assessment

Once the application for HRA approval has been made, local sites (ambulance services) can be formally invited to assess their capacity and capability to deliver the research. Factors such as whether the relevant (patient) population is seen and whether sufficient staff, equipment and processes are in place will affect whether a site can safely and effectively recruit participants to the study. It may take time to arrange these various elements, and so researchers are advised to contact sites early to avoid delays.

Nationally, researchers often approach ambulance services assuming HRA approval is sufficient, unaware of the need to work with ambulance service research departments, which can add stress to already time-sensitive projects.

Ensuring ethical practice

Research governance

Research governance is the system of oversight that ensures that the interests and rights of all involved are protected (Shaw et al., 2005). Its scope is broader than merely safeguarding the participants and researchers undertaking the research. Good governance should result in high-quality projects that meet legal, as well as ethical, standards and hit recruitment targets within a prespecified time-frame and budget. For any given project, there is no single body responsible for such oversight. For some research studies the sponsor assumes this role, but generally a number of different stakeholders have specific responsibilities with respect to approving and monitoring research projects.

Capability and capacity assessment

This is the formal assessment of a site's potential to take part in the research. The practicalities of setting up and delivering the project need to be assessed at an early stage in order that sites may identify potential barriers and arrange appropriate systems and processes to facilitate the research. The types of things that need to be considered include the number of qualified staff available to deliver the research, any additional training requirements, plans for delivery, storage and distribution of interventional products, types of data required, methods of data storage and transfer, and whether new ways of working between departments need to be put in place.

Monitoring and audit

When studies are underway, formal monitoring should be conducted to protect the well-being of participants and ensure that the research is being run in accordance with protocol and GCP standards. Studies may be audited against these and other relevant standards to ensure that their written instructions and staff's enactment of these are fit for purpose (NETSCC, 2021a). The frequency and method of monitoring are determined by the study risk assessment. Each element of the study may present a different degree of risk; the more high-risk elements might be frequently monitored or monitored by visiting the site, whereas low-risk activities might be only monitored annually or at a distance (Love et al., 2020).

Pharmacovigilance/safety reporting

In any clinical trial, it is possible that things may go wrong. Perhaps a patient has an unexpected reaction to a medicine or the study equipment fails during use. It is important to have a safety reporting mechanism in place for the detection and assessment of such 'adverse events' in order that further occurrences are prevented. The overarching term describing such mechanisms relating specifically to medicines in clinical trials of investigational medicinal products (CTIMPs) is pharmacovigilance (NETSCC, 2021b). There are differences in the way that CTIMPs and non-CTIMPs are managed. For example, reports are made to the REC for non-CTIMPs and the MHRA for CTIMPs.

Both sponsor and site teams have responsibilities regarding recording and reporting of safety information and adverse events. Assessments must be made of relatedness (to activities listed in the study protocol); expectedness (not listed as an expected effect in the study protocol); and seriousness (determining the urgency of protocol amendments if required). Where urgent safety measures need to be introduced to safeguard study participants, the sponsor must act immediately (Health Research Authority, 2022b).

Summary

Ethical tensions are ubiquitous within research. Fulfilment of ethical standards in research is wider than completion of approval processes or governance, and is underpinned by professional guidelines and legislation. When designing projects, researchers should consider the ethical behaviours underpinning their research approach, rather than merely selecting methods for convenience.

Useful resources

- Armstrong S et al. (2019). Ethical considerations in prehospital ambulance based research: qualitative interview study of expert informants. *BMC Medical Ethics*, 20: 88.
- Charlton K, Franklin J, McNaughton R (2019). Phenomenological study exploring ethics in prehospital research from the paramedic's perspective: experiences from the PARAMEDIC2 trial in a UK ambulance service. *Emergency Medicine Journal*, 36: 535–540.

Chapter 17

Involving service users in research

Sarah Black and Karl Charlton

> **Purpose of this chapter**
>
> Completion of this chapter will help you to:
> - define what is meant by patient and public involvement and engagement (PPIE) in research
> - identify best practice for PPIE activity
> - describe the benefits to research activity of PPIE, for both researcher and PPIE contributors
> - recognise common challenges and highlight methods to overcome them.

Introduction

There are several ways to describe the methods used by researchers to interact with the public around research, and while they are often used interchangeably, they are subtly different. One of the most important tasks for researchers is to be explicit about 'Why' you want to engage with service users, and 'Who' you wish to engage with. Is it to collaborate to inform and shape the design of your research project (usually termed 'involvement')? Perhaps you are aiming to inform members of the public about your findings and consult with them on how these findings can be put into practice (often described as 'engagement'). While this chapter will focus specifically on PPIE in the design of research, it will also describe some practical tips on public engagement and participation in research.

It is a core democratic principle that people affected by research have a right to a say in what and how publicly funded research is undertaken (INVOLVE, 2021). In order to deliver this, the NHS encourages all research conducted within its framework to involve service users through PPIE. PPIE in this context is defined as research carried out 'with' and 'by' members of the public rather than 'to', 'about' or 'for' them (INVOLVE, 2021). PPIE is very different from participation in research and means patients and the public act as collaborators on what the researcher intends to do and how they intend to do it. Patients and the public are directly involved in all stages of the research, from formulating the research question, through to dissemination of findings to aid translation to clinical practice, and this is discussed in more detail subsequently.

This is very much in the spirit of democratic, patient-centred healthcare (Bombak and Hanson, 2017), where research reflects the priorities and wishes of the public. It is expected that all health and social care research conducted in the UK will involve some element of PPIE, and many funding bodies, such as the National Institute for Health and Care Research (NIHR), consider PPIE to be an essential element to secure funding (NIHR, 2021a).

However, the level of PPIE described here is the gold standard and may be beyond what is possible, or indeed necessary, for small research projects. There may be different expectations for smaller scale research projects, where PPIE activities could be limited to piloting processes to determine feasibility, checking understanding of methods, survey questions or aims with end users to confirm their acceptability, or identify barriers or potential problems. Regardless of the scale of the research to be undertaken, some element of PPIE should be carried out.

Prehospital and emergency care research

Patient and public involvement and engagement is essential and applicable to research methodologies within most clinical settings, but has particular relevance to emergency care research, which can be additionally challenging.

Many emergency care studies involve patient groups who cannot provide informed consent at the point of enrolment, either because of their condition or because of the time-critical nature of the situation. This type of research not only requires research ethics approval but may also require permission from the Confidentiality Advisory Group (CAG) if patient data are going to be used without consent (see Chapter 16). Fundamental to securing CAG approval is the demonstration of robust PPIE and that the researchers have explored enrolling patients and using patient data without prior consent. PPIE can help ensure that research is ethical, practical and justified (Hirst et al., 2016).

Large prehospital trials such as PARAMEDIC2 (Perkins et al., 2018) engaged in extensive PPIE to ensure what they planned to do was acceptable to patients, their families and the wider public. However, PPIE is not only relevant to large, well-known studies, but also to more modest research projects where paramedics are the lead investigators. The responsibility lies with the researcher to demonstrate that PPIE has been undertaken and describe how this has influenced and shaped the design and methods of a study.

It should be recognised that researchers at different stages of their career might adopt different approaches to PPIE. While meaningful public involvement is both a policy imperative and a prerequisite for large-scale grant funding, approaches should be tailored to the level of study. For example, students on an undergraduate pathway might not be able to support the time and cost associated with PPIE compared with multidisciplinary research teams, so a proportionate view should be taken.

What should PPIE look like?

It is important to involve members of the public with disease-specific expertise wherever possible. This could include patients themselves, as well as their family, carers, charitable organisations and support groups. Involvement of specific groups depends on the condition or population being studied; some conditions have well-established PPIE groups (e.g. stroke) whereas other conditions such as cardiac arrests may not have such well-established groups but there are still ways to do good PPIE with relevant people (Coppola et al., 2022).

It is best practice that any patients or members of the public collaborating in a piece of research are representative of the patient group of interest. Patients are often experts in their own disease and its management, and they can provide insights into all aspects of a research idea or question, identifying potential barriers to success that the literature, a clinician or researcher may overlook. Some studies may not have an obvious PPIE population, such as studies of organisational processes, but the study may still benefit from input from advisory groups of relevant stakeholders not directly involved in the study.

Patient and public involvement and engagement should try to be diverse enough to represent wider society, allowing a broad range of perspectives to be considered. Researchers should consider, for example, including people of different ages, cultures and ethnicities when developing PPIE strategies (INVOLVE, 2012). It may be necessary to undertake groundwork to seek out relevant patient groups, particularly when these groups derive from seldom heard communities.

Examples of under-represented groups in research include patients with dementia, children and those with rare medical conditions. However, there are organisations where researchers can access PPIE for populations like these, such as the Alzheimer's Society and the Young Persons Advisory Group (YPAG). These groups, often in the independent, voluntary 'third sector', exist at regional as well as national level and projects can, and should, try to include a diverse group of service users wherever possible, although the challenges to achieving this are acknowledged.

Benefits of PPIE to research activity

Patient and public involvement and engagement can help researchers develop meaningful and appropriate studies, and as such PPIE contributors should be involved in all stages of the research, as detailed below.

The research question

Patient and public involvement and engagement is essential in helping to develop a research question that is important and relevant to patients and the public. You may have an area of interest which you think is under-researched and needs more

Chapter 17 — Involving service users in research

evidence, but this may not be reflective of or address questions that matter to patients, their relatives and carers. PPIE can help you focus on research questions that should be answered. This helps secure funding for a study, even when the project is small and funding is limited, as a project with a question of interest to patients and/or their carers is more likely to be successful, in terms of both securing funding and study delivery.

Study design and methods

Patient and public involvement and engagement is useful when deciding on the research methods to be employed. Acting as experts, PPIE contributors can help identify what will and will not work with the target population, how successful recruitment may be, what problems may be encountered and what outcomes should be set. This is of particular importance when a study requires ethical approval, as the committee (which includes lay representatives) is unlikely to provide a favourable opinion for a study involving processes or activities unacceptable to patients or the public. Collaborating on the development of participant information and consent forms can also be a key activity where PPIE contributors can add value.

Reduction in research waste

As most healthcare research is publicly funded, patients and the public have a vested interest in making sure that it delivers value for money in addition to clinical and research utility. Reducing research waste includes ensuring transparency over protocols, methods and results, and reporting all findings, including negative ones. It is also important to ensure that duplication is reduced because previous work in the area was either not reviewed or was of a poor design and conduct.

Dissemination

Patient and public involvement and engagement collaborators can assist with summarising results in a way which is accessible to a wide audience, advise about routes for dissemination of findings and help with engagement with local and national patient groups. Ensuring that the findings from research reach those who influence policy makers as well as the academic and scientific communities is another area where PPIE contributors can have impact. This is important, even in smaller pieces of research, where the researcher may want to use findings to widen the debate about a certain area of clinical practice or as the basis for further research or funding applications.

Translating findings into clinical practice

As potential users of research findings, PPIE members of the research team can be beneficial when considering how to translate research into clinical practice. PPIE collaborators may represent stakeholders or be in a position of influence with decision makers, particularly when the PPIE derives from charitable organisations. Involving PPIE collaborators in the implementation phase of research may increase the likelihood that the results are applied, increasing the impact of the findings.

Benefits of involvement for PPIE collaborators

Crocker et al. (2017) explored the views of patients and the public on their involvement in health services research. Their participants suggested a variety of perceived roles they brought to studies they had been involved with, from the expert with lived experience, able to consider the acceptability of research proposals, to being able to challenge freely and think creatively to propose solutions.

Reynolds and Beresford (2020) highlighted wider benefits to PPIE contributors, outside the research context. While participants are often approached because of their experience of a specific health condition, their narratives and motivation for taking part impacted upon other areas of their life. This intersection between the research setting, family and professional life and wider social agendas can lead to greater advocacy and renegotiation of their own perception of the value they bring as collaborators on a study.

Mathie et al. (2018) highlighted that there is often a gap in researchers giving feedback to PPIE contributors on the impact of their involvement. This can range from more passive 'acknowledgement' to specific feedback about impact, which may motivate further involvement activity and increase confidence. From the outset, it is important to understand the type of feedback that your PPIE contributors would like and ensure that the research team makes allowances both in time and costs to enable this to be meaningful.

Evaluating the impact of PPIE contributions is an expectation of larger-scale research grant funding applications, where applicants need to be explicit about the expected impact of PPIE on the proposed study. There are multiple methods for evaluating this, dependent upon the complexity of the PPIE activities. The NIHR website provides helpful guides for both researchers and patient and public members of the study team (Public Involvement Impact Assessment Framework, 2021).

Challenges to delivering PPIE

Public involvement is intrinsically felt to be of value, but meaningful PPIE may cause harm to participants and barriers exist to facilitating involvement. PPIE can benefit both researcher and participant alike – the researcher gains insightful collaboration in the design of their research while the participant has an opportunity to influence policy and practice in an autonomous way.

However, disclosing personal accounts of living with a condition or disease may be emotional or distressing, particularly when the condition or disease is burdensome or leaves participants with life challenges. Ensuring support for PPIE participants is a key responsibility of the researchers, which may be facilitated in a number of ways. Dependent upon the topic area, it may be important to signpost PPIE contributors to support services to ensure their well-being. It is appropriate at the outset to reduce the opportunity for misunderstanding by explaining common acronyms – a glossary of terms is very useful here, and PPIE members of the team can be actively engaged with this process.

By collaborating in research, PPIE participants may incur direct and indirect costs; understanding a research proposal may require the participant to undertake time-consuming familiarisation or learning activities and attending PPIE events may involve travel or parking expenses. Acknowledgement and recognition of the time and perspective of PPIE contributors are essential, and best practice states that remuneration and recognition of their contribution are essential. The NIHR produces payment guidelines for members of the public who are considering becoming involved in research (NIHR, 2023a), and researchers should familiarise themselves with these expectations. While not all PPIE collaborators will wish to be paid, it is incumbent upon researchers to highlight that if they are in receipt of welfare benefits, they may need to declare their voluntary contribution. Payment for time, skills and expertise can have implications for the tax, pension and benefits status of PPIE contributors, and this should be explored and explained.

Scientific and ethical conflicts may arise when researchers and PPIE differ (Public Involvement Impact Assessment Framework, 2021) and it can be problematic balancing the interests of the research with the perceptions and opinions of the PPIE contributors. Setting ground rules for open and honest conversations and ensuring all contributions are valued are central to meaningful debate within the research team. Researchers should anticipate and be prepared to be challenged, and flexibility in response and expectations will usually resolve such issues.

There is an assumption that small numbers of individuals may represent perspectives of diverse patient groups and members of the public. While this may be the case, researchers of all levels engaging in PPIE need to ensure that patients and public involved in research collaborations are inclusive, diverse and representative. While the policy context encourages inclusivity in PPIE activity, in practice the reality may be different. It is widely recognised that achieving diversity can be challenging, even for research teams who have access to resources to support this activity. Just as participants in clinical trials may not be representative of those most in need, so PPIE contributors may represent people who have the time and resources to participate, rather than the population of interest. In practice, PPIE may more often involve a 'hand-picked' narrow group of individuals (Coulter and Ellins, 2007; Peat et al., 2010) and consequently those with the most to gain are unfortunately the most excluded, restricting potential and limiting the opportunity to break this cycle.

Ocloo and Matthews (2016) describe PPIE as a continuum of engagement, describing barriers and facilitators to involvement, with an inverse power relationship between lay participants and paid researchers or healthcare professionals as a central challenge to true collaboration. Addressing these imbalances can include changes such as having PPIE contributors chairing meetings, although it is also recognised that these bureaucratic norms may discourage involvement from individuals who feel less comfortable with the business meeting format (Cowden and Singh, 2007).

Public and patient involvement and engagement organisations

Arguably the most well-known organisations in the UK designed to promote PPIE in health and social care research are INVOLVE and the James Lind Alliance. INVOLVE is a national advisory group funded by the NIHR, which aims to support active patient and public involvement in the NHS, public health and social care research (INVOLVE, 2021). The James Lind Alliance is a priority-setting partnership (PSP) that exists to determine unanswered questions or uncertainties that members agree are the most important. By doing this, PSPs aim to shape future research by prioritising evidence uncertainties in areas of health and social care that may be answered by research (NIHR, 2021b). They bring together patients, carers and clinicians on an equal footing, to help determine the research questions that are of most importance.

The PSPs are separated by clinical disciplines and a top 10 for each is provided. This is an example of where patients have a rare but vital say in what research is conducted and funded. Recent examples of James Lind PSPs include stroke in 2021 (James Lind Alliance, 2021) and trauma in 2023 (James Lind Alliance, 2023), both of which make direct reference to prehospital care.

Training for PPIE contributors

There is debate about the need for PPIE contributors to receive research training (healthtalk.org). Some consider that the concept of PPIE contributors as 'experts by experience' means they should not require training, which may 'professionalise' the lay perspective, making it too similar to that of researchers (Ives et al., 2012). Research teams who have evaluated the delivery of bespoke training to PPIE contributors highlight the benefits of increased confidence in participating in the research process, and autonomy at managing their own conditions by the application of research findings (Gibson et al., 2015; Miah et al., 2020). In a qualitative study, Dudley et al. (2015) explored the pros and cons of PPIE contributors' accounts of training, suggesting that training for researchers is more important than for PPIE members.

As identified above, there is debate around whether training may 'professionalise' the input from PPIE collaborators, potentially limiting their ability to provide an 'authentic patient voice'. However, NIHR standards suggest that training could be informal as well as formal, with mentorship and support in addition to feedback from lay contributors being helpful to identify areas where knowledge and confidence can be strengthened. PPIE contributors should not be expected to be expert methodologists (although some might be!), and a variety of resources are available to guide this activity such as Learning for Involvement (see useful resources).

The NIHR produces online training resources and, although many of these are aimed at the research community, some give a broad overview of what PPIE contributors can expect from involvement in health research. Several online resources specifically aimed at PPIE contributors are also available from INVOLVE, although it is recognised that these may not be accessible by lay members of a research team who experience digital exclusion due to inequalities in their IT access. Researchers should be prepared to consider other more creative and inclusive methods of making this training available when needed.

Chapter 17 — Involving service users in research

Summary

This chapter has explained the benefits of PPIE and how meaningful PPIE can enrich research projects. Whether researchers want to involve or engage with patients and the public, PPIE is feasible in all clinical research settings, regardless of the size or scope of the project. PPIE can take various forms and the approach taken can be tailored to reflect the study requirements, size and resources. Some level of PPIE should always be undertaken, and incorporating the public perspective adds value and leads to better quality research.

This chapter has highlighted some of the benefits of PPIE, as well as some of the challenges faced by researchers. Patients and the public bring with them expertise and insights that can be of benefit to researchers of all disciplines. We leave you with top tips for involving service users in research (Box 17.1).

> **Box 17.1**
>
> **Top tips for involving service users in research**
>
> - Consider who you want to be involved with your research, and why.
> - Determine if the proposed project has been identified as a research priority by conducting a review of PSPs (James Lind Alliance).
> - Contact your regional research support service (RSS) consumer panel.
> - Identify local community and charity organisations with relevance to the disease or population of interest. These may be of particular significance when the disease is rare or the population is a rarely heard community.
> - Produce a lay summary of the project idea explaining why the research is needed and what will happen to participants. This should be an easy-to-read summary and should not include jargon or clinical terms.
> - Contact your local Patient Advice Liaison Service (PALS) as they may be able to provide critical review of a research idea.
> - Ensure that any groups involved in PPIE are representative and diverse, accommodating all sexes, ethnicities, backgrounds and cultures and perspectives. In this way you can be sure the opinions you obtain reflect the wider opinion.
> - Be adaptable and responsive to different methods of communication, and consider reversing traditional 'power' balances, especially important if involving vulnerable groups.

Useful resources

- James Lind Alliance: https://www.jla.nihr.ac.uk/
- National Institute for Health Research (NIHR). Learning for involvement: www.learningforinvolvement.org.uk/

Chapter 18

Health economics: its role in health research

Jamie Miles and Peter McMeekin

> **Purpose of this chapter**
>
> Completion of this chapter will help you to:
> - develop a broad understanding of health economics
> - recognise why healthcare economics is important to prehospital care
> - understand the different types of economic evaluation
> - identify different methods of economic modelling
> - discuss how to measure uncertainty within a model.

Introduction

There are many definitions of economics, perhaps as many as there are economists. At some level, they all agree that economics is about scarcity. Everyone has limited resources and must decide how to allocate the resources at their disposal. An economist evaluates individual or societal choices to identify the best decisions. Economic evaluation is an established part of health services research, and proposals can fail if they have not considered the economic impact. This is because healthcare funding decisions are normally informed by how effectively resources are being used.

This chapter describes what an economic evaluation is, how it might be conducted and the challenges it can present in a prehospital setting.

Why is health economics important?

When we consider a new drug, intervention or service, we often view the benefit from the patient perspective, which is important. However, there are other perspectives to consider. For an intervention, new drug or any other change to be successful in the real world, it needs to be economically viable, and this is not a straightforward decision based on costs alone. It must be evaluated in the context of all the costs, benefits and losses. This could be the magnitude of patient benefit at the time versus cost of the intervention, or even the quality of life gained in later years versus the cost

Chapter 18 — Health economics: its role in health research

now. There are trade-offs in economics. A commissioner might have to evaluate a new service by looking at the whole system and the necessity to drop another service in order to fund the new one.

Think like an economist

The tools and techniques used by economists are designed to inform better decisions. They are often described in terms of four basic principles:

- The first is about the cost of anything and how it is measured. To an economist, the cost of something is what you give up for having that thing – its opportunity cost. For example, the opportunity cost of replacing a car may be a holiday forgone.

- The next principle is that incurred costs cannot be recovered regardless of future actions. Attempting to recover incurred costs, whether they be financial, time invested or effort, leads to poor decision making and inefficient use of resources.

- The third principle is the margin. Economic informed decision making is informed by the marginal, or extra, costs and benefits resulting from a choice. Where benefits and costs of alternatives are measured in the same units across choices, economists are not concerned with the absolute costs and benefits, only the differences between alternatives.

- The final economic principle is that people and organisations respond to incentives, particularly to ones that maximise their own benefit. The resulting behaviours might not be those intended by those providing the incentives. An often-quoted example of this is the Ukrainian pole-vaulter Sergey Bubka who raised the world record 35 times from 5.83 to 6.14 metres in 1 cm increments. Bubka's contract contained a clause that paid a bonus of $100,000 for breaking world records.

Economics in healthcare

Health economists face a specific set of issues when they are researching and evaluating decisions. Perhaps the most significant are how to measure the effects of alternative uses of heathcare resources, and how to value them. Compounding the issue of measurement is the level of uncertainty about the link between health and care.

This uncertainty, alongside other issues like the role of physicians and barriers to entry to potential providers of healthcare, was described in a seminal paper by Kenneth Arrow – 'Uncertainty and the welfare economics of medical care'. This paper, published in 1963, is often described as heralding the beginning of health economics as a subdiscipline. Arrow's (1963) paper made it clear that the market for 'healthcare' was unlike many others, where price transparency allowed economists to study their functioning. Instead, health economists would have to develop tools to allow them to investigate how producers and consumers of healthcare interact.

Internationally, healthcare systems differ considerably. To health economists, healthcare systems are often defined in terms of the way they are funded – the 'public/private mix'. Systems like those in the UK that are largely publicly funded differ from those with provision that is more private. The set-up of the healthcare system influences the perspective that health economists take on the choices faced by the system. Where individuals pay most of their own care costs, either indirectly or through insurances, economists are more typically concerned with efficiency and less concerned with value and affordability. Some of the concepts in this chapter are introduced in the context of the UK NHS-type model of healthcare provision, but they are still generally applicable, or generalisable, to other contexts.

It is important to note that in the majority of situations, health economic analysis is just one input into the decision-making process. Cost efficiency is not the only criterion that defines whether a particular healthcare innovation is funded.

The perfect market and the ambulance service

If we briefly step outside healthcare and into the world of economics, we find ourselves in a hypothetical marketplace full of buyers and sellers with assumptions that, if true, will create a perfect market.

A perfect market is important as the sellers can keep producing and survive, and buyers can get what they want, when they want it. It also minimises wastage within the system and is efficient. The first assumption is that there are lots of sellers with no single one having dominance over the others. There also has to be perfect knowledge for both the buyers and sellers. Everyone needs to know what's available, and at what price. There needs to be certainty in the market to allow buyers to plan ahead. There needs to be no externalities which are indirect consequences, good or bad, caused by consumption and production of products within the market. All the buyers and sellers need to be rational. All products within the market should be homogenous; so all the products are either identical or directly comparable. The final assumption is free entry and exit into and out of the market.

However, when we step back into healthcare, buyers become patients and sellers are healthcare providers. Irrespective of whether healthcare is free at the point of use or insurance provided, it becomes apparent that these assumptions do not hold true. If we take the UK model of ambulance services as an example, there is a complete lack of sellers. Each ambulance service provides all the care within a certain geography. If you had an emergency, the ambulance service is provided and not chosen.

No one has perfect knowledge. Ambulance services use intelligence to predict where and when the demand will be, and patients do not know the response time to them or the level of care they will get. This creates uncertainty for both the ambulance service and the patient.

There are lots of externalities involved in prehospital care. One example of an externality was seen during the COVID-19 pandemic when public behaviour during the initial lockdown caused a national decrease in ambulance calls (NHS England, 2023). Patients are not always rational in prehospital care, and the modern case-mix of ambulance patients is heavily tilted towards urgent care, despite only being advertised for emergencies. Ambulance services can also behave irrationally, with the vehicle type, number of responders and expertise of response not always matching what is required.

This irrationality can relate to the concept of moral hazard. Because healthcare is free in the UK, patients might not be as conscious of healthy living as they do not have to pay for care if they suffer the consequences. Furthermore, due to the lack of up-front costs, patients might be more willing to access healthcare. This is known as consumer moral hazard. Moral hazard exists in the provision of care as well. There is no direct cost to an ambulance dispatcher in sending an ambulance, or a paramedic in giving a drug, so they may make decisions that overutilise resources instead of minimising the cost. This is known as provider moral hazard.

To reduce moral hazard, the NHS uses primary care as a gateway to secondary care services, screening patients before they access them. Waiting lists are also a way to deter patients from overutilising healthcare. However, in prehospital and urgent care, there are few hurdles to reduce overutilisation, and this often means excess demand.

In summary, prehospital care is not a perfect market. It falters on all the assumptions, and this is not unique to ambulance services, as healthcare in general does not conform to these assumptions. This imperfection raises a requirement for checks and balances that can help both buyers (patients) and sellers (healthcare providers) make more efficient decisions. These are informed by specific health-related economic evaluations and, depending on the type of decision and perspective, will depend on the method of evaluation.

The perspective

Every economic analysis comes from a specific perspective, which needs to be decided prior to analysis. It provides the context of the evaluation and informs the methods to be used (Byford and Raftery, 1998). For example, an economic evaluation of healthcare insurance schemes is often undertaken from the perspective of the patient, as it informs their decision making. Xie et al. (2021) in Canada used the perspective of the public payer to evaluate their intervention of mobile integrated healthcare to provide a specialist on-site urgent care response.

In the UK, the perspective of economic evaluations is mainly that of healthcare commissioners. This means that comparison tables of different, often competing, interventions are produced, all within NHS services. Dixon et al. (2009) took the perspective of the NHS and social services when evaluating whether paramedic practitioners were a cost-effective intervention for elderly prehospital care. There is an argument, however, for a societal perspective which places the intervention under investigation in the context of all services in society and not just healthcare.

The comparator

It is important in all economic evaluations to have a comparator. This may be the counterfactual position or 'do nothing', and just describes what happens already. It may evaluate a series of interventions, comparing them all with each other and producing a league table. The choice of comparator should reflect all available options, otherwise it will decrease the validity of the analysis and lead to further issues in decision making.

Types of economic evaluation

Each of the techniques described in this section (cost-effectiveness analysis, cost-utility analysis and cost-benefit analysis) is about the evaluation of healthcare, and designed to quantify the costs and outcomes of healthcare programmes and present their results as ratios, specifically as a cost per unit of output (healthcare, health and expenditure). Each evaluation technique has its advantages, and the choice between them is often determined by who will use the results to inform their decisions.

The factor differentiating the techniques is the output (ratio denominator) used. The numerator or ratio used in each analysis is the costs, and these are always defined as the marginal costs of the healthcare being evaluated less any marginal savings that accrue because of that healthcare. For example, Hubble et al. (2008) investigated the cost-effectiveness of prehospital continuous positive airway pressure (CPAP) in the management of acute pulmonary oedema. They reported that when compared to standard care, CPAP saves an additional 0.75 lives per 1000 patients at an additional cost of $490.

Despite the numerator in economic evaluations being cost, it is not all about saving money, but rather about creating an efficient system. There are two types of economic efficiency. Technical efficiency is concerned with doing things right. It ensures that only the resources required are used, minimising wastage. An example would be stocking ambulances with the right equipment, in the right quantity. Allocative efficiency is about doing the right things. This is making sure everything in the system is of benefit and needed by the user. An example would be funding an alternative care pathway to take patients with ST-elevation myocardial infarction (STEMI) direct to a hospital that can perform primary percutaneous coronary intervention (pPCI) instead of the nearest emergency department (ED). Some techniques identified below such as cost-effectiveness and cost-minimisation analysis only concern technical efficiency, whereas cost-utility and cost-benefit also address allocative efficiency.

Cost-effectiveness analysis

Cost-effectiveness analyses are the most common form of health economics analyses. They are concerned with technical efficiency, or the effectiveness with which inputs are used to produce outputs. The most technically efficient healthcare treatment is the one that produces the most outcomes with a given set of inputs, or a specified set of outputs with the minimum inputs. Cost-effectiveness analyses measure healthcare, rather than health. Examples of outcome measures could be cost per non-conveyance, cost per specialist paramedic, cost per drug.

The comparators in a cost-effectiveness analysis are used to generate a summary statistic called an incremental cost-effectiveness ratio (ICER). This summarises the difference in cost and benefit. The equation for an ICER looks like this:

$$ICER = \frac{C1-C0}{E1-E0}$$

where $C1$ is the total intervention costs, $C0$ is the total control costs, $E1$ is the total intervention benefit and $E0$ is the total control benefit

As an illustrative example, imagine a new drug was being proposed that all paramedics could use to treat pain without having to put a cannula in the patient and which would be successful first time, every time. All the costs of the new drug would be added together to total the intervention costs of, say, £40 per patient ($C1$ = £40). The patients receiving the new drug report an average reduction in pain of 6 out of 10 ($E1$ = 0.6). Now we take all the costs of providing intravenous (IV) analgesia (cannulation kit, IV drugs, extra skillset of staff, extra costs for failure to cannulate) which cost £60 per patient ($C0$ = £60). IV analgesia might have a reduction in pain of 5 out of 10 ($E0$ = 0.5). The ICER in this example would be (40 − 60) / (0.6 − 0.5) = (−20) / (0.1) = −200. This means there is a cost saving of £200 for every one unit decrease in pain score using the new intervention per patient.

Another example comes from Snooks and colleagues, who undertook an economic evaluation of paramedic assessment of older adults who had fallen (Snooks et al., 2017). Their analysis took place alongside a randomised controlled trial and found that, for an additional cost ($23), subsequent calls to the ambulance service were reduced in the six months following the index fall. They observed no reduction in future care costs.

Pilbery et al. (2022) also undertook a cost-effectiveness analysis into what impact specialist paramedics had on appropriate non-conveyance. They found that there was a saving of £615 per appropriate non-conveyance for the intervention group compared to the control, and a cost-effectiveness ratio of £1759 per percentage increase in appropriate non-conveyance.

Cost-utility analysis

Cost-effectiveness analyses estimate value for money. As such, they have a limited role in informing the decisions providers of healthcare face, between alternate uses of limited resources where the outcomes are different, for example, between a programme of assessment to reduce recurrent falling and the use of CPAP to manage acute pulmonary oedema. To make valid comparisons, decision makers need a common unit of outcome instead of healthcare – that unit of outcome is health.

Measuring health

There are a range of methods that can be used to measure health. The numerous methods are a consequence of the many ways in which health is viewed, for

Types of economic evaluation

example in terms of freedom from illness or the benefits it brings to enjoy life. This subsection describes one approach that is typically used in the UK. It reflects the way in which healthcare is funded in the UK and is known as the quality-adjusted life year (QALY).

The QALY is a composite measure of the length and quality of life. It assumes that the effects of any healthcare on health can be measured in terms of its effect on mortality and morbidity. A one QALY gain represents one additional year lived in full health, half a QALY represents either an additional six months lived at full health, or an additional year lived in half of full health, or any combination in between. As a hypothetical example, imagine a trauma patient who did not call for help. Figure 18.1 shows what would happen to their quality and quantity of life. In contrast, imagine that they called for help and received an ambulance. The ambulance has prevented a further decrease in morbidity and lengthened the time to eventual mortality. Notice how the person never fully recovers to perfect health and the graph accounts for this. However, a significant amount of QALYs are gained in the intervention. Mortality effects are straightforward to estimate (x-axis). The challenge is how to estimate health states as a proportion of full health (y-axis).

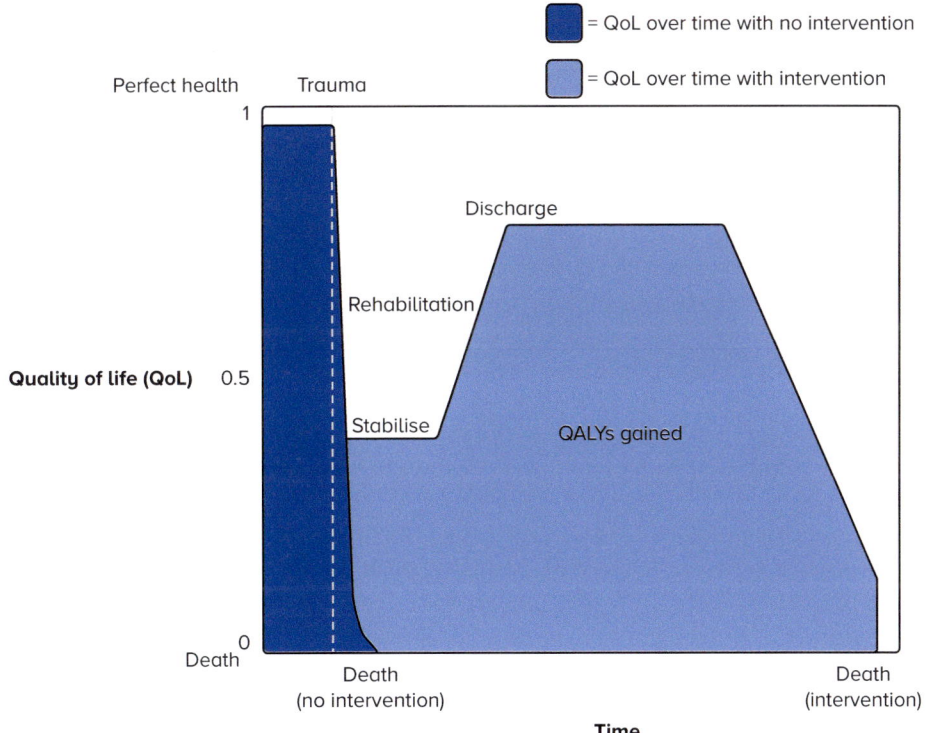

Figure 18.1 QALY gain example.

Early measures of morbidity simply asked people to rate their current health-related quality of life on a scale between zero and one. While this subjective measure of morbidity had advantages (primarily people were free to use their own

Chapter 18 — Health economics: its role in health research

interpretation of health), its value to decision makers was limited. Therefore, a measure of health-related quality of life was developed in terms of five domains: mobility, self-care, usual activities, pain and discomfort, anxiety and depression. Any health state can be described in terms of levels of these attributes. This instrument is known as EQ-5D and is available in many languages and versions for adults and children (Rabin and Charro, 2001). The EQ-5D has a value set that consists of population-specific preference weights. These are used to assign utility values to different health states defined by the EQ-5D. You can explore this further at www.euroqol.org. Each possible state described by EQ-5D corresponds to a value between death (zero) and full health (one).

Achana and colleagues analysed the use of adrenaline for out-of-hospital cardiac arrest and found that each additional QALY in the adrenaline arm of their trial cost £1.7 million (Achana et al., 2020). Different organisations will have a cost-effectiveness threshold for each additional QALY. For example, the National Institute for Health and Care Excellence (NICE) sets a QALY threshold of between £20,000 and £30,000 for consideration of implementation in the NHS (NICE, 2013). Dixon et al. (2009) undertook a cost-effectiveness analysis into whether paramedic practitioners improved the care of elderly people (measured in QALYs). They found that there was a cost difference between usual care (£77 per patient) and paramedic practitioners (£73 per patient) but the benefit was negligible. Paramedic practitioners equated to 0.0003 fewer QALYs. However, because of the difference in cost, the intervention fell within the NICE threshold of £20,000 per QALY.

Cost-benefit analysis

In a cost-benefit analysis, everything is turned into a monetary value. This is straightforward for the costs of an intervention, but there is more subjectivity in valuing benefit.

There are numerous ways of placing monetary value on a benefit that is under investigation. Some are crude yardsticks such as the Human Capital Approach (HCA) which uses a person's wages to estimate the benefits of an intervention. If intervention A extends a person's life by 10 years, the benefit can be calculated by multiplying a person's wages by 10. This method is not robust to gender, age or social deprivation and is often inappropriate to use in healthcare. More commonly, a method known as stated preferences is used, which tests people's willingness to pay for an intervention by asking questions such as 'Would you prefer to pay for an air ambulance or three road ambulances?' or 'How much would you be willing to pay to have a specialist critical care ambulance in your area?'. Because it transforms benefits into monetary values, it obtains a sense of appetite from the consumer, allowing this method to address allocative efficiency.

Snooks et al. (1996) undertook a cost-benefit analysis of the Helicopter Emergency Medical Services (HEMS) in England. They found that compared to road ambulances, there were marginal health benefits that were only actualised in specific scenarios. However, the costs were significantly higher than the road ambulances.

Modelling in economic evaluation

The type of economic evaluation stipulates which denominator is used to measure efficiency. The methods involved in economic evaluation describe how to undertake an economic evaluation. This section will describe from start to finish how economic modelling is undertaken.

Premodelling assumptions

In economic modelling, it is important to determine certain conditions that act as the 'settings' for an economic model. Once the perspective is decided, the type of analysis can be chosen. The type of evaluation may be dictated by what data are available or feasible to collect. Large clinical trials often have an economic section and this tends to be a cost-effectiveness analysis. The limitation in choosing a cost-effectiveness analysis is that it only allows for direct comparison with other similar interventions, whereas a cost-utility analysis can have broader comparators. This ties in with the perspective required.

Time

Time is an important factor. In economic modelling, there is a time horizon to consider, which is the length of time spent in measuring the costs and benefits in the evaluation. In cancer studies, for example, the horizon might go all the way to eventual mortality. There can be a lag between upfront costs of an intervention and when the benefits are eventually realised, such as childhood vaccination programmes or smoking cessation. To account for this lag, economic models must discount future years using a discount rate. This in effect penalises interventions with a long time to benefit, as there is a strong preference to have the benefits now as opposed to later. The industry standard is to apply a uniform discount rate to each year up to the time horizon. In the UK, NICE recommends a discount rate of 3.5% applied to costs and benefits (NICE, 2013).

In prehospital care, the time horizon is often short due to the length of time spent with patients. Modern research extends the horizon to inpatient outcomes, but this is still short compared to public health interventions. The Rapid Analgesia for Prehospital hip Disruption (RAPID) study by Jones et al. (2019) examined the benefit of paramedics performing a fascia iliac compartment block (FICB) in the case of patients with fractured neck of femur. They used inpatient bed days as one of the outcome measures. Due to the short time horizon, there is little value for discount rates, which can be beneficial. Conversely, shorter time horizons create a challenge for generating accurate QALYs in a cost-utility analysis. This can make prehospital interventions inappropriate for comparison with wider health interventions.

Modelling methods

Undertaking an economic model is a specialist skill, and it would always be advisable to consult with a health economist before commencing such a task. There are numerous ways of creating and analysing the model once you have all the costs, benefits and premodelling assumptions.

Chapter 18 — Health economics: its role in health research

Decision trees

The simplest form of economic model is a decision tree. This is a flow diagram which maps out the costs and benefits of an intervention along with the probabilities at each split. It consists of decision nodes, chance nodes and terminal nodes. As an example, Figure 18.2 shows a decision tree for the cost of treating epileptic patients in the ambulance service. The costs (Curtis, 2013; NHS Improvement, 2018), benefits and probabilities (Dickson et al., 2016, 2017a, 2017b) have been taken from the literature.

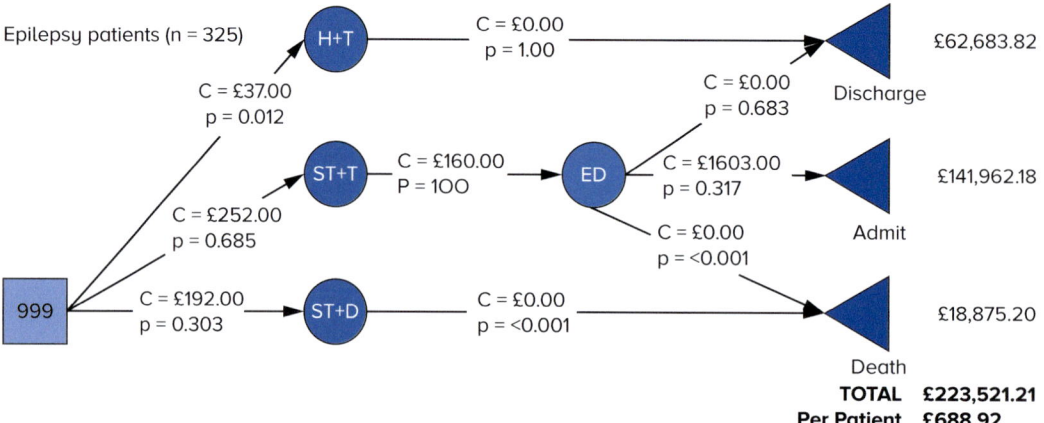

Key: H+T: Hear and Treat, ST+T: See, Treat and Transport ST+D: See, Treat and Discharge, ED: Emergency Department

Figure 18.2   Decision tree model for epilepsy patients in the ambulance service.

The limitation with decision trees is they do not always reflect true practice. Patients cannot enter at different points, or re-enter once they have reached a terminal node. It is viewing the whole situation as if it was embedded in a block of ice.

Markov models

Markov models are similar to decision trees, except they account for patients moving between health states. They can also be modelled to indicate how a population moves through each state over time. Probabilities are no longer just linear but also loop for staying in the same state and moving back into a previously entered state.

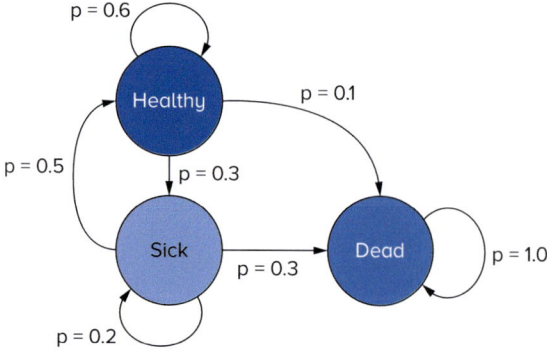

Figure 18.3   Markov model example.

Modelling in economic evaluation

Figure 18.3 is a high-level Markov model example with three states. Markov models are more complicated in their design as it can be a challenge to identify probabilities of moving through states. However, they are useful in ambulance service modelling even outside the economic context, as demonstrated by Li et al. (2021) who used a Markov model to determine ambulance destinations when the service was experiencing offload delay.

Discrete event simulation (DES)

One of the limitations of both the decision tree and the Markov model is that they map a cohort of patients into the model. All patients entering the model have the identical probability of each state transition. However, this is not what happens in the real world. Both time and probability differ per patient on random events that often cannot be controlled. It would be more realistic to create a simulation as close to real life as possible, where individuals are followed through the system. This is what a DES does.

Figure 18.4 is a simplified example of a patient journey from calling for help, through to handover at ED. The input is an entity generator, which in this example creates a patient every time someone calls 999. These are then held in a queue until they can move into the next part of the simulator. The circles (S1, S2 and S3) are known as 'servers'. These hold the patient for a certain amount of time before releasing them to the next step. Once the patient is transported to ED, they are held in another queue to hand over. The simulation ends once they are handed over. There are numerous parts in the simulation that would not make sense to have as fixed values (such as in a decision tree or Markov model). The rate of 999 calls and the server times all take different amounts of time per patient. The on-scene time changes with every patient, for example. To account for this, a DES uses a method of random sampling known as a Monte Carlo simulation. This creates a probability distribution via random sampling over each variable, and patients going through will have a different length of time on scene depending on the distribution.

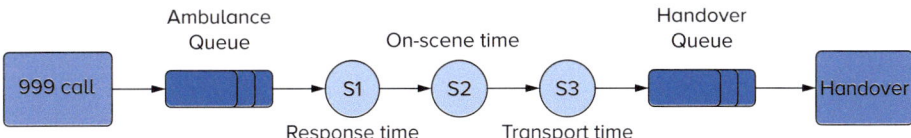

Figure 18.4 Discrete event simulation.

This type of modelling particularly suits the prehospital environment, as most of the functions can be divided into discrete events. Wei Lam et al. (2013) published a DES modelling different strategies to reduce ambulance response times. They were able to make inferences that are more useful because of the level of detail a DES provides. They could conclude that adding 10 ambulances and staggering shift times gave the greatest improvement. However, more ambulances also resulted in a decrease in utilisation.

The base-case and the sensitivity analysis

Modelling uncertainty is important in health economics because a model will not be useful if the margin for cost-effectiveness is slim. The concept of how to model

Chapter 18 — Health economics: its role in health research

uncertainty is quite simple. Create a base-case which is the default model and is the one that was optimised through modelling. Then perform a sensitivity analysis, where variables are tweaked and the model re-evaluated. This can be done one variable at a time (univariate analysis) or the values taken to the extreme (extreme-case analysis). The most useful sensitivity analysis is the stochastic analysis. Like the Monte Carlo method above, this creates a distribution of probabilities for the point estimates in the base-case. This can then be used to represent cost-effectiveness graphically at different values.

Reporting a health economic study

Like many disciplines, a range of standards have been developed to ensure the consistency and quality of health economics analyses. These standards are a key resource for individuals and groups planning economic evaluations. For example, the Consolidated Health Economic Evaluation Reporting Standards (CHEERS) statement provides reporting guidance (Husereau et al., 2013). In the UK, NICE has published a reference case that 'details methods for assembling and synthesising evidence on the technology being appraised in order to estimate its clinical and cost effectiveness' to ensure that decision-makers can interpret the results and understand the applicability to their own context (NICE, 2013).

Summary

Health economics is an important part of the research process and accounting for all the costs, benefits and losses of an intervention is valuable information for stakeholders. The research question, and available data, will steer the type of analysis to be undertaken. It is preferable to create models that can account for the uncertainty and randomness that occur in the real world. Reporting health economic models using recognised guidelines will help with interpretation and comparison with other models.

Chapter 19
Sharing research findings

James Yates and Pete Gregory

Purpose of this chapter

Completion of this chapter will help you to:
- understand why it is important to share research findings
- identify the best ways to share research findings
- recognise and create the messages to be shared
- identify the optimum time within which findings should be shared

Introduction

Research is of no use unless it gets to the people who need to use it.
(Professor Chris Whitty)

Part 1 of this chapter covers six fundamental issues to consider when sharing your research:

- Why are you engaging in dissemination?
- Who is the target of your dissemination?
- What are the messages to be disseminated?
- How will you disseminate your findings?
- When should dissemination occur?
- Evaluating whether the strategy met its aims.

Part 2 of this chapter provides a detailed look at various media that can be used to share research:

- Platforms for dissemination
- Academic journals

Chapter 19 — Sharing research findings

- Conference presentations
- Posters and poster presentation
- Social media
- Podcasts.

Part 1: Fundamentals of dissemination

Sharing research findings through a carefully considered and targeted dissemination strategy is a vital component of any research project. While your work may result in important findings and conclusions, unless these reach people who can act upon them, the project will fail to make any impact. An effective dissemination strategy should ensure that your research reaches the right people, in the right format, to enable it to be used to its greatest effect.

Good dissemination used to mean publication in a high-impact journal, but this approach limited the audience to a small group of academics and clinicians, disregarding large cohorts of people that might benefit from the work. Now researchers can, and arguably should, be more innovative in their approach. Social media and open access websites have become increasingly popular with podcasts, blog posts and the #FOAMed (free open access medical education) movement representing some of the newer methods for dissemination. Platforms for engagement and knowledge-sharing continue to evolve and, to generate the maximum impact, researchers must remain conversant with the most effective means to communicate with their chosen audiences. While many options exist, none should be viewed in isolation but rather as components of a complete and varied strategy. Used appropriately, the researcher can reach a large and diverse audience, allowing individuals to access, understand and act upon their work.

Creating a dissemination strategy can easily be overlooked when designing a research proposal, but it is essential to consider this early. Ideally, the strategy will be composed during development of the study protocol. Publishing findings only once the research is complete misses a world of opportunity to engage with audiences as the project progresses. Planning a robust and varied dissemination strategy may also form an integral component of an application for funding, without which it may fail. The time constraints and costs involved in dissemination also need to be considered.

Despite the evolution in options for dissemination, there remain six fundamental questions which need to be considered in the formulation of a robust strategy. Though each question is presented in isolation, they are fundamentally linked to each other, with each topic influencing others.

1. Why are you engaging in dissemination?

When establishing a dissemination strategy, it is essential to consider what you want to achieve from sharing your work. Do you want to reach a wider, non-academic audience? Do you want to generate discussion or stimulate more research on a topic? Or maybe you want to influence clinical practice. Whatever the purpose, having clearly defined aims is a vital first step, as it will influence many subsequent decisions. Key measures of success and how they will be appraised also need to be identified to enable evaluation to be undertaken. This is discussed further in the evaluation section.

2. Who is the target of your dissemination?

Your target audience will be heavily influenced by the aims identified in step 1. Appreciating who the audiences are represents a critical step in the success of the strategy, as this will guide how to reach them and what is communicated to them. Consider who needs to hear about your work to meet the aims of the dissemination strategy.

Who will be influenced by your work or who will find your work valuable? There may only be one audience, such as 'paramedics working for the NHS', but often there are multiple audiences who can be categorised into primary and secondary groups. Primary audiences are those who can directly act upon your work, whereas secondary audiences can influence the actions and decisions of the primary audience. Engaging both primary and secondary audiences is a powerful way to maximise the impact of your work. It is important to consider each group separately, however, as they will have different needs, abilities to understand research and levels of engagement with the various platforms for dissemination. It is also worth considering that audiences are not uniform and there may be diversity within each group.

3. What are the messages to be disseminated?

Key messages need to be identified within your work which are clear, succinct and relatable. These messages must be targeted to each of your audiences, ensuring they are both relevant and appropriate in terms of the language and terminology used. Consider the needs and abilities of the audience with regard to accessing and understanding research. A useful approach is to consider what the audience wants to hear from you and not what you want to tell them. Depending on the type of research undertaken, it may be appropriate to make recommendations on how the findings could be used, for example following a systematic review. Alternatively, a researcher engaged in primary research should focus on making the research available and accessible, allowing the wider healthcare community to decide how to assimilate the findings into current knowledge and practice.

4. How will you disseminate your findings?

Decisions about the right platforms for dissemination and the style you adopt will be highly influenced by the identified objectives, the audiences and the time and resources available. Careful consideration of which platforms to use is essential, because no matter how beautifully created and well thought out your strategy, if the target audience does not engage with the platform chosen, then it will be useless. Determine where your audience looks for information and then ensure that the style of presentation is appropriate to that platform.

You may have identified more than one audience, each requiring a different approach. Consider your colleagues; some will be active on social media, others will

Chapter 19 — Sharing research findings

enjoy attending conferences while others will subscribe to journals. A multifaceted approach is often very effective and avoids over-reliance on one form of media. Publication in a peer-reviewed journal remains essential for validation of research processes and findings, but articles can be augmented with other forms of non-traditional dissemination to amplify the reach and impact of your work.

Publishing a manuscript often puts research behind a paywall, limiting the audience to subscribers of the journal, students and academics with institutional access or those willing to pay to read your work. Some journals offer open-access publication for a limited period, or indefinitely, while others exclusively publish open access articles. Open-access publication, which is becoming more common and often a requirement of the funder, generally involves a higher cost to the author, although organisations or professional societies may subsidise these costs. Huang et al. (2024) suggest that open-access articles are viewed more often and receive more diverse citations, although there needs to be further examination of these metrics over time.

Non-traditional methods of dissemination are almost limitless and, to some degree, are only restricted by the resources, imagination and creativity of the authors. However, as an example of the breadth of options available and how these can be assimilated to create a powerful dissemination strategy, AIRWAYS-2 (2024) serves as an excellent case study. This trial will be discussed throughout the remainder of this section to highlight good dissemination practice.

AIRWAYS-2 was published in August 2018 (Benger et al., 2018), but in the preceding three years there was significant activity from the research team, demonstrating the power of a staged approach, discussed in the next section. During this time, an official AIRWAYS-2 account and hashtag was created on Twitter (now 'X') which was used to share updates on issues such as the training of trial paramedics, recruitment targets and dissemination events. While the account had a modest number of followers, the power of Twitter/X and social media in general is that the audience can act as an amplifier for your messages, sharing and tagging in their feeds, while also feeling engaged by the research team and therefore more interested in the results.

Podcasts have seen significant growth recently as they offer a flexible, accessible and often free means of accessing research and wider medical education. If the target audience for the dissemination strategy is matched to the right podcast, with listeners of a similar demographic, then researchers can increase the reach of their work significantly while also allowing explanation of their work and therefore increasing its accessibility. The AIRWAYS-2 team integrated podcasts into their strategy, pre-recording interviews with The Resus Room and FOAMfrat (an online learning platform) podcasts which were released simultaneously with the journal article.

Conferences have provided a means to share research for many years, either through formal presentation or via submission of abstracts to poster competitions. Preparation for these events can be time-consuming and with their reach often being limited to the delegates present (even if it is an online conference), it is worth considering the impact these events can have. The potential to engage with your audience and network with colleagues should not be overlooked. Some conferences may offer the benefit of being recorded, with the content subsequently available online, while others may offer publication of the abstracts accepted. Accepting the limited exposure available from a conference, the AIRWAYS-2 team presented at multiple conferences and submitted a variety of different abstracts to others. It is important to be aware of the convention that the same abstract should not be submitted more than once.

If your work is of interest to the public, or may affect them, then attracting the interest of the media with press releases should be part of your strategy. The AIRWAYS-2 team used two strategically-timed press releases – at the start of the recruitment phase, describing the trial and its aims, and then simultaneously with the journal article, describing the findings in lay terms. There are many templates available online to assist with creating a press release, but major stakeholders such as funders should always be consulted to determine how they want to be acknowledged and whether there are any key messages they want highlighted. There are risks with engaging with the wider media as results can be misinterpreted or misrepresented and maintaining control of the 'story' may be challenging.

Another option for knowledge-sharing is infographics. These are visual representations of the research process and the findings, produced with attractive designs and clear, concise messaging. Many large research projects in recent times, including AIRWAYS-2, have produced infographics, which are easily shared through social media, websites or printed press. Videos can also be created which open up further platforms for dissemination, such as YouTube.

5. When should dissemination occur?

Dissemination should not necessarily be left until the research is complete and all the findings are available. The AIRWAYS-2 trial serves as an excellent example of how a staged approach can be utilised, releasing information consistently throughout the project. This can help to raise awareness of a project early on, provide feedback and updates on progress throughout the research process and then highlight achievements and findings once the project is complete. A staged approach also opens up the potential for bidirectional conversations between the audience and the researchers, depending on the platforms used. This can be a powerful way to create engagement with your work.

A formal method of staged release, and an example of transparent research practice, is publishing your research protocol (Perkins et al., 2016; Price et al., 2019; Mitra et al., 2021). This allows the audience to appreciate the underpinning methodology while anticipating the release of the results. As with any strategy, a staged approach needs to be well considered and carefully structured. This structure can be derived from identifying key points of your work that will trigger the next release alongside looking for windows of opportunity such as conferences.

6. Evaluate whether the strategy met its aims

The aim of creating a dissemination strategy is to ensure that your work reaches the right audience, in the right format, at the right time for maximum impact. As with all aspects of practice, reflection on performance is essential to identify strengths and learning points for the future. Therefore, evaluating your dissemination efforts is essential to determine whether your strategy has been successful. Reflect back on the aims from step 1 and the key measures of success you identified. Have these aims been met?

Success can be measured both quantitatively and qualitatively, depending on the nature of the aims and outcomes. Quantitative measures of success include parameters such as the number of citations a paper receives, the number of likes and interactions a message gets on social media, and the number of unique visitors to the project's website or views of video media. Qualitative measures often take the form of feedback from target audiences, such as interviews, focus groups or questionnaires.

Summary of Part 1

In conclusion, planning how to disseminate your work is a vital component of your project regardless of its size or complexity. Early consideration of dissemination will allow a staged approach to information release and ensure maximum impact. Identifying key aims for your dissemination strategy is the first step from which the rest of the structure will cascade, as well as allowing for evaluation of the strategy subsequently. Determining your audiences and the messages you want to convey to them will play a significant role in choosing how you communicate those messages. The options available for dissemination are diverse, and integrating multiple platforms in a carefully considered approach can increase the reach and accessibility of your work.

Part 2: Platforms for Dissemination

The range of options available to researchers can be overwhelming. While various platforms have been discussed in the preceding section, understanding how to get the most out of each is a skill. This section aims to provide tips and tricks to maximise the impact of your work.

Academic journals

For many who work in academia, writing for an academic journal is part of the job and it remains an important method of dissemination for research. Unfortunately, getting articles published holds many challenges and can be time-consuming and frustrating. The following tips will not guarantee publication, but they should help:

- Decide early which journals are likely to reach your target audience and have the impact you are seeking. Planning early is essential – if a journal requires you to use a specific reporting statement, for example those from the EQUATOR network, it may be too late to accommodate this once you have completed your study.
- High impact factor journals may look good on your CV, but does your target audience read those journals?
- Investigate the editorial policies – what are they interested in and does your work meet their priorities? If not, look elsewhere.

- Download the author guidelines and follow them to the letter.
- Read articles from the targeted journal to formulate your paper – mirror the successfully submitted articles.
- Write clearly, succinctly and at a level appropriate to the anticipated readership.
- Ensure that your referencing meets the journal's requirements.
- Ensure any collaborators have seen and agree with the work being submitted – make sure all named authors meet the ICJME guidelines for authorship (ICJME, 2024).
- Ask a critical friend to peer-review your work before you submit.
- Allow time to upload your submission – the process often takes longer than expected.
- Be prepared for rejection and the notorious 'reviewer two' comments.
- Act on feedback from reviewers and show how you have addressed any requested changes. If you do not agree with suggested changes, respond with a clear explanation of why.
- Have back-up plans in case your chosen journal rejects your submission.
- If you need to move to plan B, make sure that you amend your article to meet their requirements. This can take time, but could make the difference between acceptance and rejection. Rejection from multiple journals does not mean that you should give in, it just means that you may need to change your approach. Your project may be considered too small for the high-impact journals, or it may not meet their commercial aspirations; if that's the case, look to a different journal.

Oral presentations

Creating a presentation for a conference is about engaging the audience and keeping them interested. The last thing you want to see is people checking their mobile phones or leaving the room (unless they are posting about your presentation, of course!). Many presentations are via a PowerPoint slide set and so considering the content and format of these slides is essential.

Work by Blome et al. (2017) provides insight on how to give a medical research presentation at a scientific conference and we present some of those key points here (Box 19.1).

Box 19.1

Key points in presentations

Know your audience and adapt your slides and presentation. What do they already know about your topic, what are their expectations and interests? How do you best communicate your message to the attendees?

Slides

- Keep slides simple – include the key points and talk around them. Don't overload slides with words and/or diagrams.
- Consider the key messages you want to get across and create a logical flow.
- Slides should augment the story you are telling. The story shouldn't be led by the slides.
- A well-designed graphic can be more effective than a word-heavy slide.
- Consider the size of text and graphics – it is frustrating when the presenter says 'I know you won't be able to read everything that's on this slide …'.
- Check whether the event organisers have specific requirements for formatting.
- Consider the font – it needs to be readable and convey the right tone.
- Use animations cautiously! They can be useful to emphasise a point but used overenthusiastically, they can be distracting and annoying.
- Keep your presentation clear and to the point. Remember you want to keep the audience engaged, not lose them in the fine detail.
- End with a summary slide to review what you have discussed.

Preparation for delivery

- Practise your presentation so you are comfortable with the sequence and know what you are going to say. Try not to read from the slides or a manuscript, as this suggests that you don't know your subject well enough and is likely to disengage the audience.
- Practise to ensure that your timings fit within the limits given to you by the event organisers. Always leave yourself with a few minutes spare to reduce the pressure on you during the day and to answer questions.
- Ensure you know your topic thoroughly. This will increase your confidence, and it will avoid any awkward moments in the Q&A at the end.
- In addition, to increase the impact of your presentation you may want to:
  - upload your slides to a repository and add a DOI to your presentation
  - schedule posts before and during the presentation that use the conference hashtag to publicise your talk or poster
  - add information about your contribution to email out-of-office messages.

Presentation style

- Make eye contact with delegates. This shows that you are speaking to them and they matter.
- Vary your tone of voice to avoid a monotonous delivery.

- Don't speak too fast; allow the audience to keep up and appreciate each of your key points.
- Be enthusiastic; this will help create an interesting and engaging presentation style. Tell your story, don't just deliver a lecture.

Posters and poster presentations

A poster offers an opportunity to present your research findings succinctly at a conference. They require you to condense your aims, methods, results and discussion into a single poster that should allow delegates to understand your work without you being there. Sometimes, posters are presented, and you will have a short time (3–5 minutes) to highlight your work to an audience. Even without formal presentation, submitting a poster to a conference is a great opportunity to meet colleagues, spread the word about your work and gain valuable feedback. Creating a striking and informative poster can be difficult but, following some key pointers, it is eminently achievable.

Poster preparation

- If you have not prepared a poster before, ask for support from somebody who has. They may have a template that would fit your requirements or provide examples of their work. Look online for poster presentations to get a feel for what works.
- Consider your audience and your key messages.
- Ensure that you know the formatting requirements and adhere to them – for example, the orientation of the poster or the expected dimensions.
- PowerPoint allows you to create the poster on one slide by adjusting the size of the slide under 'Page setup'.
- A poster should contain all the elements you would expect from a scientific paper, but condensed.
- Posters need to be eye-catching and laid out in a clear fashion with enough detail to allow the reader to understand the subject.
- Lay out the poster so that the reader intuitively flows through the poster's content.
- Aspects of formatting are listed below.
    - The poster should be clean, clear and uncluttered.
    - In contrast to conference presentations, the poster should have a light background and dark font.
    - Make the font as large as possible.
    - Leave some clear space to help declutter the poster.
    - Appropriate use of graphics/graphs can replace many words.
    - Research shows that delegates scan the title, introduction and conclusions, so ensure that these sections are well considered in their content and formatting.

Chapter 19 — Sharing research findings

- Be available! Stand by your poster throughout the break periods to interact with delegates and discuss your work.
- Be welcoming. Stand to the side of your poster and maintain an open body language.
- Smile and introduce yourself to delegates and invite them to read your work and ask any questions they may have.
- Have a short and clear 'elevator pitch' which covers what your research topic was, what you found and why this is important.

Social media

Social media platforms have become an increasingly important means of disseminating research both within and beyond academic circles. In January 2024, Statista (2024) reported that Facebook had 3.049 billion users, Twitter/X 619 million users and Instagram 2 billion users. As such, social media can allow rapid and easy sharing of information to a much wider audience than traditional methods of communication. It transcends traditional and national barriers and opens a whole new channel for research dissemination.

Maximising the benefits of any social media platform requires work and takes time. For example, creating your network of followers requires effort and may take a while to establish. However, with the right preparation and when used correctly, social media can significantly enhance your research profile and promote the work you are doing. Interested parties will comment and share your messages so that their network can see your work and this process can continue creating an exponential spread of your work.

It is important, however, not to see social media in isolation. Peer-reviewed papers are still the cornerstone of accepted, reliable research dissemination, but consider how you can combine social media with publication. For example, social media can generate interest in the build-up to publication and then raise awareness and generate discussion when publication is live. Additionally, using social media at your conference or poster presentation can take the messages beyond the confines of the event.

Tips for using social media

- Split your personal and professional profiles on social media but remember that your personal social media may still be linked back to your professional profile.
- Use social media to engage with users, answer questions and generate discussion.
- Social media requires regular input. Posting and forgetting will not generate the same level of engagement as regular updates and conversations.
- Consider preparing and scheduling social media posts, using a platform such as Hootsuite so that there is a considered, sequential release of information.

- Time social media posts so that they coincide with the highest-traffic times.
- Consider current trending topics to see whether you can piggyback onto a hashtag.
- Create various messages with different angles, interpretations and language to engage different users.
- On a long post, only the top section is seen, so make the introductory sentence short and interesting to draw readers in.
- Use website links to encourage readers to click through and read your work in more depth.
- Pictures can be very useful to quickly and clearly describe findings, or indeed summarise an entire paper. Infographics are quickly becoming a must-have for disseminating research output.
- Don't take on too much. Consider your platforms and your audience. Social media requires work so choose a handful of platforms and commit to them.

Podcasts

Podcasts are an increasingly popular source of FOAMed, allowing people to consume educational content in their own time and at their convenience. Many podcasts exist, and choosing the right one will require insight into the number of listeners, their demographic and the reach of the podcast. Podcasts have many benefits, but primarily offer you the opportunity to discuss your work, allowing listeners to understand and navigate some of the complexities that otherwise may be a barrier to them. Podcasts also allow for discussion of how the findings of your work may be translated into practice, bridging the gap between research and evidence-based medicine.

Tips for using podcasts

- Choose the podcast or podcasts you want to talk on with due consideration to your topic and the audience of the podcast.
- Consider the key messages you want to get across during the episode.
- Creating a template for the episode can help with the flow and prevent repetition, but avoid scripting the content as this can result in a stilted and unnatural conversation.
- Remain professional but also be yourself. Listeners want to hear your personality come through during the episode. A monotonous, dry delivery of a topic will have listeners switching off!
- Avoid moving around, tapping and fidgeting during the recording, particularly if using a professional microphone as it will pick up all the little sounds. And make sure your phone is on silent.
- If using a professional microphone with a POP filter, then keep your mouth uncomfortably close to the filter for the best-quality sound.

Chapter 19 — Sharing research findings

Summary of Part 2

Part 2 offers practical guidance for researchers to effectively disseminate their work across various platforms. It starts with tips for publishing in academic journals, emphasising strategic selection, adherence to editorial policies and incorporating feedback. The section then covers oral presentations, stressing clear delivery and engaging slide design. Posters are also discussed, focusing on effective content organisation and engagement with attendees. Social media's role in dissemination is highlighted, along with strategies for maximising impact. Lastly, podcasts are recognised as a valuable medium for sharing research, with advice on episode preparation and delivery.

Overall, Part 2 equips researchers with actionable strategies to maximise the impact and reach of their work.

Useful resources

- Equator Network: www.equator-network.org/

Chapter 20

Developing a successful research proposal

Janette Turner and Andy Newton

> **Purpose of this chapter**
>
> Completion of this chapter will help you to:
> - understand why a research proposal is important
> - identify what factors make a good proposal
> - recognise key items that need to be included
> - avoid common mistakes.

Introduction

A research proposal provides an explicit written account of an intended project and how it will be carried out. The term 'research proposal' is often used interchangeably with 'research protocol'. However, there are some subtle differences between the two – for example, a protocol may not include details of funding required, whereas a proposal will – but overall, the component parts are essentially the same. Proposals will also differ in terms of size and scope – much more information will be needed to describe a multicentre, multimillion pound randomised controlled trial than a small-scale local pilot study but, again, the main components are the same, with the only difference being the number of items and complexity of detail required for each component part. In this chapter, these component parts will be introduced to provide a template that can be used as a guide for any type of proposal.

What is a research proposal used for?

For any research project, there will come a point in its development where a proposal is needed that sets out a plan for the research. It is used to support applications for:

- funding
- academic projects (undergraduate and postgraduate dissertations and doctoral programmes)

Chapter 20 — Developing a successful research proposal

- research ethics and governance approvals
- organisational support and approval.

The proposal is a working document that is used throughout the lifetime of a project to provide a framework for the different activities that need to be carried out and for writing up reports. A research proposal can go through many iterations as an original draft is refined over time by various members of the research team.

What makes a good research proposal?

At the most basic level, a research proposal is a means of selling an idea. It needs to persuade and convince a funding body, ethics committee or academic supervisor that the research is trying to answer an important question, has been robustly designed to achieve this and those conducting the research have the skills and experience to complete the project. This means it needs to tell a story that conveys:

- why this research is important
- what is the question you want to answer
- how you plan to do this.

To achieve this, there are some basic principles that lay the foundations for a good research proposal.

First, it needs to be clear and easy to read for a mixed audience. For funding and ethics committees, even though many members will be healthcare professionals and/or have academic expertise, they will come from a wide range of backgrounds and may not be familiar with the particular topic area. Increasingly, these committees involve lay members to represent patients and the general public. It is therefore important to describe the problem you are trying to address using terms and language that make sense to a non-expert, be it another professional or a potential or actual service user. Using simple, plain language is a good habit to develop as it will help engage and pique the interest of any reader. Clarity helps a proposal to stand out – a critical factor for funding applications in particular, as there will be huge competition from numerous, equally capable research teams.

Second, it needs to be succinct but have sufficient detail to be replicable. A proposal should tell a story and follow a logical sequence which mirrors the research process itself. The balance between succinctness and detail can seem daunting, but it provides good training for developing a clear and focused style of writing. The key is precision, keeping it factual and avoiding the use of lots of extraneous words or complex descriptions. It is perfectly acceptable to use bullet points or numbered lists, tables or charts (for example, flow diagrams) to describe some elements, and these often help with clarity and can convey far more information than blocks of text.

Third, look at any guidance provided about the structure of a research proposal from target organisations. Most major funding bodies, including the National Institute for Health and Care Research (NIHR) and charities, will have clear instructions and advice about what needs to be included in an application, including word or character limits for each section (these follow the standard list of components for a proposal described in the next section).

Main components of a research proposal

In this section, the common components of research proposals are described in more detail. Depending on what the proposal is being used for, not every component will be necessary but the majority will be, particularly those concerned with background and rationale, research question and methods.

Introduction, background and rationale

This component sets the scene and context for a project and has three key elements:

- A description of the topic area which sets out the problem being addressed. This might be, for example, a specific health condition (e.g. trauma); a population or general service issue (e.g. response types); or staffing (e.g. skills and education). It needs to explain why the topic area is important and what the consequences of problems are (morbidity, mortality, inadequate service provision, staff recruitment and retention). It should be factual, explained from a non-expert perspective (e.g. define what a category 1 call is) and wherever possible include numbers to illustrate scale, such as how many people are affected. If there is an international perspective, make this clear. Make sure to reference sources.

- What is the current evidence and where are the gaps? This should not be an exhaustive literature review but highlight the key publications in the area with a critical appraisal of the evidence. There should also be an assessment of the potential benefits of generating new evidence to fill these gaps. For NIHR funding bodies in particular, a very important criterion they assess is the benefit for patients or the NHS, so this needs to be spelled out. However, it is important that benefits are described as potential; there are no givens and if there were, there would be no need for the research. Avoid trying to pre-empt the findings of research and making statements that X or Y will be achieved. When done well, this should seamlessly lead into the next element.

- Which knowledge gap is this research trying to address? This should lead to an explicit statement about the research question the proposal is attempting to answer. For more discussion about formulating research questions, see Chapter 7. It is worth reiterating that the question needs to be clear, important and achievable by the research design that subsequently follows.

It is important to keep this section concise. A common mistake (particularly where there are no word limit restrictions) is to write the background section as a comprehensive literature review that then takes up more than half of the proposal.

Chapter 20 — Developing a successful research proposal

This balance is wrong as the bulk of a proposal should be describing the planned work in detail as it is this that is under scrutiny. A good rule of thumb is to keep this section to no more than two sides of A4 paper.

Aims and objectives

The terms 'aims' and 'objectives' are often used interchangeably, but a useful distinction is to think of the aim or aims as a description of the overall intention of the project while objectives set out how this will be achieved. Objectives can then be stated using 'action' terms such as 'measure', 'assess', 'compare', 'estimate'. Stating objectives as actionable tasks helps keep focus when describing the research methods, as these can be linked to specific objectives. This is particularly helpful in complex studies that include several work packages, as each can be associated with an objective and it keeps the proposal coherent. See Chapter 7 for more information on aims and objectives.

Plan of investigation (methods)

This is the core part of a proposal and should comprise the bulk of the text. It should describe how the research will be conducted and contain sufficient detail that another researcher could read the proposal and replicate the study.

Table 20.1 identifies the critical elements that should be included. Depending on the project, not all items will be relevant, but it provides items that should be considered. It is worth structuring this part of the proposal in a logical order that will follow how the research will be conducted, for example data cannot be collected until participants have been recruited. Using this logical sequence helps a reader to understand how things will happen and at what point during the research. Think of this section like a recipe in a cookbook that provides step-by-step instructions on what ingredients are needed, how much and what to do with them to achieve a finished product. Of course, the recipe could be ignored, and some butter, sugar, eggs and flour could just be put into a saucepan and put on the hob — it will never be a Victoria sponge though. If catastrophe strikes, someone else should be able to use the 'recipe' in the proposal and achieve the same end-product.

This list can seem daunting, and it is true that a lot of information needs to be included, but that does not mean it has to be very lengthy. If the text is precise and factual then much of the necessary information can be provided in relatively few words. It is basically a list of tasks that will be carried out.

Patient and public involvement

There is an expectation that health service research studies will involve patient and public representation so that their views and ideas are included to help steer research that is meaningful to those who will be the end users (see Chapter 17). This can start early with input into the development of a research question and study design and continue as participation in the research process itself. If required, describe how patients or the public have been involved, what changes were made due to their involvement, who has participated up to the proposal stage and what plans there are to involve them during the conduct and final dissemination of the study.

Table 20.1 Plan of investigation.

Plan of investigation components	Factors to include
A short overview including the research design	Briefly summarise what will happen. Describe the research design to be used (randomised trial; observational controlled or uncontrolled; cohort; mixed methods; qualitative interview, etc.) and why this is the best choice. For large studies where there may be a number of discrete but linked components, a flow diagram can convey a message far more effectively than lots of text and link each component to the study objectives.
Population/ subjects and setting	Identify clearly who or what the research is including and where the research will take place. If patients – is it a specific disease, condition, symptom? A type of 999 call? If a service – which service: 999 ambulance, NHS111, response type (helicopter, non-conveyed, falls). If staff – which staff: specialist, registered HCP, student. Setting – clinical (responding), Emergency Operations Centre, hospital, station. How will potential subjects be identified and selected – records; on scene; professional groups/organisations.
Recruitment	Describe how potential participants will be recruited. How will they be approached? How will consent be obtained? For surveys or interviews, how many attempts will be made to request a response?
Inclusions and exclusions	List any inclusions and/or exclusions as bullet lists. For example: Age – specific age ranges included or excluded. Time – in hours or out of hours; weekdays or weekends; since onset of symptoms; waiting times. Call types – specific call categories; response types (hear and treat, conveyed or not conveyed; managed at home). Condition – co-morbidities; specific injuries; specific physiological parameters. Staff – educational level; length of service.
Intervention	If an intervention study, describe it in detail and make clear how this differs from current standard operation. An intervention might be a treatment but also a new way of patient assessment, a service change (e.g. how calls are prioritised, introducing electronic records, co-delivery with a community service), an online educational package, etc.

(Continued)

Chapter 20 — Developing a successful research proposal

Table 20.1 (*Continued*).

Plan of investigation components	Factors to include
Instruments and outcome measures	Describe any instruments that will be used (surveys; patient satisfaction and experience tools; pain scales; diagnostic tools; quality of life tools). Describe any outcome measures (death, survival, pain, times – response, to treatment, etc.); call volumes; hospital admission; admission avoidance; satisfaction; resource savings; staff absence; well-being and quality of life, etc.
Data collection	Describe which data will be collected, the source(s) of data and when they will be collected. Distinguish between primary data (new data being collected for this study) and secondary data (using data from existing datasets). For survey studies, describe how the questionnaire will be designed, tested and administered. This should link to items described in the section on instruments and outcome measures. For complex studies with multiple data sources measured at different times, a table is a good way of setting this out, outlining data, source and when they will be captured. These can be linked back to the objectives. Describe how data will be handled, for example by constructing a database, what software package will be used, how numerical and text data will be recorded and stored. For qualitative studies, describe development of topic guides for interviews; methods for recording observation; recording; transcribing, etc. Describe processes for keeping data secure.
Economic evaluation	If a study includes an economic evaluation, describe how this will be conducted. Key things to specify are: Type – cost consequence, cost-effectiveness, cost-benefit. Data sources – if these will be derived locally by the research teams or if standard NHS reference costs will be used. Outcome measures used for cost-effectiveness studies, such as quality of life measures. How the economic data will be analysed (including any sensitivity analyses) and presented.
Statistics and sample size	If a study needs a sample size calculation to enable effects to be measured, describe how the sample size has been calculated and which outcome measure(s) have been used. If a statistical analysis will be undertaken, describe which statistical methods and tests will be used to address each of the objectives, for example if two groups are being compared for differences, changes over time using a time series analysis or association between characteristics using regression methods.

Main components of a research proposal

Table 20.1 (*Continued*).

Plan of investigation components	Factors to include
Analyses	For some quantitative studies, this will be a continuation or subsection of the statistics and sample size description. For all studies, there needs to be a description of how data will be analysed. This should link back to the objectives and be explicit. If comparisons between groups are being made (before and after, control and intervention), describe what these will be – for example, measure if there is a reduction in conveyance, an increase in satisfaction, a reduction in mortality, an association between frequent calls and deprivation, an increase in job satisfaction. For surveys, there may be some quantitative comparisons and more qualitative analyses of text responses. Describe how text responses will be analysed and reported. For qualitative studies, describe what type of qualitative analysis will be used and how this will be conducted in detail. Cite references where appropriate to support analytical methods. For mixed methods studies, describe how the different component parts will be integrated to address the study aims and objectives. Remember the rule that someone should be able to read a proposal and replicate the study. One reason for unsuccessful proposals is insufficient detail in this section. It is not enough to just put a sentence saying 'appropriate descriptive and statistical tests will be conducted' or 'the interviews will be analysed using framework analysis' with no further expansion about *how* this will be done.

Strengths of the research team

This is an important section as funding bodies in particular want to be assured that their money will not be wasted, and that the research team has the skills, expertise and track record to see a study through to completion. If specialist input is needed (e.g. statisticians, health economists, modellers, clinical expertise), list these. Give brief examples of successful projects that members of the team have already conducted. Describe any organisational support available. Briefly describe how the project will be managed, for example using project management groups and study steering groups that provide some external support and oversight.

Ethical considerations and approval

Not every study will require ethical approval – for example, systematic reviews or secondary data analytical studies that use databases already in the public domain – but if it is expected that ethical approval and research governance permissions will be needed, describe what permissions/approvals will be sought (see Chapter 16) and outline any potential ethical issues that may arise. This could, for example, involve gaining informed consent from patients at scene or accessing personal data.

Methods of dissemination and implementation

The findings of any health services research are only of value if they reach beyond the research team. This means they need to be communicated to those who can use the findings – patients, staff, organisations – so new knowledge and information are shared and acted on (see Chapter 19).

Traditionally, dissemination meant academic journal papers and conference presentations. These are still important, but reach a very limited audience. In the digital world there are many more effective ways to reach a wider audience. Short research summaries and leaflets in simple language that highlight the key aspects of a study are far more likely to be read than a huge research report or academic paper. Increasingly, slide sets and short films are being used for dissemination through NHS Trust websites, patient groups and professional organisations (such as the College of Paramedics). Social media platforms have hugely increased the capacity to spread a message to diverse groups of potential readers globally. Think creatively and provide a short description of any plans for developing materials to help communicate important messages and recommendations generated by the study.

Timetable and project milestones

Provide a timetable as a Gantt chart or table that sets out when the different phases of the study will take place (with dates) and key milestones when components are expected to be completed (e.g. literature review, data collection). Include sufficient time to write up the study once analyses are complete – this is often forgotten and can take much longer than anticipated depending on the size and scope of a study.

Justification of support

This section is used in proposals that are part of a funding application. There will usually be a separate section where all the financial costs requested are entered and split by different types of expense. A brief description of costs is used as part of the proposal for members of funding committees or peer reviewers who will not see the detailed cost breakdown. A summary should be provided that sets out requested costs for broad groups, such as staffing, equipment, travel and expenses, consumables, PPIE payments, and so on. Be guided by the groups of costs in the costing form.

Potential challenges

It is worth highlighting briefly any potential difficulties that might be encountered (few health research studies are straightforward and problem-free) and how they might be mitigated. This demonstrates that some of the practical limitations and risks have already been thought about. This can include, for example, issues around recruitment (if it is slow, can anything be done to increase the potential pool of participants?); obtaining informed consent; compliance (for intervention studies); obtaining data – particularly if they must come from an external source such as NHS Digital or an NHS trust; how missing data can be managed.

Characteristics of a 'good' research proposal

A research proposal is an important document. It is a vital step in the research process and is necessary to secure funding, approvals and permissions and academic or organisational support. It is the point at which a research idea becomes crystallised into a clear question and a plan is formulated to set out how this question can be answered.

In the first instance, it has to 'sell' this idea and convince a range of people that it is important, achievable, has the potential to produce benefits and is worth investing in. If successful, it then becomes the template or framework that will guide a study through to completion. Box 20.1 lists the characteristics of a good research proposal.

> **Box 20.1**
>
> ### Characteristics of a good research proposal
>
> - Write in clear, simple, unambiguous language and make no assumptions about the knowledge of someone reading it. The proposal should be understandable and pique the interest of a lay member, academic or clinical reader who is not familiar with the topic area or a topic expert. Explain terminology that will not be obvious to a non-expert.
> - Be enthusiastic for the topic area and the potential benefits if a knowledge gap is explored. Competition for funding is tough, so a proposal needs to stand out. Do not make promises that cannot be kept, but do emphasise why it is important.
> - Have a logical sequence that tells the story of this study from establishing a need through to a step-by-step guide to how the research will be conducted.
> - Ensure you have a clear and explicit question with aims and objectives that summarise the intention or purpose.
> - The plan of investigation should be detailed, precise, replicable and achievable. Use lists, tables and diagrams to help simplify descriptions. Keep it factual and avoid complicated and verbose explanations. Regularly link descriptions of research methods back to the objectives so the relationship between the two is reinforced.
> - Read and comply with any guidance about how a proposal should be constructed and any word limits. Failure to do this creates a bad impression and sows a seed of doubt about ability to see a plan through.

Summary

Writing a research proposal can be daunting, particularly for the first time. If possible, get involved in writing parts of a proposal being led by someone else, as this provides support and feedback. Create drafts and ask other people (particularly non-experts)

Chapter 20 — Developing a successful research proposal

to read and feed back on whether they understand what the proposal is describing. In academic institutions, there will often be access to proposals written by students or academics in previous years. These can be a good resource as examples. Many larger-scale research studies now publish the study protocol. If these have been published in the same topic area, read them as they will provide a very helpful description about study design, data collection and analyses. Funding bodies also publish successful proposals/protocols, so it is worth seeking these out for projects in the same study area. The NIHR website is useful for this and can be searched for relevant prehospital or ambulance related research.

One final word of wisdom — proposal writing is part art, part science. It gets easier and the quality gets better as the number completed increases. Keep going!

Useful resources

- McCombes S and George T (2023). How to write a research proposal. www.scribbr.com/dissertation/research-proposal/
- Sudheesh K, Duggappa DR and Nethra SS (2016). How to write a research proposal? *Indian Journal of Anaesthesia*, 60(9): 631–634.

Chapter 21

Obtaining research funding: hints and tips

Graham McClelland and Fiona Bell

> **Purpose of this chapter**
>
> Completion of this chapter will help you to:
> - identify key considerations when applying for grant funding
> - choose appropriate funders and relevant funding streams
> - recognise the importance of accurate costings for research
> - build an appropriate research grant application team
> - prepare a successful grant application.

Introduction

Research takes time, often longer than anticipated, and money buys time and resources, including staff, so the ability to source and secure funding is a vital skill for a researcher. Small research projects can be completed without funding, but these often rely on people committing time above and beyond other roles to progress, but for larger projects, and generally any project beyond level 7 (master's), funding of some sort is normally required. Securing funding is time-consuming and often requires considerable work developing the idea for the project and a plan to deliver the study before you can apply for the funding.

For healthcare research in the UK, the National Institute for Health and Care Research (NIHR) (Davies et al., 2016) is one of the largest and most visible funders and supports the delivery of research in the NHS through a variety of schemes. The range of research funding available is broad: small projects; internships; personal awards such as PhD or postdoctoral fellowships; feasibility studies; single-site studies; or large programmes of work with multiple sites over multiple years. Funding awarded in open competition is very competitive, and grant applications can have a low rate of success. In 2022, of 49 applications to round 1 of the Doctoral Clinical and Practitioner Academic Fellowship (DCAF), formerly the Clinical Doctoral Research Fellowship (CDRF), 18 (37%) fellowships were awarded (NIHR DCAF Chairs Report, 2023).

Chapter 21 – Obtaining research funding: hints and tips

The NIHR is not the only source of funding; bodies such as the Medical Research Council (MRC) fund a broad range of research, whereas charities and organisations such as the Stroke Association or the Resuscitation Council fund more targeted research.

To be successful, a funding application needs to demonstrate the value to science and society, the feasibility and the impact of the planned research. Any proposal should demonstrate that the problem you seek to address is relevant to the funder, involves a clearly-defined population and that you are the right person/team to answer the question. It is also important that a proposed project is achievable, will answer the research question and ideally, from a paramedic perspective, that the results will inform and/or influence patient care or paramedic practice.

The tips written below, and expanded upon later, assume that the reader already has an idea of the type of project they may be working towards developing for a funding application (see Chapter 7).

1. Don't wait for competitions or grant funding calls to be announced.
2. Do your background research.
3. Make sure what you propose matches the funder's priorities and interests.
4. Talk to the funder.
5. Good ideas need to demonstrate impact and numbers.
6. Consider where you are in your career and what sort of funding is available.
7. Building a grant application is a team effort.
8. Track records matter.
9. There's a fine line between promising the earth and making a project attractive.
10. Accurately cost your proposal.
11. Get feedback early and often.
12. Everything takes longer than you think.
13. Be resilient.

Tips for developing a successful grant application

1. Don't wait for competitions or grant funding calls to be announced

Many grants are announced around the same time each year and have the same sort of application window, which can be quite short. This means you can anticipate when a grant call might come out and develop your idea in advance. Prospective applicants are advised to be proactive and begin working on an application before the call is announced, as preparing a high-quality grant application takes time. Not all

> **Box 21.1**
>
> **Examples of funding bodies**
>
> - Government – in the UK the NIHR funds project, personal and programme awards.
> - Regional bodies such as the Applied Research Collaboratives (ARCs) or the Health Innovation Networks (HINs) and the Community for Allied Health Professions Research (CAHPR).
> - Charities – for a national or international disease specialty, or local charities.
> - Professional bodies – College of Paramedics, Royal College of Emergency Medicine, Royal College of Nursing.
> - Higher education institute funding arrangements, including for fellowships.
> - Commercial companies – either in the capacity of an investigator approaching the company to support their project, or from a commercial company funding and sponsoring the research or charitable foundations associated with commercial companies.

funding works like this and there will be some opportunities that unexpectedly arise in response to a situation (e.g. COVID) or priority-setting exercise.

There are few funders specifically supporting paramedic-led research. Different types of funders may support research led by paramedics or focused on the prehospital setting, or if you are ambitious then funding from multiple sources can be sought for a single project, but this can introduce complications in terms of balancing competing demands. Some funding bodies to consider are identified in Box 21.1.

Horizon-scanning for opportunities should include investigating the types of bodies funding research in your area of interest, considering how other projects have been funded and exploring upcoming prospects via networks. Knowing what type of funding is normally supported can help narrow the number of potential funders – for example, not all funders will support personal fellowships. Once potential funders and schemes are identified, maximising the chance of seeing opportunities by using social media, signing up for mailing lists from relevant funders, and working with the NIHR Research Support Service (RSS) will ensure opportunities are not missed.

A prospective or active researcher should consider the timing of any upcoming calls in relation to current and planned commitments and the anticipated project start date. This planning should include consideration of fit with career plans and other commitments, including the potential need to apply to multiple funders or rounds of competition if you are unsuccessful at the first attempt.

2. Do your background research

Look into what has previously been funded by the organisation you want to apply to. Speak to people involved in previous funding rounds if possible. If you can get hold of previous applications, both successful and unsuccessful, preferably with feedback from the funder, these can be useful to help you see how previous applicants have structured applications and may identify areas you hadn't thought about. While previous applications are useful, funders do change their priorities and requirements so always make sure you look at the latest guidance and forms.

3. Make sure what you propose matches the funder's priorities and interests

You might have the best idea in the world but if it doesn't match the funder's interests and priorities then your chances are slim. Most large funding bodies will publish their research priorities and previously-funded projects, and they will have clear and defined aims for a funding call. This information will provide useful insight into the funder's priorities, interests and types of projects they are likely to support. Ensuring that the proposal meets the funder's remit and is costed within the available funds means time is not wasted preparing and reviewing projects that are unsuitable for the competition. Make sure you show the funder very clearly in any proposal how your research addresses their aims.

4. Talk to the funder

Funders want to support the best research and will normally engage with you as a researcher if you approach them about an idea. If you have questions about the application process or anything related to the funding call, you are better off contacting the funder and discussing it as opposed to hoping for the best and potentially jeopardising your chances. Contacting a funder does not have to be in response to a specific funding call; if you have an idea that aligns with a funder's area of interest but there are no calls out, it may still be worth contacting them to see what may be in the pipeline.

5. Good ideas need to demonstrate impact and numbers

Make sure you know the size of the population you are talking about and/or the scale of the problem you are trying to address. If you can evidence how your study directly addresses the impact of the disease/condition/population then this is useful to include in a grant application. You need to clearly justify why this project is necessary and important. When considering impact, you need to include how you will disseminate your findings to maximise the outputs for the funder's investment in your project. Impact can be achieved in many ways including changing patient care, contributing to future research and influencing guidelines.

6. Consider where you are in your career and what sort of funding is available

If you are at the start of your career, then developing an application for a multi-million pound grant is probably not the best use of your time. There are career development grants and personal fellowships and other smaller grants that allow you to complete a project, gain skills and build a CV. Apply for smaller grants at the start of your research journey and build a track record that positions you to apply for bigger grants. Success with smaller grants will build a network of contacts that you will need when applying for bigger grants. Success leads to success in this type of endeavour.

7. Building a grant application is a team effort

Use your contacts! Don't ignore advice from people like the RSS (NIHR RSS, 2023), university support services or ambulance service research departments. Accessing expertise from these types of services will improve the chances of success.

Don't forget to involve and cost in specialist skills like statisticians and health economists if these are needed. The RSS can help with the identification and costing of specialists if engaged early in the proposal development. You don't want to be in the position of getting a grant then having to go back to the funder as you forgot to cost something; this looks unprofessional and there is no obligation on the funder to give you any more money.

With the project outline defined, and funding type or even a funder in mind, an investigator should begin identifying the collaborations that will be required for success. Identifying and demonstrating engagement with stakeholders and collaborators in the application will reassure the funder that your project is feasible. Consider the research setting to identify clinicians, academics, clinical services, patients, and local R&D teams who will be key to success.

Discussions with key collaborators may identify a need to generate preliminary data to support the application. Applying for smaller grants to support preliminary work may be beneficial before working up to the larger project. Smaller related grants and outputs signal commitment to, and understanding of, the area of research that may be viewed favourably by the funding committee.

Preliminary work may include engagement with stakeholders relevant to the project. Early, relevant stakeholder involvement (see Chapter 17) should be demonstrated in an application, as professional and lay members of funding committees will want to be satisfied that involvement is demonstrated in both the development and delivery of the project. Ongoing involvement for the life of the project may be demonstrated through including suitable stakeholders as co-applicants, or by identifying specific activities where patient and public representatives will be asked to participate. PPIE advisory groups and individuals can be engaged through existing groups, and there may be opportunities to access funding to support this activity through specific grants from organisations like the NIHR RSS.

Individuals, organisations and services who may not be directly involved with the delivery of the project may write letters of recommendation to include in the application that demonstrate and support the need for the project.

8. Track records matter

Sometimes having the right support on a grant application makes the difference. Don't just add the name of an eminent professor or leading researcher in your field if they don't bring anything to the project, especially if you must pay for a percentage of their time. However, there is value in mentorship, contacts, support and other less easily quantifiable benefits that having well-known researchers on your grant application brings. In addition, funding bodies may be more confident in funding you if they see that you are supported by a well-known name with a track record of delivering projects.

Organisations which fund research will fund projects, but they also fund people. Investing in an up-and-coming researcher who will go on to lead research over their career is a more attractive proposition than someone who will deliver a single project then move into a different area of practice. Demonstrating that you are on a trajectory to becoming a research leader of the future makes you an attractive investment. To signal your trajectory to a research funder, you can allude to future work or studies that the current grant may lead on to, but don't lose the focus on the current project. If you don't get the current grant, then the follow-up projects don't matter.

Making yourself an attractive investment for a grant funder is about showing how your interests and ambitions align with theirs, in the short and longer terms. A track record of delivering on previous projects may improve the credibility of the proposal for a research-funding body.

Early career researchers should consider mentorship and support as part of the application, and for personal awards, supervision or mentorship by more senior or experienced researchers is often required.

In larger-scale applications, expertise matters and having the correct subject matter or methodological expertise included in the proposal development can make all the difference. Existing contacts and networks should be engaged to identify suitable collaborations and co-applicants. This should be done at the project development stage, but inclusion in an application should not be tokenistic, instead demonstrating a clear and defined role with appropriate responsibilities; for example, there may be a requirement to demonstrate that statistical support has been sought or will be a part of the study delivery team.

9. There's a fine line between promising the earth and making a project attractive

Grants are competitive and therefore you need to be ambitious in what you propose. However, if you promise the earth on a tiny budget, then funding bodies are unlikely to take you seriously. The opposite also applies – if you ask for millions of pounds and only propose a small project which could be delivered for much less, don't expect to get funded. Better to underpromise and overdeliver than vice versa. Each step of the process often takes longer than you think, such as the time required for gaining the requisite research governance approvals.

Tips for developing a successful grant application

The people who sit on grant-funding bodies have probably been in the position you find yourself in as an applicant, and may have reviewed tens if not hundreds of similar proposals and outputs, so they will have an idea of what is achievable and what isn't.

Always give some indication, or at least have it in the back of your head in case you get asked at interview, of where you will go next or what the logical next steps are after this project you are planning.

Chapter 20 provides specific guidance on developing proposals. Ensure that feedback is sought early and acted upon. It may be that some preliminary data gathering or generation is required to demonstrate the need for the project, potential impacts or feasibility. If data are required, then smaller development grants may be appropriate (e.g. local RSS-funded PPIE grants or other local funding).

10. Accurately cost your proposal

Funders are looking for value for money, and to be confident that their financial investment in the project will return potential benefits. Therefore, the expected outputs and impact of these should be clearly stated, alongside demonstrating that the project will deliver its objectives to time and within budget. You should also consider the time needed to prepare the outputs and any costs for conference or publication fees, or events such as workshops or presentations to stakeholders if applicable.

There is a fine line between overselling yourself and your project and not being ambitious enough in a grant proposal. Realistic projects are more likely to get funding than wildly ambitious projects with very little chance of succeeding or delivering on time. Make sure you cost in the support, skills and time you will need, as well as any materials (consumables, specified computer programs for data analysis) or services (translation of study materials).

The value in the project will depend on the funder, the size of the grant and your career stage. Some schemes are looking to develop you as a researcher and the 'value' to the funder may come from raising the profile of their area of interest, the skills and experience you develop over the course of the grant and where this will take you in the future, and it should be clear in the proposal how you will demonstrate this development.

Small grants may not be sufficient to cover everything that happens during the project, and you may have to contribute time or find support or additional funding from other sources. If the success of a grant or project depends on securing other funding then this makes getting the funding more difficult and the value may be more difficult to demonstrate.

Funders expect researchers to deliver good value for money. If a funder gives money to you then they aren't funding another project, so there is a need to show that you have considered how best to use the money. If you ask for funding to travel to the other side of the world, make sure the value of the trip is crystal clear and show how you will maximise the value that these opportunities afford you.

11. Get feedback early and often

Discuss your idea with people and see what they say. Spending time planning and discussing with a range of people will help you to refine your project and will improve the clarity and focus of the proposal.

Discuss your idea with people outside your clinical field as they may see things in a different light and give you a different perspective on a project. Discuss your idea with patients, or people not involved in research or the medical professions, as many grant funders will have lay people on the committees and summaries in lay, or plain, English form part of many applications. Record what people say as you may need to show how your idea evolved and how you incorporated feedback into your study. PPIE feedback and support is very important in many grant applications.

12. Everything takes longer than you think

Funding deadlines are normally fixed dates and you should treat them as such. If you need to get signatures, make sure the people you need to get them from don't have two weeks' holiday planned just before the submission deadline – give them plenty of notice.

Developing a good grant application is a time-consuming process and you should give it the time it deserves. Ideas can take time to evolve, and getting feedback and input and polishing an application all take time. Don't assume people with their own priorities and jobs will turn something around immediately just because you are up against a deadline.

13. Be resilient

Writing grant applications is a skill like any other, and you should get better with practice. If you want a career as a researcher, you may have to write many grant applications over the course of your career. The reality of grant applications is that not all will be funded. Don't give up after the first rejection if you believe in the project. There are normally ways in which a project can be changed to suit a different funding scheme, or improved based on the feedback you received and resubmitted to the next round of funding from the same funder you originally applied to.

Summary

Do not be afraid to change things – this process is iterative. Do not give up if unsuccessful at your first attempt. Take the feedback, get more advice and plan your next move to resubmit either to the same place or elsewhere or try something else!

Useful resources

- AcoRD: www.gov.uk/government/publications/guidance-on-attributing-the-costs-of-health-and-social-care-research
- Clinical Trials Toolkit: www.ct-toolkit.ac.uk/routemap/funding-proposal/

Useful resources

- Community for Allied Health Professions Research (CAHPR): https://cahpr.csp.org.uk/
- NIHR Applied Research Collaborations (ARCs): www.nihr.ac.uk/explore-nihr/support/collaborating-in-applied-health-research.htm
- Medical Research Council (MRC): www.ukri.org/councils/mrc/
- Health Innovation Networks (HIN): https://thehealthinnovationnetwork.co.uk/

Chapter 22

Research careers for paramedics

Kim Kirby and Graham McClelland

> **Purpose of this chapter**
>
> Completion of this chapter will help you to:
> - understand the range of research careers for paramedics
> - identify what you need to be successful in research
> - get started in research
> - explore doctorate options
> - recognise the importance of publishing, presenting and networking.

Introduction

All healthcare professionals have a role to play in research, from being effective consumers of research through to developing robust research studies and leading its development as a chief investigator. There are many opportunities to engage in paramedic research and sometimes it is difficult to know where to start.

What is the range of research careers for paramedics?

Research as a career choice for paramedics is a relatively new option, and only recently has much been published on the role of the research paramedic (McClelland, 2013; Whitley and Wilson, 2022; Wilson et al., 2022b; Runacres et al., 2024). There are probably fewer paramedics working in research than in the other pillars (clinical, education, leadership) and research roles are more likely to be short-term and externally funded. Having said this, there are an increasing number of paramedics demonstrating that research is a viable career option.

All paramedics are expected to have some level of research knowledge (HCPC, 2023) and at higher levels of practice, being able to source and critically appraise evidence and having a greater understanding of how research works and affects practice is part of most roles.

Chapter 22 — Research careers for paramedics

Many research roles start off short-term, and some paramedics will gain some research skills and understanding, then go back to clinical practice or on to non-research roles where the skills and experience they picked up doing research will be useful. Other paramedics will develop longer-term research careers, and there are options and support available for people who wish to pursue this path. The National Institute for Health and Care Research (NIHR) has multiple schemes (NIHR, 2024) and a distinct career ladder for AHPs which paramedics can apply for, including:

- internships
- predoctoral clinical academic fellowships
- clinical and non-clinical doctorates
- advanced fellowships
- professorships.

This career ladder provides a neat framework and insight into academic hierarchies and where a research-focused career could go. The College of Paramedics has its own career framework (College of Paramedics, 2023) which represents another perspective on what a research career may look like. In addition to schemes for qualified paramedics, there are opportunities for undergraduate students to get involved in research while studying, such as the INSIGHT: Inspiring Students into Research Scheme (NIHR, 2023b).

Many trusts employ research paramedics who tend to focus on delivery of a particular study or group of studies. These roles are very good starting points and, while they present a steep learning curve, they are a good vehicle for learning about research. Some trusts employ research fellows or senior research paramedics whose role includes more responsibility for developing research ideas and proposals, publishing and presenting research and supporting other paramedics and clinicians who are interested in research. Beyond this, there are research governance and management roles and university posts with research responsibilities. Some research roles may not require clinical qualifications. The governance and management of healthcare research require more generalisable knowledge and there are roles for paramedics with research skills outside the ambulance service. Joint appointments between NHS Trusts and universities are rare, but emerging as a model for paramedics and other clinicians, which enable people to pursue clinical and academic development without having to leave the NHS.

If you want to develop a research career, then partnership with a university is highly beneficial and probably required for more senior roles and development. Paramedics working in education in universities are in a good position to pursue research if time can be found in their busy timetables. The top of the research career tree is probably the professorial role which is a university-awarded title as opposed to an ambulance service rank. Few paramedics reach this level, but these rare individuals are leading lights in developing and driving forward paramedic and prehospital research. More professors with a paramedic background are needed, and the emergence of these roles will be a sign of a healthy research community.

What do you need to be successful in research?

What you need to be successful in research depends on how you define success. Is success having a long and rewarding career, becoming a professor, earning lots of money, positively affecting care or all of the above and more? Being a successful researcher is not just about raw intelligence; many other qualities are needed, plus a sprinkling of good luck doesn't hurt!

Many established researchers say that perseverance is a key quality due to the long-term investment of time that is needed for any research. Research does not happen fast, and coming from a paramedic background where time is measured in jobs which often take less than an hour, the extended timelines involved in any research project can feel quite alien.

A thick skin and the ability to handle rejection are other skills that you either need to be successful in research or that you develop by working in the field. Research is full of rejection – it might be the idea you take to your supervisor, the paper you submitted to a journal or a grant you applied for. The ability to deal with rejection, learn from it and move on is a key skill for a long career in research.

Finding a good mentor, or mentors, can be very helpful. At the start of a research career, having someone to offer support, guidance and initial opportunities sets you up to be successful in the future. Later in your career, having trusted mentors with whom you can discuss issues and from whom to secure sound advice is also very useful.

Getting started

The common route to getting started in research as a paramedic is through the research paramedic role. This role often requires little prior knowledge of research, and focuses on delivery of a study developed and supported by another more senior researcher or research team. Research paramedic positions are excellent opportunities to learn about research, but are often temporary, which can be useful as it allows you to try research but not commit to it in the long term. The short-term nature of many of these roles does mean that if you want to carry on working in research then you may need to string together multiple short-term positions or secure a more permanent research post, which can be challenging.

The research paramedic role is not the only way to get started in research. Undergraduate paramedic training increasingly offers some insight into research, and there are opportunities to build on these foundations if research is of interest by moving on to a Master's level qualification which will involve more research. These academic qualifications then serve as a good platform for moving across into a more clinical research role. Organisations such as the NIHR offer support for undergraduate students interested in research (NIHR, 2023b).

There are also more formal schemes such as the HEE/NIHR research internship. These internships are competitive schemes that offer a small amount of funding to novice researchers to backfill normal duties and allow the intern to spend time with an established researcher, team or department where they will learn about research and complete a small project. These internships are the first rung on the clinical academic ladder offered by the NIHR, and serve as excellent stepping stones to the next level, which is the predoctoral clinical and practitioner academic fellowship (PCAF).

Different routes to getting a doctorate

A doctorate is often seen as a major milestone in a research career. A doctorate is viewed as a training scheme or apprenticeship in academia, and completion of one establishes that you have some of the skills and characteristics needed to develop as an independent academic. Having said this, you do not need a doctorate to be involved in research, but if you want to lead research studies, apply for large pots of funding and build a long-term career, which will in all likelihood involve more formal links with a university, then a doctorate is probably on your radar.

What is a doctorate, though? A doctoral degree is the highest level of academic qualification available, mapping to level 8 on the UK academic scale. A doctorate normally involves three years of full-time study, or four-plus years of part-time study, and it traditionally concludes with publication of a thesis that makes an original and novel contribution to the pool of knowledge, which the student must defend. The route described is often the traditional route to a doctor of philosophy (PhD) but there are other ways to achieve a PhD, for example by publication, or you can look at equivalent qualifications such as a professional doctorate (DProf).

If you are going to study for three or more years, then you are likely to need some way of funding this. You could self-fund if you have the resources, you could apply for an advertised PhD opportunity with a student stipend or you could secure external funding. Organisations such as the NIHR, the Wellcome Trust and charities offer funded fellowships which allow you to complete a doctorate, often with additional benefits such as training, mentorship and additional funding for expenses. These fellowships are incredibly competitive but can be major career steps if awarded.

Importance of publishing, presentations and networking

'Publish or perish' is a phrase associated with working in academic research, and can be quite intimidating to a novice researcher. Publishing is undoubtedly an important part of being a researcher, in terms of sharing of knowledge, allowing others to build on your work and the peer review process, but it is also an important part of developing as a researcher and building a CV.

Writing for publication is a skill that can be learned, practised and polished to a fine art. Working in research requires different styles of writing for a variety of audiences, and writing for publication is one part of this skillset. Condensing a five-year project into a single 3000 word article is a tricky task. Writing takes time, with most papers going through multiple drafts and rounds of revisions, especially when multiple authors are involved, while submitting your paper to a journal for publication can be a time-consuming, and sometimes bruising, process.

Despite efforts to change the culture, academics are often judged and measured on publications, so learning about the publishing business is part of developing as a researcher and academic. One note of caution for novice researchers is to beware of unsolicited invites to publish with a journal you have never heard of, especially if there is a publication fee or article-processing charge involved. There is a whole industry preying on unsuspecting academics, known as predatory publishing (Elmore and Weston, 2020). Having access to people you can trust such as mentors, ambulance trust research departments, university research support services or senior academics in your field will help you navigate these hazards.

Publishing in a journal is not the only way of communicating your research and building your CV. Presenting at conferences is another way of achieving these goals. Standing up in front of your peers and colleagues can be a daunting prospect, and presenting your research opens you up to challenge and question in a very real and immediate fashion. However, if you attend conferences where research is presented, you will hopefully see presentations that bring a project to life, challenge your practice and leave you inspired. You will also see presentations which do none of the above. Presenting, like writing, is a skill that can be learned, practised and polished and overcoming your fear of presenting to a live audience is a worthwhile task. There is no point doing research if you don't tell people about it, and presenting live is one method of doing that.

Conferences are not only opportunities to present your research and practise your presentation skills, but they also offer the chance to hear about other research in your field and to meet and talk to people working in fields similar to yours or that you are interested in. Conferences that are face-to-face rather than virtual offer a valuable opportunity to meet people in person, exchange stories over coffee and spark up conversations that may lead to future projects and collaborations down the line. Conferences also help you to feel part of a research community, as they offer a rare opportunity for people focused on a particular topic or field but who may work in geographically distinct locations to meet, mingle and interact. Conferences do normally require some funding for things like entry, travel and accommodation, which can be a barrier to attendance if resources are limited.

Longer-term research careers

If research is the career direction that you want to follow, then there is growing recognition that clinical academics are valuable, and that this is a viable career choice for paramedics. Physicians and other NMAHP professions have been making clinical academic careers an option and have more established pathways, but there are few paramedics who have gone down this pathway at the time of writing.

In order to sustain a research career, you will need funding, and therefore you must make yourself attractive to funders. There are multiple aspects to being fundable, including having a clear career trajectory where you are on track to become one of the research leaders of the future, having good ideas that match the funder's aims and address recognised challenges in your field and working with the right people who may be experts in a particular field or methodology.

Chapter 22 — Research careers for paramedics

Building a good track record and CV is part of developing a sustainable research career. Successful completion of small projects and being awarded small grants set you up for larger grants and projects. You are unlikely to be awarded a million-pound grant if you don't have a good track record. Research can also be both collaborative and competitive. You need to collaborate if you want to develop, and collaboration with good people brings lots of benefits. However, there is also a competitive element to research as most funders have limited pots of money, so researchers have to compete for funding. Sometimes you may have a really good idea but the funder just doesn't have enough money to fund all the really good applications they receive, which can be disheartening. If you have a good idea, then you may need to apply to multiple funders or schemes, but hopefully you will get useful feedback from rejections that allows you to improve the idea for the next submission.

More senior research-based career opportunities for paramedics within ambulance services are starting to emerge, but these are few and far between and may involve moving into management or governance-based roles. Universities provide a more natural home for academic careers, but the institutions that train paramedics are not always the ones with active research departments. In an ideal world, some form of joint role shared between an ambulance trust and a university may offer the best of both worlds and the space where paramedic clinical academics can maximise their impact.

Top tips for 'making it' in research

- *Find a topic you are interested in.* If you are doing a doctorate then you are looking at a minimum of three years on one topic. Other projects may involve more or less time, and if you get a doctorate in a particular area then the chances are you will have opportunities to continue working in that area, so find a topic that interests you and you can imagine yourself still working on in a few years. This doesn't mean that whatever topic you choose for your first research project will set the direction for your whole career and you can't change, but think ahead when committing to large pieces of work.

- *Find your people.* Research can be a very solitary pursuit, but it can also involve large teams of people. Find the people who share your interest and your enthusiasm, your pain and your problems. Feeling part of the research community may help you sustain a career in research, and it also gives you people who you can bounce ideas off, potential collaborators and sources of inspiration and motivation. The paramedic research community will always be a relatively small grouping within the profession, but finding these people will help you in the long run. Your tribe may extend outside the paramedic profession as paramedics are part of the wider NMAHP family, and also the wider NHS and researchers can find common ground in many ways, not just professional background. Some problems with research will be very generic, and you may be able to learn from a physiotherapist clinical academic or a research nurse who may have used a methodology you are interested in, so don't be afraid to talk to other people.

Top tips for 'making it' in research

- *Find good mentors (more than one, change over time).* Good mentors or supervisors are worth their weight in gold, especially when you are first starting out in research. Research can be baffling, with a whole new language to learn, regulations to adhere to and processes to follow, so having an experienced hand to guide and support you is very helpful when you start out. Your relationship with your mentor may change, and you may change mentors as you require different types of support at different stages of your career. At some point, you may become a mentor to other people, which involves a whole new skillset.

- *You can't do everything, so be selective.* You will have many opportunities to get involved in other projects, interesting-sounding papers, organising conferences and other activities, all of which may be valuable but will take up some of your time. It can be tempting to say yes to every opportunity that comes along for fear of missing out as it is difficult, if not impossible, to tell which projects and partnerships will pay dividends in the long run. Saying yes to one thing often means saying no to another, or reduces your valuable time, so concentrating on activities that work towards your main goal or contribute towards the qualification you are working on need to be prioritised, and sometimes you will have to say no even to projects you want to be involved in.

- *Collaborate.* Research can be seen as a solitary activity but the more you get into research, the more you realise that this isn't true. Research involves collaborating with a wide range of people and the larger the project, the more people you will need to work with. A good network of contacts is a valuable resource and while you may not be an expert in statistics or health economics, you may know somebody who is who can help you.

- *Be kind to yourself.* There are many challenges with working in research, especially if you are trying to balance this with clinical work as well. Academia celebrates the successful, and there can be pressure to work extra hours and constantly push yourself forward on a never-ending treadmill of grants and publications. One common challenge researchers face is imposter syndrome, where you feel you don't fit in or shouldn't be in the position you are in. There are other aspects of research that may cause you sleepless nights or distress, so remember to be kind to yourself and look after yourself.

- *Persevere.* Research for most people is about incremental gains and long-term development of the evidence base, so perseverance is vital. Many researchers will work on projects that either don't pan out as expected or fail completely, grant applications that have taken months of blood, sweat and tears will be rejected, and supervisors will send lovingly polished drafts back covered in red pen. Through these challenges you need to keep going as they are part of the business of research.

- *Don't forget about the patient.* At the end of the day, we do research to improve patient care. Your project may seem many steps removed from direct patient care, but this is what we work towards in the long term. The big projects that you hear about and that you see changing and influencing care

Chapter 22 — Research careers for paramedics

delivered by paramedics will often be the end-results of years of work, lots of training, many challenges and rejections and a series of small projects that led to bigger projects.

Summary

Research may be a niche career choice for paramedics, but it is a viable career for some individuals. People can benefit from a short-term role in research and learn valuable skills to take onto other roles, or they can build a long career, with a portfolio of studies, and go on to lead research that influences practice across the profession. Finding that initial opportunity to get involved in research can be challenging, so resilience is a key attribute if this is your chosen path. There is support out there and people who are interested in research or doing research. Connect with these people as they will probably be very happy to talk to you about their research. There is a career ladder to follow, which might end up taking you in directions you never intended to go when you joined the ambulance service, but this can be an exciting part of the process.

The paramedic profession needs people to push the boundaries, develop the evidence and improve patient care, and research is one way to pursue all these goals.

Useful resources

- Community for Allied Health Professions Research: https://www.ahpf.org.uk/CAHPR.htm

Chapter 23

Conclusion: next steps

Graham McClelland and Julia Williams

In the introduction, we outlined the purpose of this book. We discussed the intended audience and the challenges posed by the evolving nature of the profession, making concise definitions challenging. Nearly 30 years ago Callaham described the 'scanty science of prehospital emergency care' and painted a bleak picture of EMS practice and research (Callaham, 1997). EMS and the paramedic profession have come a long way since 1997, and the fact that a book like this is needed and could be written illustrates the development of the research underpinning the science of prehospital care.

The paramedic profession continues to change, and we have moved from delivering research for other people, to collaborating on the research, to now where paramedics are leading research. This book will hopefully help more paramedics feel comfortable with research and support them to get involved in research.

Unlike a novel, a book like this is not designed to be read cover-to-cover from start to finish, so thank you for making it this far. While thought was given to the order of the chapters and how earlier content supports later content, this book is written so you can dip in to the bits you need. Section 1 introduced concepts and ideas and gave a broad overview of research as a field. Section 2 covered the major quantitative and qualitative approaches to research and gave more detail on specific methods. Section 3 covered additional things to think about when considering how to do research in real life like funding, ethics and what it might mean for your career. Each chapter in this book represents the tip of the iceberg in terms of content, material and learning, and many resources are signposted throughout. Research is a vast field, and prehospital research is a rapidly-growing part of that field.

In a way, writing this book has felt very similar to completing a major research project. There was the initial idea, putting a team together, working out what it would look like and how to do it, a very long timeline, concerns that it was going completely off the rails, results (chapters) eventually coming together and then pulling it all together into a document with the hope that somebody would read it. Looking back over this book, like looking back over a research project, there are always questions about what could have been done better, what to do differently next time and what we learned from the process. We have learned a great deal over

Chapter 23 — Conclusion: next steps

the process of writing this book and we hope there is something valuable in here for you the reader.

At the end of the day, as with any good piece of research, the conclusion must be 'more research is needed'. So, ask questions, find your fellow paramedic researchers, use the tools in this book, read widely, and hopefully we can drive practice forward and deliver ever better care to the patients we have the privilege of looking after.

References

Abelsson A and Lindwall L (2012). The prehospital assessment of severe trauma patients performed by the specialist ambulance nurse in Sweden – a phenomenographic study. *Scandinavian Journal of Trauma, Resuscitation and Emergency Medicine*, 20: 67.

Achana F et al. (2020). Cost-effectiveness of adrenaline for out-of-hospital cardiac arrest. *Critical Care*, 24(1): 579.

Agee J (2009). Developing qualitative research questions: a reflective process. *International Journal of Qualitative Studies in Education*, 22(4): 431–447.

Aggarwal R and Ranganathan P (2019). Study designs: Part 4 – Interventional studies. *Perspectives in Clinical Research*, 10(3): 137–139.

Agich GJ (2001). Ethics and innovation in medicine. *Journal of Medical Ethics*, 27: 295–296.

Ahern KJ (1999). Ten tips for reflexive bracketing. *Qualitative Health Research*, 9(3): 407–411.

Ahmed R et al. (2018). A comparison of smartphone and paper data-collection tools in the Burden of Obstructive Lung Disease (BOLD) study in Gezira state, Sudan. *PLoS One*, 13(3):e0193917.

AIRWAYS-2 (2024). Airway management in cardiac arrest patients. Available at: https://airways2.blogs.bristol.ac.uk/

Alam N et al. (2018). Prehospital antibiotics in the ambulance for sepsis: a multicentre, open label, randomised trial. *Lancet Respiratory Medicine*, 6(1): 40–50.

Al-Busaidi ZQ (2008). Qualitative research and its uses in health care. *Sultan Qaboos University Medical Journal*, 8(1): 11–19.

Alderson P (1998). Theories in health care and research: the importance of theories in health care. *BMJ*, 317(7164): 1007–1010.

Althubaiti A (2016). Information bias in health research: definition, pitfalls, and adjustment methods. *Journal of Multidisciplinary Healthcare*, 9: 211–217.

Angrosino M (2007). *Doing Ethnographic and Observational Research*. Los Angeles: Sage.

Appleton JP et al. (2019). Ambulance-delivered transdermal glyceryl trinitrate versus sham for ultra-acute stroke: rationale, design and protocol for the Rapid Intervention with Glyceryl trinitrate in Hypertensive stroke Trial-2 (RIGHT-2) trial (ISRCTN26986053). *International Journal of Stroke*, 14(2): 191–206.

Arksey H and O'Malley L (2007). Scoping studies: towards a methodological framework. *International Journal of Social Research Methodology*, 8(1): 19–32.

Armstrong S et al. (2017). Assessment of consent models as an ethical consideration in the conduct of prehospital ambulance randomised controlled clinical trials: a systematic review. *BMC Medical Research Methodology*, 17(1): 142.

Arrow KJ (1963). Uncertainty and the welfare economics of medical care. *American Economic Review*, 53(5): 941–973.

References

Avis M (2003). Do we need methodological theory to do qualitative research? *Qualitative Health Research*, 13(7): 995–1004.

Bahm AJ (1993). *Axiology: The Science of Values*. Atlanta: Rodopi.

Ball L (2005). Setting the scene for the paramedic in primary care: a review of the literature. *Emergency Medical Journal*, 22(12): 896–900.

Baptiste I (2001). Qualitative data analysis: common phases, strategic difference. *Forum Qualitative Sozialforschung*, 2(3): article 22.

Barbour RS (2001). Checklists for improving rigour in qualitative research: a case of the tail wagging the dog? *BMJ*, 322: 1115–1117.

Bärnighausen T et al. (2017). Quasi-experimental study designs series – paper 4: uses and value. *Journal of Clinical Epidemiology*, 89: 21–29.

Barrett D and Heale R (2020). What are Delphi studies? *Evidence Based Nursing*, 23(3): 68–69.

Bauer M et al. (2020). Mortality in sepsis and septic shock in Europe, North America and Australia between 2009 and 2019 – results from a systematic review and meta-analysis. *Critical Care*, 24(1): 239.

Baxter P and Jack S (2008). Qualitative case study methodology: study design and implementation for novice researchers. *Qualitative Report*, 13(4): 544–559.

Beauchamp TL and Childress JF (2019). *Principles of Biomedical Ethics*, 8th edn. Oxford: Oxford University Press.

Beecher HK (1966). Ethics and clinical research. *New England Journal of Medicine*, 274(24): 1354–1360.

Bell F and Fitzpatrick D (2016). Pre-hospital hypoglycaemia referral pathways. *British Paramedic Journal*, 1(3): 29–31.

Benger JR et al. (2018). Effect of a strategy of a supraglottic airway device vs tracheal intubation during out-of-hospital cardiac arrest on functional outcome: the AIRWAYS-2 randomized clinical trial. *JAMA*, 320(8): 779–791.

Bernal JL, Cummins S and Gasparrini A (2017). Interrupted time series regression for the evaluation of public health interventions: a tutorial. *International Journal of Epidemiology*, 46(1): 348–355.

Bernard C (1957). *An Introduction to the Study of Experimental Medicine*, vol 400. New York: Courier Corporation.

Bernard SA et al. (2010). Prehospital rapid sequence intubation improves functional outcome for patients with severe traumatic brain injury: a randomised controlled trial. *Annals of Surgery*, 252(6): 959–965.

Bertero C (2012). Grounded theory methodology – has it become a movement? *International Journal of Qualitative Studies on Health and Well-being*, 7(1): 18571.

Berwick DM (2008). The science of improvement. *JAMA*, 299(10): 1182–1184.

Bhaskar R (1975). *A Realist Theory of Science*. London: Routledge.

Bhaskar R (2009). *Scientific Realism and Human Emancipation*. London: Routledge.

Bhaskar R (2014). *The Possibility of Naturalism: A Philosophical Critique of the Contemporary Human Sciences*. London: Routledge.

Biesta GJJ and Burbules NC (2003). *Pragmatism and Educational Research*. Washington: Rowman and Littlefield Publishers.

Bigham B and Welsford M (2015). Applying hospital evidence to paramedicine: issues of indirectness, validity and knowledge translation. *Canadian Journal of Emergency Medicine*, 17(3): 281–285.

Blome C, Sondermann H and Augustin M (2017). Accepted standards on how to give a medical research presentation: a systematic review of expert opinion papers. *GMS Journal of Medical Education*, 34(1): Doc11.

Bombak AE and Hanson HM (2017). A critical discussion of patient engagement in research. *Journal of Patient-Centred Research and Reviews*, 4(1): 39.

References

Bonell C et al. (2018). Are randomised controlled trials positivist? Reviewing the social science and philosophy literature to assess positivist tendencies of trials of social interventions in public health and health services. *Trials*, 19: 1–12.

Booker MJ et al. (2018). 'Primary care sensitive' situations that result in an ambulance attendance: a conversation analytic study of UK emergency '999' call recordings. *BMJ Open*, 8(11): e023727.

Booth A (2017). Finding the evidence. In: Hoffmann T, Bennett S and Del Mar C (eds) *Evidence Based Practice Across the Health Professions*, 3rd edn. Oxford: Elsevier, pp. 34–48.

Bootland D (2017). *Critical Appraisal from Papers to Patient: A Practical Guide*. Oxford: Taylor and Francis Group.

Bordage G (2009). Conceptual frameworks to illuminate and magnify. *Medical Education*, 43(4): 312–319.

Boswell C and Cannon S (2020). Connection between research and evidence based practice. In: Boswell C and Cannon S (eds) *Introduction to Nursing Research – Incorporating Evidence-Based Practice*, 5th edn. Burlington: Jones and Bartlett Learning, pp. 1–30.

Bourhis J (2017). Narrative Literature Review. In: Allen M (ed.) *The Sage Encyclopaedia of Communication Research Methods*. London: Sage, pp. 1076–1077.

Bowles KA et al. (2024). A scoping review of out-of-hospital research in Ireland from 2000 to 2022. *Paramedicine*, 21: 6.

Bradshaw C, Atkinson S and Doody O (2017). Employing a qualitative description approach in health care research. *Global Qualitative Nursing Research*, 4(1): 1–8.

Brandt AM (1978). Racism and research: the case of the Tuskegee syphilis study. *Hastings Centre Report*, 8(6): 21–29.

Braun V and Clarke V (2021a). *Thematic Analysis: A Practical Guide*. London: Sage.

Braun V and Clarke V (2021b). To saturate or not to saturate? Questioning data saturation as a useful concept for thematic analysis and sample-size rationales, *Qualitative Research in Sport, Exercise and Health*, 13: 201–216.

Bressers G, Brydges M and Paradis E (2020). Ethnography in health professions education: slowing down and thinking deeply. *Medical Education*, 54(3): 225–233.

British Educational Research Association (2018). *Ethical Guidelines for Educational Research*, 4th edn. London: British Educational Research Association.

British Psychological Society (2021). *Code of Ethics and Conduct*. Leicester: British Psychological Society.

British Sociological Association (2017). *Statement of Ethical Practice*. Durham: British Sociological Association.

Brotsky S and Giles D (2007). Inside the 'Pro-Ana' community: a covert online participant observation. *Eating Disorders*, 15: 93–109.

Brown MEL and Dueñas AN (2020). A medical science educator's guide to selecting a research paradigm: building a basis for better research. *Medical Science Educator*, 30(1): 545–553.

Brydges M (2022). Fractured: a study of intraprofessional paramedic dynamics on professionalization in Ontario, Canada. Unpublished thesis. https://macsphere.mcmaster.ca/handle/11375/27995

Brydges M and Batt AM (2023). Untangling the web: the need for theory, theoretical frameworks, and conceptual frameworks in paramedic research. *Paramedicine*, 20(4): 89–93.

Bryman A (2006). Integrating quantitative and qualitative research: how is it done? *Qualitative Research*, 6(1): 97–113.

Burger HU et al. (2021). The use of external controls: to what extent can it currently be recommended? *Pharmaceutical Statistics*, 20(6): 1002–1016.

Burges Watson DL et al. (2011). Evidence from the scene: paramedic perspectives on involvement in out-of-hospital research. *Annals of Emergency Medicine*, 60(5): 641–650.

References

Burnard P et al. (2008). Analysing and presenting qualitative data. *British Dental Journal*, 204(8): 429–432.

Burrell G and Morgan G (2019). *Sociological Paradigms and Organisational Analysis: Elements of the Sociology of Corporate Life*, 2nd edn. London: Routledge.

Byford S and Raftery J (1998). Perspectives in economic evaluation. *BMJ*, 316(7143): 1529–1530.

Caelli K, Ray L and Mill J (2003). 'Clear as mud': toward greater clarity in generic qualitative research. *International Journal of Qualitative Methods*, 2(2): 1–23.

Callaham M (1997). Quantifying the scanty science of prehospital emergency care. *Annals of Emergency Medicine*, 30(6): 785–790.

Carr W and Kemmis S (2003). *Becoming Critical: Education Knowledge and Action Research*. London: Routledge.

Carroll DL et al. (1997). Barriers and facilitators to the utilization of nursing research. *Clinical Nurse Specialist*, 11(5): 207–212.

Cavanagh N et al. (2023). Looking back to inform the future: a review of published paramedicine research. *BMC Health Services Research*, 23(1): 108.

Centre for Reviews and Dissemination (2009). *Systematic Reviews: CRD's Guidance for Undertaking Reviews in Healthcare*. York: Centre for Reviews and Dissemination/University of York.

Chamberlain K (2000). Methodolatry and qualitative health research. *Journal of Health Psychology*, 5(3): 285–296.

Charlton K, Franklin J and McNaughton R (2019). Phenomenological study exploring ethics in prehospital research from the paramedic's perspective: experiences from the PARAMEDIC2 trial in a UK ambulance service. *Emergency Medicine Journal*, 36(9): 535–540.

Charmaz K (2006). *Constructing Grounded Theory: A Practical Guide Through Qualitative Analysis*. London: Sage.

Charmaz K (2014). *Constructing Grounded Theory*. London: Sage.

Clark LV et al. (2021). Mental health, well-being and support interventions for UK ambulance services staff: an evidence map, 2000 to 2020. *British Paramedic Journal*, 5(4): 25–39.

Cochrane AL (1972). *Effectiveness and Efficiency: Random Reflections on Health Services*. London: Nuffield Provincial Hospitals Trust.

Cochrane AL (1989). Foreword. In: Chalmers I, Enkin M, Keirse MJNC (eds) *Effective Care in Pregnancy and Childbirth*. Oxford: Oxford University Press, p. iii.

Cohen J (1988). *Statistical Power Analysis for the Behavioural Sciences*, 2nd edn. Hillsdale: Erlbaum.

College of Paramedics (2023). *Post Registration Career Framework*, 5th edn. Bridgwater: College of Paramedics.

Collins B (2018). *Adoption and Spread of Innovation in the NHS*. London: King's Fund.

Colorafi KJ and Evans B (2016). Qualitative descriptive methods in health science research. *Health Environments Research and Design Journal*, 9(4): 16–25.

Commission Directive 2005/28/EC of 8 April 2005 laying down principles and detailed guidelines for good clinical practice as regards investigational medicinal products for human use, OJ L 91, 9.4.2005, pp. 13–19.

Coppola A et al. (2022). Patient and public involvement and engagement with cardiac arrest survivors. *British Paramedic Journal*, 7(1): 29–35.

Corbin JM and Strauss AL (2015). *Basics of Qualitative Research: Techniques and Procedures for Developing Grounded Theory*, 4th edn. Los Angeles: Sage.

Cormack S (2022). Development of a behavioural marker system for the non-technical skills used by paramedics managing an out-of-hospital cardiac arrest. Unpublished PhD thesis, Coventry University. https://pureportal.coventry.ac.uk/en/studentTheses/development-of-a-behavioural-marker-system-for-the-non-technical-

References

Corrigan O (2003). Empty ethics: the problem with informed consent. *Sociology of Health and Illness*, 25(3): 768–792.

Coulter A and Ellins J (2007). Effectiveness of strategies for informing, educating and involving patients. *BMJ*, 335: 24–27.

Couper K et al. (2024). Route of drug administration in out-of-hospital cardiac arrest: a protocol for a randomised controlled trial (PARAMEDIC-3). *Resuscitation Plus*, 17: 100544.

Cowden S and Singh G (2007). The 'user': friend, foe or fetish? A critical exploration of user involvement in health and social care. *Critical Social Policy*, 27(1): 5–23.

Crabtree BF and Miller WL (1999). *Doing Qualitative Research*. London: Sage.

CRASH-3 Trial Collaborators (2019). Effects of tranexamic acid on death, disability, vascular occlusive events and other morbidities in patients with acute traumatic brain injury (CRASH-3): a randomised, placebo-controlled trial. *Lancet*, 394(10210): 1713–1723.

Creswell JW (2014). *A Concise Introduction to Mixed Methods Research*. Los Angeles: Sage.

Creswell JW (2016). *Qualitative Inquiry and Research Design: Choosing Among Five Approaches*. Los Angeles: Sage.

Creswell JW et al. (2003). Advanced mixed methods research designs. In: Tashakkori A and Teddlie C (eds) *Handbook of Mixed Methods in Social and Behavioural Research*. Thousand Oaks: Sage, pp. 209–240.

Crocker JC et al. (2017). Is it worth it? Patient and public views on the impact of their involvement in health research and its assessment: a UK-based qualitative interview study. *Health Expectations*, 20(3): 519–528.

Crotty M (1998). *Foundations of Social Research: Meaning and Perspective in the Research Process*. London: Sage.

Curtis B and Curtis C (2011). *Social Research*. Los Angeles: Sage.

Curtis L (2013). *Unit Costs of Health and Social Care 2013*. Canterbury: PSSRU.

Cutcliffe JR (2003). Reconsidering reflexivity: introducing the case for intellectual entrepreneurship. *Qualitative Health Research*, 13(1): 136–148.

Cutcliffe JR and McKenna HP (1999). Establishing the credibility of qualitative research findings: the plot thickens. *Journal of Advanced Nursing*, 30(2): 374–380.

Cypress BS (2017). Rigor or reliability and validity in qualitative research: perspectives, strategies, reconceptualization, and recommendations. *Dimensions of Critical Care Nursing*, (36)4: 253–263.

Davies SC et al. (2016). The NIHR at 10: transforming clinical research. *Clinical Medicine*, 16(6): 501–502.

Davis DP et al. (2003). The effect of paramedic rapid sequence intubation on outcome in patients with severe traumatic brain injury. *Journal of Trauma*, 54(3): 444–453.

Deeks J et al. (2003). Evaluating non-randomised intervention studies. *Health Technology Assessment*, 7(27): iii–173.

Denzin N and Lincoln Y (eds) (2000). *Handbook of Qualitative Research*, 2nd edn. Thousand Oaks: Sage.

Department of Health (2008). *High Quality Care for All. NHS Next Stage Review Final Report*. London: Stationery Office.

Department of Health (2010). *Building the Evidence Base in Prehospital Urgent and Emergency Care: A Review of Research Evidence and Priorities for Future Research*. London: Stationery Office.

Des Jarlais DC et al. (2004). Improving the reporting quality of nonrandomized evaluations of behavioral and public health interventions: the TREND statement. *American Journal of Public Health*, 94(3): 361–366.

Dickson JM et al. (2016). Cross-sectional study of the prehospital management of adult patients with a suspected seizure (EPIC1). *BMJ Open*, 6(2): e010573.

References

Dickson JM et al. (2017a). An alternative care pathway for suspected seizures in pre-hospital care: a service evaluation. *British Paramedic Journal*, 2(2): 22–28.

Dickson JM et al. (2017b). Cross-sectional study of the hospital management of adult patients with a suspected seizure (EPIC2). *BMJ Open*, 7(7): e015696.

Dixon S et al. (2009). Is it cost effective to introduce paramedic practitioners for older people to the ambulance service? Results of a cluster randomised controlled trial. *Emergency Medicine Journal*, 26: 446–451.

Dixon-Woods M et al. (2011). Problems and promises of innovation: why healthcare needs to rethink its love/hate relationship with the new. *BMJ Quality and Safety*, 20(Suppl 1): i47–51.

Donabedian A (1966). Evaluating the quality of medical care. *Milbank Memorial Fund Quarterly*, 44(3): 166–206.

Draper J (2015). Ethnography: principles, practice and potential. *Nursing Standard*, 29(36): 36–41.

Dudley L et al. (2015). A little more conversation please? Qualitative study of researchers' and patients' interview accounts of training for patient and public involvement in clinical trials. *Trials*, 16: 190.

Dumas F et al. (2014). Is epinephrine during cardiac arrest associated with worse outcomes in resuscitated patients? *Journal of the American College of Cardiology*, 64(22): 2360–2367.

Eaton G (2024a). Using realist approaches to explain and understand the optimal use of paramedics in primary care. Unpublished PhD thesis, University of Oxford. http://dx.doi.org/10.5287/ora-jnbpqrey5

Eaton G (2024b). An introduction to ethics. In: Eaton G (ed.) *Law and Ethics for Paramedics*, 3rd edn. Bridgwater: Class Professional Publishing, pp. 19–34.

Eaton G, Mahtani K and Catterall M (2018). The evolving role of paramedics – a NICE problem to have? *Journal of Health Services Research and Policy*, 23(3): 193–195.

Eaton G et al. (2020). Contribution of paramedics in primary and urgent care: a systematic review. *British Journal of General Practice*, 70(695): e421–e426.

Eaton-Williams P et al. (2020). A national survey of ambulance paramedics on the identification of patients with end of life care needs. *British Paramedic Journal*, 5(3): 8–14.

Economic and Social Research Council (2022). *Framework for Research Ethics*. Swindon: Economic and Social Research Council.

Egly J et al. (2011). Assessing the impact of prehospital intubation on survival in out-of-hospital cardiac arrest. *Prehospital Emergency Care*, 15(1): 44–49.

Elmore SA and Weston EH (2020). Predatory journals: what they are and how to avoid them. *Toxicologic Pathology*, 48(4): 607–610.

Emmanuel EE, Wendler D and Grady C (2000). What makes clinical research ethical? *JAMA*, 283(20): 2701–2711.

Emond K, Furness S and Deacon-Crouch M (2015). Undergraduate paramedic students' perception of mental health using a pre-and post-questionnaire. *Australasian Journal of Paramedicine*, 12(5): 1–6.

Eschmann NM et al. (2010). The association between emergency medical services staffing patterns and out-of-hospital cardiac arrest survival. *Prehospital Emergency Care*, 14(1): 71–77.

Feilzer MY (2010). Doing mixed methods research pragmatically: implications for the rediscovery of pragmatism as a research paradigm. *Journal of Mixed Methods Research*, 4(1): 6–16.

Feldman A et al. (2015). Randomised controlled trial of a scoring aid to improve Glasgow Coma Scale scoring by emergency medical services providers. *Annals of Emergency Medicine*, 65(3): 325–329.

Fetters MD, Curry LA and Creswell JW (2013). Achieving integration in mixed methods designs – principles and practices. *Health Services Research*, 48(6 Pt 2): 2134–2156.

References

Finlay L (2003). The reflexive journey: mapping multiple routes. In: Finlay L and Gough G (eds) *Reflexivity: A Practical Guide for Researchers in Health and Social Sciences*. Oxford: Blackwell Science, pp. 3–20.

First S, Tomlins L and Swinburn A (2012). From trade to profession – the professionalisation of the paramedic workforce. *Journal of Paramedic Practice*, 4(7): 378–381.

Flyvbjerg B. (2006). Five misunderstandings about case-study research. *Qualitative Inquiry*, 12(2): 219–245.

Foley G and Timonen V (2014). Using grounded theory method to capture and analyze health care experiences. *Health Services Research*, 50(4): 1195–1210.

Ford-Jones PC (2019). Mental health and psychosocial calls in the prehospital setting in Ontario: a qualitative case study. Unpublished PhD thesis, York University, Toronto. https://hdl.handle.net/10315/37469

Fothergill RT et al. (2013). Does use of the recognition of stroke in the emergency room stroke assessment tool enhance stroke recognition by ambulance clinicians? *Stroke*, 44(11): 3007–3012.

Fouche PF et al. (2019). The association of paramedic rapid sequence intubation and survival in out-of-hospital stroke. *Emergency Medicine Journal*, 36(7): 416–422.

Frieden TR (2017). Evidence for health decision making – beyond randomized, controlled trials. *New England Journal of Medicine*, 377(5): 465–475.

Gale NK et al. (2013). Using the framework method for the analysis of qualitative data in multi-disciplinary health research. *BMC Medical Research Methodology*, 13: 117.

Gans HJ (1962). *The Urban Villagers: Group and Class in the Life of Italian-Americans*. New York: Free Press.

Gates S et al. (2015). Mechanical chest compression for out of hospital cardiac arrest: systematic review and meta-analysis. *Resuscitation*, 94: 91–97.

Gaw A (2009). *Trial by Fire: Lessons from the History of Clinical Trials*. Edinburgh: SA Press.

Gehlbach H and Artino AR (2018). The survey checklist (Manifesto). *Academic Medicine*, 93(3): 360–366.

Gehlbach H, Artino AR and Durning SJ (2010). AM last page: survey development guidance for medical education researchers. *Academic Medicine*, 85(5): 925.

General Medical Council (2013). *Good Practice in Research and Consent to Research*. London: GMC.

Gibson A et al. (2015). Exploring the impact of providing evidence-based medicine training to service users. *Research Involvement and Engagement*, 1: 10.

Given LM (ed.) (2008). *The SAGE Encyclopedia of Qualitative Research Methods*, vols 1 and 2. Los Angeles: SAGE.

Glaser B (2002). Constructivist grounded theory? *Forum: Qualitative Social Research*, 3(3): Art 12.

Glaser BG and Holton J (2004). Remodelling grounded theory. *Forum: Qualitative Social Research*, 5(2): Art 4.

Glaser BG and Strauss AL (1967). *The Discovery of Grounded Theory: Strategies for Qualitative Research*. Oxford: Routledge.

Goldman AI (2001). Social routes to belief and knowledge. *Monist*, 84(3): 346–367.

Goldstein J (2013). The assessment of frailty in community-dwelling older adults: a feasibility and validation study. Unpublished PhD thesis, Dalhousie University Halifax, Nova Scotia. https://DalSpace.library.dal.ca//handle/10222/56651

Goldstein T et al. (2014). When qualitative research meets theater: the complexities of performed ethnography and research-informed theater project design. *Qualitative Inquiry*, 20(5): 674–685.

Gorelick PB (2019). The global burden of stroke: persistent and disabling. *Lancet Neurology*, 18(5): 417–418.

References

Grady D, Cummings SR and Hulley SB (2013). Alternative clinical trial designs and implementation issues. In: Hulley SB et al. (eds) *Designing Clinical Research*, 4th edn. Philadelphia: Lippincott Williams and Wilkins, pp. 151–170.

Grant BM and Giddings LS (2002). Making sense of methodologies: a paradigm framework for the novice researcher. *Contemporary Nurse*, 13(1): 10–28.

Grbich C (2013). *Qualitative Data Analysis*. London: Sage.

Green J and Thorogood N (2018). *Qualitative Methods for Health Research*, 4th edn. Los Angeles: Sage.

Greenhalgh T (2019). *How to Read a Paper: The Basics of Evidence-based Medicine and Healthcare*, 6th edn. London: Wiley-Blackwell.

Greenhalgh T et al. (2004). Diffusion of innovations in service organizations: systematic review and recommendations. *Millbank Quarterly*, 82(4): 581–629.

Grimshaw JM et al. (2012). Knowledge translation of research findings. *Implementation Science*, 7(1): 50.

Grochowska A, Gawron A and Bodys-Cupak I (2022). Stress-inducing factors vs. the risk of occupational burnout in the work of nurses and paramedics. *International Journal of Environmental Research and Public Health*, 19(9): 5539.

Guba EG and Lincoln YS (1994). Competing paradigms in qualitative research. In: Denzin LK and Lincoln YS (eds) *Handbook of Qualitative Research*. Thousand Oaks: Sage, pp. 105–117.

Guetterman TC, Fetters MD and Creswell JW (2015). Integrating quantitative and qualitative results in health science mixed methods research through joint displays. *Annals of Family Medicine*, 13: 554–561.

Gupta R et al. (2011). Pain management policy formulation at a tertiary care teaching institute in India: a prospective observational study. *Perspectives in Clinical Research*, 2(3): 109–112.

Guyatt GH (1991). Evidence based medicine. *American College of Physicians Journal Club*, 114(suppl. 2): A–16.

Häikiö K et al. (2023). Reduced quality of life, more technical challenges, and less study motivation among paramedic students after one year of the COVID-19 pandemic – a survey study. *BMC Medical Education*, 23(1): 136.

Hall WA and Callery P (2001). Enhancing the rigor of grounded theory: incorporating reflexivity and relationality. *Qualitative Health Research*, 11(2): 257–272.

Hallett RE and Barber K (2014). Ethnographic research in a cyber era. *Journal of Contemporary Ethnography*, 43(3): 306–330.

Hamm RM (1988). Clinical intuition and clinical analysis: expertise and the cognitive continuum. In: Dowie J and Elstein A (eds) *Professional Judgment: A Reader in Clinical Decision Making*. Cambridge: Cambridge University Press, pp. 78–108

Hammersley M (1992). *What's Wrong with Ethnography?* London: Routledge.

Hammersley M and Atkinson P (1995). *Ethnography: Principles in Practice*, 2nd edn. London: Routledge.

Hanif MA, Kaji AH and Niemann JT (2010). Advanced airway management does not improve outcome of out-of-hospital cardiac arrest. *Academic Emergency Medicine*, 17(9): 926–931.

Hansen M et al. (2016). Understanding the value of mixed methods research: the Children's Safety Initiative-Emergency Medical Services. *Emergency Medicine Journal*, 33: 489–494.

Hariton E and Locascio JJ (2018). Randomised controlled trials – the gold standard for effectiveness research: study design: randomised controlled trials. *British Journal of Obstetrics and Gynaecology*, 125(13): 1716.

Harris J, Grafton K and Cooke J (2020). Developing a consolidated research framework for clinical allied health professionals practising in the UK. *BMC Health Services Research*, 20(1): 852.

Harrison H et al. (2017). Case study research: Foundations and methodological orientations. *Forum: Qualitative Social Research*, 18(1).

Health and Care Professions Council (2023). *Paramedics. Standards of Proficiency*. London: Health and Care Professions Council.

Health Foundation (2014). *Improvement collaboratives in health care*. Available at: www.health.org.uk/publications/improvement-collaboratives-in-health-care

Health Foundation (2015). *Evaluation: What to Consider. Commonly Asked Questions about How to Approach Evaluation of Quality Improvement in Health Care*. London: Health Foundation.

Health Foundation (2021). *Quality Improvement Made Simple*. London: Health Foundation.

Health Research Authority (2018a). *Is my study research?* Available at: www.hra-decisiontools.org.uk/research/

Health Research Authority (2018b). *Do I need NHS REC approval?* Available at: www.hra-decisiontools.org.uk/ethics/

Health Research Authority (2020a). *Confidentiality Advisory Group*. Available at: https://www.hra.nhs.uk/about-us/committees-and-services/confidentiality-advisory-group/

Health Research Authority (2020b). *Governance arrangements for research ethics committees*. Available at: www.hra.nhs.uk/planning-and-improving-research/policies-standards-legislation/governance-arrangement-research-ethics-committees/

Health Research Authority (2022a). *Online booking service*. Available at: www.hra.nhs.uk/about-us/committees-and-services/online-booking-service/

Health Research Authority (2022b). *Safety reporting*. Available at: www.hra.nhs.uk/approvals-amendments/managing-your-approval/safety-reporting/

Health Research Authority (2023a). *HRA approval*. Available at: www.hra.nhs.uk/approvals-amendments/what-approvals-do-i-need/hra-approval/

Health Research Authority (2023b). *UK Policy Framework for Health and Social Care Research*. Available at: www.hra.nhs.uk/planning-and-improving-research/policies-standards-legislation/uk-policy-framework-health-social-care-research/

Health Services Research Team (2021). *999 EMS Research Forum – Annual Conference*. Available at: www.999emsresearch.co.uk/annual-conference

Hewitt CE et al. (2010). Assessing the impact of attrition in randomized controlled trials. *Journal of Clinical Epidemiology*, 63(11): 1264–1270.

Higgs J and Llewellyn G (1998). *Framing the Research Question*. Denver: Hampden Press.

Higgs R (2006). On telling patients the truth. In: Kuhse H and Singer P (eds) *Bioethics: An Anthology*, 3rd edn. Oxford: Blackwell Publishing, pp. 621–628.

Hildebrand DL (2011). Pragmatic democracy: inquiry, objectivity, and experience. *Metaphilosophy*, 42(5): 589–604.

Hirst E, Irving A and Goodacre S (2016). Patient and public involvement in emergency care research. *Emergency Medicine Journal*, 33(9): 665–670.

Houser J (2015). The importance of research as evidence in nursing. In: Houser J (ed.) *Nursing Research – Reading, Using, and Creating Evidence*. Burlington: Jones and Bartlett Learning, pp. 3–27.

Howard I et al. (2019). Improving the prehospital management of ST elevation myocardial infarction: a national quality improvement initiative. *BMJ Open Quality*, 8: e000508.

Hsia RY, Krumholz H and Shen YC (2020). Evaluation of STEMI regionalization on access, treatment, and outcomes among adults living in nonminority and minority communities. *JAMA Open Network*, 3: e2025874.

Huang CK et al. (2024). Open access research outputs receive more diverse citations. *Scientometrics*, 129: 825–845.

References

Hubble MW, Richards ME and Wilfong DA (2008). Estimates of cost-effectiveness of prehospital continuous positive airway pressure in the management of acute pulmonary edema. *Prehospital Emergency Care*, 12(3): 277–285.

Hulley S, Cummings SR and Newman TB (2013). Designing cross-sectional and cohort studies. In: Hulley SB et al. (eds) *Designing Clinical Research*, 4th edn. Philadelphia: Lippincott Williams and Wilkins, pp. 85–96.

Human Tissue Act 2004 (c. 30). London: The Stationary Office.

Human Tissue (Scotland) Act 2006 (asp 4). Edinburgh: The Stationery Office.

Husereau D et al. (2013). Consolidated Health Economic Evaluation Reporting Standards (CHEERS) statement. *BMJ*, 346: f1049.

Hutchinson LC et al. (2021). The role of lifestyle on NHS ambulance workers' wellbeing. *Journal of Workplace Behavioral Health*, 36(2): 159–171.

International Committee of Medical Journal Editors (ICMJE) (2024). *Defining the Role of Authors and Contributors*. Available at: https://www.icmje.org/recommendations/browse/roles-and-responsibilities/defining-the-role-of-authors-and-contributors.html

International Council for Harmonisation (ICH) (2023). *E6(R3) Good Clinical Practice: Consolidated Guideline 2023*. Available at: www.ich.org/

INVOLVE (2012). *Inclusion supplement*. Available at: www.invo.org.uk/current-work/diversity-and-inclusion/

INVOLVE (2021). *Briefing Notes for Researchers: Involving the Public in NHS, Public Health and Social Care Research*. Eastleigh: INVOLVE.

Ives J, Damery S and Redwood S (2012). PPI, paradoxes and Plato: who's sailing the ship? *Journal of Medical Ethics*, 39(3): 181–185.

James Lind Alliance (2021). *Stroke*. Available at: https://www.jla.nihr.ac.uk/priority-setting-partnerships/stroke

James Lind Alliance (2023). *Major Trauma (International) PSP*. Available at: https://www.jla.nihr.ac.uk/priority-setting-partnerships/major-trauma-international

Jenn NC (2006). Common ethical issues in research and publication. *Malaysian Family Physician*, 1(2–3): 74–76.

Jimenez O (2023). *Metaphors for qualitative research*. Available at: www.andrews.edu/~freed/qualmetaphor.htm

Johnson CO et al. (2019). Global, regional, and national burden of stroke, 1990–2016: a systematic analysis for the Global Burden of Disease Study 2016. *Lancet Neurology*, 18: 439–458.

Johnson JL, Adkins D and Chauvin S (2020). A review of the quality indicators of rigor in qualitative research. *American Journal of Pharmaceutical Education*, 84(1): 7120.

Johnson RB, Onwuegbuzie AJ and Turner LA (2007). Toward a definition of mixed methods research. *Journal of Mixed Methods Research*, 1: 112–133.

Joint Royal Colleges Ambulance Liaison Committee, Association of Ambulance Chief Executives (2013). *JRCALC Clinical Guidelines 2013*. Bridgwater: Class Professional Publishing.

Joint Royal Colleges Ambulance Liaison Committee, Association Of Ambulance Chief Executives (2016). *JRCALC Clinical Guidelines 2016*. Bridgwater: Class Professional Publishing.

Jones JK et al. (2019). Rapid Analgesia for Prehospital hip Disruption (RAPID): findings from a randomised feasibility study. *Pilot and Feasibility Studies*, 5(1): 1–13.

Kahlke RM (2014). Generic qualitative approaches: pitfalls and benefits of methodological mixology. *International Journal of Qualitative Methods*, 13(1): 37–52.

Kallio H (2016). Systematic methodological review: developing a framework for a qualitative semi-structured interview guide. *Journal of Advanced Nursing*, 72(12): 2954–2965.

References

Keeling P et al. (2003). Safety and feasibility of prehospital thrombolysis carried out by paramedics. *BMJ*, 327(7405): 27–28.

Keen L et al. (2018). Use of scratchcards for allocation concealment in a prehospital randomised controlled trial. *Emergency Medicine Journal*, 35(11): 708–710.

Kelly M (2010). The role of theory in qualitative health research. *Family Practice*, 27(3): 285–290.

Kemmis S and McTaggart R (2005). Participatory action research. Communicative action and the public sphere. In: Denzin NK and Lincoln YS (eds) *Handbook of Qualitative Research*. Los Angeles: Sage, pp. 559–603.

Kenny M and Fourie R (2015). Contrasting classic, Straussian, and constructivist grounded theory: methodological and philosophical conflicts. *Qualitative Report*, 20(8): 1270–1289.

Keunecke JG et al. (2019). Workload and influencing factors in non-emergency medical transfers: a multiple linear regression analysis of a cross-sectional questionnaire study. *BMC Health Service Research*, 19(1): 812.

Khan WAA et al. (2020). Sleep and mental health among paramedics from Australia and Saudi Arabia: a comparison study. *Clocks and Sleep*, 2(2): 246–257.

Krusenvik L (2016). *Using case studies as a scientific method: advantages and disadvantages*. Unpublished dissertation, Halmstad University, Halmstad. Available at: https://urn.kb.se/resolve?urn=urn:nbn:se:hh:diva-32625

Kuhn TS (1994). *The Structure of Scientific Revolutions*, 2nd edn. Chicago: University of Chicago Press.

Kvale S and Brinkmann S (2009). *Interviews: Learning the Craft of Qualitative Research Interviewing*. London: Sage.

LaDonna KA, Taylor T and Lingard L (2018). Why open-ended survey questions are unlikely to support rigorous qualitative insights. *Academic Medicine*, 93(3): 347–349.

Laine C (2009). Evidence based drug utilization. In: Waldman S et al. (eds) *Pharmacology and Therapeutics*. Philadelphia: W.B Saunders, pp. 41–50.

Lally J et al. (2020). Paramedic experiences of using an enhanced stroke assessment during a cluster randomised trial: a qualitative thematic analysis. *Emergency Medicine Journal*, 37(8): 480–485.

Langley GJ et al. (2009). *The Improvement Guide, A Practical Approach to Enhancing Organisational Performance*. San Francisco: Jossey-Bass.

Law GR and Pascoe SW (2013). *Statistical Epidemiology*. Wallingford: CABI.

Lazarus J, Iyer R and Fothergill R (2019). Paramedic attitudes and experiences of enrolling patients into the PARAMEDIC2 adrenaline trial: a qualitative survey within the London Ambulance Service. *BMJ*, 9(11).

Lewis TL et al. (2016). Ambulance smartphone tool for field triage of ruptured aortic aneurysms (FILTR): study protocol for a prospective observational validation of diagnostic accuracy. *BMJ Open*, 6(10): e011308.

Li M et al. (2021). Determining ambulance destinations when facing offload delays using a Markov decision process. *Omega*, 101: 102251.

Liamputtong P and Serry T (2013). Making sense of qualitative data. In: Liamputtong P (ed.) *Research Methods in Health: Foundations for Evidence-Based Practice*. Melbourne: Oxford University Press, pp. 365–379.

Lincoln YS and Guba E (1985). *Naturalist Inquiry*. Beverly Hills: Sage.

LoBiondo-Wood G and Haber J (2022). *Nursing Research: Methods and Critical Appraisal for Evidence-Based Practice*, 10th edn. St Louis: Elsevier.

Long T and Johnson M (2000). Rigour, reliability and validity in qualitative research. *Clinical Effectiveness in Nursing*, 4: 30–37.

References

Love S, Grumett J and Corkhill A (2020). Monitoring clinical trials during the COVID-19 pandemic. R&D Forum Symposia. Available at: rdforum.nhs.uk/wp-content/uploads/formidable/22/Sharon-Love-Joanne-Grumett-Andrea-Corkhill.pdf

Lund H et al. (2016). Towards evidence based research. *BMJ*, 355: i5440.

Maanen JV (1979). The fact of fiction in organizational ethnography. *Administrative Science Quarterly*, 24(4): 539.

MacQuarrie S (2018). *Fit for duty: context and correlates of paramedic health status and job performance*. Unpublished PhD thesis, Charles Sturt University, Bathurst. Available at: https://researchoutput.csu.edu.au/files/71941964/Alexander_MacQuarrie_Thesis.pdf

Mahta A et al. (2021). Short- and long-term opioid use in survivors of subarachnoid hemorrhage. *Clinical Neurology and Neurosurgery*, 207: 106770.

Malterud K (2001). Qualitative research: standards, challenges, and guidelines. *Lancet*, 358(9280): 483–488.

Mann CJ (2003). Observational research methods. Research design II: cohort. cross sectional, and case-control studies. *Emergency Medicine Journal*, 20: 54–61.

Mansour T et al. (2022). International comparison of injury care structures, processes, and outcomes between integrated trauma systems in Québec, Canada, and Victoria, Australia. *Injury*, 53(9): 2907–2914.

Mansournia MA (2018). Case–control matching: effects, misconceptions, and recommendations. *European Journal of Epidemiology*, 33(1): 5–14.

Maso I (2003). Necessary subjectivity: exploiting researchers' motives, passions and prejudices in pursuit of answering 'true' questions. In: Finlay L and Gough B (eds) *Reflexivity: A Practical Guide for Researchers in Health and Social Sciences*. Oxford: Blackwell Science, pp. 39–51.

Mason S et al. (2007). Effectiveness of paramedic practitioners in attending 999 calls from elderly people in the community: cluster randomised controlled trial. *BMJ*, 335(7626): 919.

Mason S et al. (2012). A pragmatic quasi-experimental multi-site community intervention trial evaluating the impact of emergency care practitioners in different UK health settings on patient pathways (NEECaP Trial). *Emergency Medicine Journal*, 29(1): 47–53.

Mathie E et al. (2018). Reciprocal relationships and the importance of feedback in patient and public involvement: a mixed methods study. *Health Expectations*, 21(5): 899–908.

Mausz J (2022). *A role identity perspective on paramedic mental health*. Unpublished PhD thesis, McMasters University, Hamilton. Available at: https://macsphere.mcmaster.ca/handle/11375/27823

May C (2003). Where do we stand in relation to the data? In: Latimer J (ed.) *Advanced Qualitative Research for Nursing*. Oxford: Blackwell, pp. 17–31.

Mays N and Pope C (1995). Rigour and qualitative research. *BMJ*, 311: 109–112.

McClelland G (2013). The research paramedic: a new role. *Journal of Paramedic Practice*, 5(10): 582–586.

McClelland G, Limmer M and Charlton K (2023). The RESearch PARamedic Experience (RESPARE) study: a qualitative study exploring the experiences of research paramedics working in the United Kingdom. *British Paramedic Journal*, 7(4): 14–22.

McCombes S (2023). Writing Strong Research Questions | Criteria & Examples. Available at: www.scribbr.com/research-process/research-questions/

McDonnell A, Wilson R and Goodacre S (2006). Evaluating and implementing new services. *BMJ*, 332(7533): 109–112.

McErlean M et al. (2023). The reporting standards of randomised controlled trials in leading medical journals between 2019 and 2020: a systematic review. *Irish Journal of Medical Science*, 192(1): 73–80.

McInnes MDF et al. (2018). Preferred reporting items for a systematic review and meta-analysis of diagnostic test accuracy studies: the PRISMA-DTA Statement. *JAMA*, 319(4): 388–396.

McManamny T et al. (2014). Mixed Methods and its application in prehospital research: a systematic review. *Journal of Mixed Methods Research*, 9: 214–231.

McNiff J and Whitehead J (2010). *You and Your Action Research Project*. London: Routledge.

Meats E et al. (2009). Evidence based medicine teaching in UK medical schools. *Medical Teacher*, 31(4): 332–337.

Medical Research Council (2014). *Good Research Practice: Principles and Guidelines*. London: Medical Research Council.

Medical Research Council (2021). *Involving Children in Research: MRC And ESRC Joint Guidance*. London: Medical Research Council.

Medicines for Human Use (Clinical Trials) (Amendment) (EU Exit) Regulations 2019 (SI 2019/744). London: The Stationery Office.

Meinefeld W (2004). Hypothesis and prior knowledge in qualitative research In: Flick U, von Kardorff E and Steinke I (eds) *A Companion to Qualitative Research*. Los Angeles: Sage, pp. 153–158.

Merriam SB and Tisdell EJ (2009). *Qualitative Research: A Guide to Design and Implementation*. San Francisco: Jossey-Bass.

Meyer J (2000). Qualitative research in health care: using qualitative methods in health related action research. *BMJ*, 320(7228): 178–181.

Miah J et al. (2020). Evaluation of a research awareness training programme to support research involvement of older people with dementia and their care partners. *Health Expectations*, 23(5): 1177–1190.

Miake-Lye IM et al. (2016). What is an evidence map? A systematic review of published evidence maps and their definitions, methods, and products. *Systematic Reviews*, 5(1): 1–21.

Michelet F et al. (2023). Randomised controlled trial of analgesia for the management of acute severe pain from traumatic injury: study protocol for the paramedic analgesia comparing ketamine and morphine in trauma (PACKMaN). *Scandinavian Journal of Trauma, Resuscitation and Emergency Medicine*, 31(1): 84.

Miles M (1979). Qualitative data as an attractive nuisance: the problem of analysis. *Administrative Science Quarterly*, 24(4): 560–601.

Miles MB and Huberman AM (1994). *Qualitative Data Analysis: An Expanded Sourcebook*, 2nd edn. Los Angeles: Sage.

Mills J and Fitzgerald M (2008). The changing role of practice nurses in Australia: an action research study. *Australian Journal of Advanced Nursing*, 26(1): 16–20.

Mitra B et al. (2021). Protocol for a multicentre prehospital randomised controlled trial investigating tranexamic acid in severe trauma: the PATCH-Trauma trial. *BMJ Open*, 11: e046522.

Modayil PC, Panchikkeel RK and Alex N (2009). Audit in clinical practice. *Indian Journal of Otolaryngology, Head and Neck Surgery*, 61: 109–111.

Montalescot G et al. (2014). Prehospital ticagrelor in ST-segment elevation myocardial infarction. *New England Journal of Medicine*, 371(11): 1016–1027.

Moore C et al. (2014). Paramedic-supplied 'take home' naloxone: protocol for cluster randomised feasibility study. *BMJ Open*, 4(3): e004712.

Moore GF et al. (2015). Process evaluation of complex interventions: Medical Research Council guidance. *BMJ*, 350: h1258.

Morrell-Scott NE (2018). Using diaries to collect data in phenomenological research. *Nurse Researcher*, 25(4): 26–29.

Morrison LJ et al. (2009). The Toronto Prehospital Hypertonic Resuscitation-Head Injury and Multi-Organ Dysfunction Trial (TOPHR HIT) – methods and data collection tools. *Trials*, 10: 105.

Morse J (2001). Situating grounded theory within qualitative inquiry. In: Schreiber RS and Stern PN (eds) *Using Grounded Theory in Nursing*. New York: Springer, pp. 1–16.

References

Motulsky H (1995). *Intuitive Biostatistics*. Oxford: Oxford University Press.

Mueller RA (2019). Episodic narrative interview: capturing stories of experience with a methods fusion. *International Journal of Qualitative Methods*, 18.

Munro SF et al. (2018). The use and impact of 12-lead electrocardiograms in acute stroke patients: a systematic review. *European Heart Journal Acute Cardiovascular Care*, 7: 257–263.

Murphy-Jones G and Timmons S (2016). Paramedics' experiences of end-of-life care decision making with regard to nursing home residents: an exploration of influential issues and factors. *Emergency Medicine Journal*, 33(10): 722–726.

Myers R (1998). Prehospital management of acute myocardial infarction: electrocardiogram acquisition and interpretation, and thrombolysis by prehospital care providers. *Canadian Journal of Cardiology,* 14(10): 1231–1240.

Nakao JH et al. (2014). Jolt accentuation of headache and other clinical signs: poor predictors of meningitis in adults. *American Journal of Emergency Medicine*, 32(1): 24–28.

NASMeD (2014). NASMeD set out future clinical priorities for Ambulance Services in England. *Association of Ambulance Chief Executives (AACE)*. Available at: https://aace.org.uk/news/nasmed-set-future-clinical-priorities-ambulance-services-england/

National Institute for Health and Care Research (NIHR) (2021a). *Good Clinical Practice (GCP)*. Available at: www.nihr.ac.uk/career-development/clinical-research-courses-and-support/good-clinical-practice

National Institute for Health and Care Research (2021b). *Trauma and Emergency Care and the James Lind Alliance*. Available at: www.jla.nihr.ac.uk/

National Institute for Health and Care Research (2024). *Research Support Service*. Available at: www.nihr.ac.uk/explore-nihr/support/research-support-service/

NETSCC (2021a). *Clinical Trials Toolkit: Audit*. Available at: www.ct-toolkit.ac.uk/routemap/audit/

NETSCC (2021b). *Clinical Trials Toolkit: Pharmacovigilance*. Available at: https://www.ct-toolkit.ac.uk/routemap/pharmacovigilance

Neubauer BE, Witkop CT and Varpio L (2019). How phenomenology can help us learn from the experiences of others. *Perspectives on Medical Education*, 8(2): 90–97.

Newman TB et al. (2013). Designing case-control studies. In: Hulley SB et al. (eds) *Designing Clinical Research*, 4th edn. Philadelphia: Lippincott Williams and Wilkins, pp. 97–117.

Newton A, Hunt B and Williams J (2020). The paramedic profession: disruptive innovation and barriers to further progress. *Journal of Paramedic Practice* 12(4): 138–148.

NHS England (n.d.). *Clinical audit*. Available at: https://www.england.nhs.uk/clinaudit/

NHS England (2023). *Ambulance quality indicators*. Available at: www.england.nhs.uk/statistics/statistical-work-areas/ambulance-quality-indicators/

NHS Improvement (2018). Reference Costs 2017/18. Available at: https://webarchive.nationalarchives.gov.uk/ukgwa/20200501111106/https://improvement.nhs.uk/resources/reference-costs/

NICE (2013). *Guide to the methods of technology appraisal [PMG9]*. Available at: www.nice.org.uk/process/pmg9/chapter/foreword

NICE (2020). Acute Coronary Syndromes NG185. London: National Institute for Health and Care Excellence.

NICOR (2024). *Myocardial Ischaemia National Audit Project (MINAP)*. Available at: www.nicor.org.uk/national-cardiac-audit-programme/heart-attack-audit-minap/

Oakley A et al. (2006). Process evaluation in randomised controlled trials of complex interventions. *BMJ*, 332(7538): 413–416.

O'Cathain A, Murphy E and Nicholl J (2007). Integration and publications as indicators of 'yield' from mixed methods studies. *Journal of Mixed Methods Research*, 1: 147–163.

References

O'Cathain A, Murphy E and Nicholl J (2008). The quality of mixed methods studies in health services research. *Journal of Health Services Research and Policy*, 13(2): 92–98.

O'Cathain A, Murphy E and Nicholl J (2010). Three techniques for integrating data in mixed methods studies. *BMJ*, 341: c4587.

O'Cathain A and Thomas KH (2004). 'Any other comments?' Open questions on questionnaires – a bane or a bonus to research? *BMC Medical Research Methodology*, 4: 25.

O'Cathain A et al. (2013). What can qualitative research do for randomised controlled trials? A systematic mapping review. *BMJ Open*, 3(6): e002889.

Ocloo J and Matthews R (2016). From tokenism to empowerment: progressing patient and public involvement in healthcare improvement. *BMJ Quality and Safety*, 16(25): 626–632.

Olaussen A et al. (2017). Paramedic literature search filters: optimised for clinicians and academics. *BMC Medical Informatics and Decision Making*, 17(1): 146.

O'Leary Z (2018). *Little Quick Fix: Research Question*. Los Angeles: Sage.

Omery A and Williams RP (1999). An appraisal of research utilization across the United States. *Journal of Nursing Administration*, 29(12): 50–56.

Ostadal P et al. (2023). Extracorporeal membrane oxygenation in the therapy of cardiogenic shock: results of the ECMO-CS randomized clinical trial. *Circulation*, 147(6): 454–464.

Ottrey E, Jong J and Porter J (2019). Authors' response. *Journal of the Academy of Nutrition and Dietetics*, 119(1): 31–32.

Ozdemir BA et al. (2015). Research activity and the association with mortality. *PLoS One*, 10(2): e0118253.

Pacifico Silva H et al. (2018). Introducing responsible innovation in health: a policy-oriented framework. *Health Research Policy and Systems*, 16(1): 90.

Page MJ et al. (2021). The PRISMA 2020 statement: an updated guideline for reporting systematic reviews. *BMJ*, 372: n71.

Pannucci CJ and Wilkins EG (2010). Identifying and avoiding bias in research. *Plastic and Reconstructive Surgery*, 126(2): 619–625.

Paramedic PhD (2021). *Statistics*. Available at: www.paramedicphd.com/statistics

Park Y, Konge L and Artino A (2020). The positivism paradigm of research. *Academic Medicine*, 95(5): 690–694.

Patino M and Ferreira JC (2018). Internal and external validity: can you apply research study results to your patients? *Jornal Brasileiro de Pneumologia*, 44(3): 183.

Paulus T, Lester J and Dempster P (2014). *Digital Tools for Qualitative Research*. Los Angeles: Sage.

Peat M et al. (2010). Scoping review and approach to appraisal of interventions intended to involve patients in patient safety. *Journal of Health Services Research and Policy*, 15(Suppl 1): 17–25.

Pedley DK et al. (2003). Prospective observational cohort study of time saved by prehospital thrombolysis for ST elevation myocardial infarction delivered by paramedics. *BMJ*, 327(7405): 22–26.

Perera N et al. (2023). 'If you miss that first step in the chain of survival, there is no second step' – emergency ambulance call-takers' experiences in managing out-of-hospital cardiac arrest calls. *PLoS One*, 18(3): e0279521.

Perkins GD et al. (2015). Mechanical versus manual chest compression for out-of-hospital cardiac arrest (PARAMEDIC): a pragmatic, cluster randomised controlled trial. *Lancet*, 385(9972): 947–955.

Perkins GD et al. (2016). Pre-hospital assessment of the role of adrenaline: measuring the effectiveness of drug administration in cardiac arrest (PARAMEDIC2): trial protocol. *Resuscitation*, 108: 75–81.

Perkins GD et al. (2018). A randomized trial of epinephrine in out-of-hospital cardiac arrest. *New England Journal of Medicine*, 379(8): 711–721.

References

Phillips AW, Reddy S and Durning SJ (2016). Improving response rates and evaluating nonresponse bias in surveys: AMEE Guide No. 102. *Medical Teacher*, 38(3): 217–228.

Phillips MR et al. (2021). Risk of bias: why measure it, and how? *Eye*, 36(2): 346–348.

Pilbery R (2018) How do paramedics learn and maintain the skill of tracheal intubation? A rapid evidence review. *British Paramedic Journal*, 3(2): 8–15.

Pilbery R, Young T and Hodge A (2022). The effect of a specialist paramedic primary care rotation on appropriate non-conveyance decisions (SPRAINED) study: a controlled interrupted time series analysis. *British Paramedic Journal*, 7(1): 9–18.

Pitt K (2002). Prehospital selection of patients for thrombolysis by paramedics. *Emergency Medicine Journal*, 19(3): 260–263.

Platt A (2020). A service evaluation of transport destination and outcome of patients with post-ROSC STEMI in an English ambulance service. *British Paramedic Journal*, 5(1): 32–36.

Plsek PE and Greenhalgh T (2001). The challenge of complexity in health care. *BMJ*, 323(7313): 625–628.

Pope C and Mays N (1995). Qualitative research: reaching the parts other methods cannot reach: an introduction to qualitative methods in health and health services research. *BMJ*, 311: 42–45.

Pope C and Mays N (2009). Critical reflections on the rise of qualitative research. *BMJ*, 339: b3425.

Pope C et al. (2013). Using computer decision support systems in NHS emergency and urgent care: ethnographic study using normalisation process theory. *BMC Health Service Research*, 13: 111.

Porter A et al. (2020). Electronic health records in ambulances: the ERA multiple-methods study. *Health Services and Delivery Research*, 8(10).

Pourhoseingholi MA, Baghestani AR and Vahedi M. (2012). How to control confounding effects by statistical analysis. *Gastroenterology and Hepatology from Bed to Bench*, 5(2): 79–83.

Pratt B (2021). Achieving inclusive research priority-setting: what do people with lived experience and the public think is essential? *BMC Medical Ethics*, 22: 117.

Price CI et al. (2019). Paramedic Acute Stroke Treatment Assessment (PASTA): study protocol for a randomised controlled trial. *Trials*, 20(1): 121.

Price CI et al. (2020). Effect of an enhanced paramedic acute stroke treatment assessment on thrombolysis delivery during emergency stroke care: a cluster randomized clinical trial. *JAMA Neurology*, 77(7): 840–848.

Pringle J, Hendry C, McLafferty E (2011). Phenomenological approaches: challenges and choices. *Nurse Researcher*, 18(2): 7–18.

Public Involvement Impact Assessment Framework (PiiAF) (2021). *PiiAF Resources*. Available at: http://piiaf.org.uk/resources.php

Pyone T et al. (2015). Data collection tools for maternal and child health in humanitarian emergencies: a systematic review. *Bulletin of the World Health Organization*, 93(9): 648–658A.

Rabin R and Charro F (2001). EQ-SD: a measure of health status from the EuroQol Group. *Annals of Medicine*, 33(5): 337–343.

Rabinow P (1985). Discourse and power: on the limits of ethnographic texts. *Dialectical Anthropology*, 10: 1–13.

Reason P and Bradbury-Huang H (2007). *The SAGE Handbook of Action Research: Participative Inquiry and Practice*. London: Sage.

Reed B (2023). *What is the relationship between professional registration, identity and professionalisation in Australian Paramedics?* Unpublished thesis, University of Wollongong. Available at: https://ro.uow.edu.au/theses1/1676

Rees N et al. (2018). Paramedics' perceptions of the care they provide to people who self-harm: a qualitative study using evolved grounded theory methodology. *PLoS One*, 13(10): e0205813.

Reeves S, Kuper A and Hodges BD (2008). Qualitative research methodologies: ethnography. *BMJ*, 337(7668): 512–514.

References

Regulation (EU) No 536/2014 of the European Parliament and of the Council of 16 April 2014 on clinical trials on medicinal products for human use, OJ L 158, 27.5.2014, p. 1–76.

Renshaw J (2019). Medical research. In: Eaton G. (ed.) *Law and Ethics for Paramedics*. Bridgwater: Class Professional Publishing, pp. 213–233.

Reynolds J and Beresford R (2020). 'An active, productive life': narratives of and through participation on public and patient involvement in health research. *Qualitative Health Research*, 30(14): 2265–2277.

Rice TW (2008). The historical, ethical, and legal background of human-subjects research. *Respiratory Care*, 53(10): 1325–1329.

Ritchie J and Lewis J (2003). *Qualitative Research Practice: A Guide for Social Science Students and Researchers*. London: Sage.

Roberts I et al. (2013a). The CRASH-2 trial: a randomised controlled trial and economic evaluation of the effects of tranexamic acid on death, vascular occlusive events and transfusion requirement in bleeding trauma patients. *Health Technology Assessment*, 17(10): 1–79.

Roberts L et al. (2013b). The challenges of gaining ethics approval for ethnographic research in the pre-hospital setting. *Journal of Psychiatric and Mental Health Nursing*, 20(4): 374–378.

Rolfe U, Pope C and Crouch R (2020). Paramedic performance when managing patients experiencing mental health issues – exploring paramedics' presentation of self. *International Emergency Nursing*, 49: 100828.

Ross S and Naylor C (2017). *Quality Improvement in Mental Health*. London: King's Fund.

Rosser M (2012). Evidence based practice in paramedic practice. In: Griffiths P and Mooney GP (eds) *The Paramedic's Guide to Research*. Maidenhead: Open University Press, pp. 25–39.

Rostami P, Ashcroft DM and Tully MP (2018). A formative evaluation of the implementation of a medication safety data collection tool in English healthcare settings: a qualitative interview study using normalisation process theory. *PLoS One*, 13(2): e0192224.

Runacres J et al. (2024). Paramedics as researchers: a systematic review of paramedic perspectives of engaging in research activity from training to practice. *Journal of Emergency Medicine*, 66(6): e680–689.

Sackett D et al. (1996). Evidence based medicine: what it is and what it isn't: it's about integrating individual clinical expertise and the best external evidence. *BMJ*, 312(7023): 71–72.

Samarkandi OA et al. (2018). Research utilization barriers for emergency medical technicians in Saudi Arabia. *Advances in Medical Education and Practice*, 9: 519–526.

Samuel N, Steiner IP and Shavit I (2015). Prehospital pain management of injured children: a systematic review of current evidence. *American Journal of Emergency Medicine*, 33(3): 451–454.

Sandelowski M (2000). Whatever happened to qualitative description? *Research in Nursing and Health*, 23: 334–340.

Sandelowski M (2010). What's in a name? Qualitative description revisited. *Research in Nursing and Health*, 33(1): 77–84.

Scholz KH et al. (2020). Long-term effects of a standardized feedback-driven quality improvement program for timely reperfusion therapy in regional STEMI care networks. *European Heart Journal: Acute Cardiovascular Care*, 10(4): 397–405.

Schoonenboom J and Johnson RB (2017). How to construct a mixed methods research design. *Kölner Zeitschrift für Soziologie und Sozialpsychologie*, 69(Suppl 2): 107–131.

Schulz KF, Altman DG and Moher D (2010). CONSORT 2010 statement: updated guidelines for reporting parallel group randomised trials. *BMJ*, 340: c332.

Schulz KF and Grimes DA (2002). Case–control studies: research in reverse. *Lancet*, 359(9304): 431–434.

Scott A et al. (2020). Exempting low-risk health and medical research from ethics reviews: comparing Australia, the United Kingdom, the United States and the Netherlands. *Health Research Policy and Systems*, 18(1): 11.

References

Selwyn N (2014). 'So what?'... a question that every journal article needs to answer. *Learning, Media and Technology*, 39(1): 1–5.

Shannon B (2023). *What are the experiences of health service providers introducing alternative care pathways in a community setting?* Unpublished PhD thesis, Monash University, Melbourne. Available at: https://doi.org/10.26180/23647050.V1

Shapiro E (2019). A video analysis of clinical handovers between paramedics and emergency care staff. *British Paramedic Journal*, 4(1): 44.

Shaw L et al. (2011). Paramedic Initiated Lisinopril For Acute Stroke Treatment (PIL-FAST): study protocol for a pilot randomised controlled trial. *Trials*, 31(12): 1–11.

Shaw S, Boynton PM and Greenhalgh T (2005). Research governance: where did it come from, what does it mean? *Journal of the Royal Society of Medicine*, 98(11): 496–502.

Shea M (2020). Forty years of the four principles: enduring themes from Beauchamp and Childress. *Journal of Medicine and Philosophy*, 45(4–5): 387–395.

Short TH (1999). Media Highlights. *College Mathematics Journal*, 30(5): 413.

Shuster E (1997). Fifty years later: the significance of the Nuremberg Code. *New England Journal of Medicine*, 332(20): 1436–1440.

SIGN (2016). *Acute Coronary Syndrome Guidance. SIGN 148*. Edinburgh: Healthcare Improvement Scotland.

Silverman D (2000). *Doing Qualitative Research: A Practical Guide*. Thousand Oaks: Sage.

Slade SC, Philip K and Morris ME (2018). Frameworks for embedding a research culture in allied health practice: a rapid review. *Health Research Policy and Systems*, 16(1): article 29.

Slowther A, Boynton P and Shaw S (2006). Research governance: ethical issues. *Journal of the Royal Society of Medicine*, 99(2): 65–72.

Smith PLT (2021). *Decolonizing Methodologies: Research and Indigenous Peoples*, 3rd edn. London: Bloomsbury.

Snooks HA et al. (1996). The costs and benefits of helicopter emergency ambulance services in England and Wales. *Journal of Public Health*, 18(1): 67–77.

Snooks HA et al. (2017). Paramedic assessment of older adults after falls, including community care referral pathway: cluster randomized trial. *Annals of Emergency Medicine*, 70(4): 495–505.

Stake RE (2006). *Multiple Case Study Analysis*. New York: Guilford.

Standing M (2008). Clinical judgement and decision-making in nursing – nine modes of practice in a revised cognitive continuum. *Journal of Advanced Nursing*, 62(1): 124–134.

Starks H and Brown Trinidad S (2007). Choose your method: a comparison of phenomenology, discourse analysis, and grounded theory. *Qualitative Health Research*, 17(10): 1372–1380.

Statista (2024). *Most popular social networks worldwide as of January 2024, ranked by number of monthly active users*. Available at: www.statista.com/statistics/272014/global-social-networks-ranked-by-number-of-users/

Stevelink SAM et al. (2020). The mental health of emergency services personnel in the UK Biobank: a comparison with the working population. *European Journal of Psychotraumatology*, 11(1): 1799477.

Stiell IG et al. (2003). The Canadian C-spine rule versus the NEXUS low-risk criteria in patients with trauma. *New England Journal of Medicine*, 349(26): 2510–2518.

Strauss AL and Corbin JM (1990). *Basics of Qualitative Research: Techniques and Procedures for Developing Grounded Theory*. London: Sage.

Sullivan-Bolyai S, Bova C and Harper D (2005). Developing and refining interventions in persons with health disparities: the use of qualitative description. *Nursing Outlook*, 53(3): 127–133.

Swanson JA, Schmitz D and Chung KC (2010). How to practice evidence-based medicine. *Plastic and Reconstructive Surgery*, 126(1): 286–294.

References

Tanious R and Onghena P (2019). Randomized single-case experimental designs in healthcare research: what, why, and how? *Healthcare*, 7(4): 143.

Tashakkori A and Teddlie C (2010). *Sage Handbook of Mixed Methods in Social and Behavioral Research*. Thousand Oaks: Sage.

Tavares W, Bowles R and Donelon B (2016). Informing a Canadian paramedic profile: framing concepts, roles and crosscutting themes. *BMC Health Services Research*, 16(1): 477.

Taylor B and Francis K (2013). *Qualitative Research in the Health Sciences: Methodologies, Methods and Processes*. London: Routledge.

Teddlie C and Tashakkori A (2009). *Foundations of Mixed Methods Research: Integrating Quantitative and Qualitative Approaches in the Social and Behavioral Sciences*. Thousand Oaks: Sage.

Tedlock B (2000). Ethnography and ethnographic representation. In: Denzin N and Lincoln Y (eds) *Handbook of Qualitative Research*. Thousand Oaks: Sage, pp. 455–486.

Teherani A et al. (2015). Choosing a qualitative research approach. *Journal of Graduate Medical Education*, 7(4): 669–670.

Thorlund K et al. (2020). Synthetic and external controls in clinical trials – a primer for researchers. *Clinical Epidemiology*, 12: 457–467.

Thorne S, Kirkham SR and MacDonald-Emes J (1997). Interpretive description: a noncategorical qualitative alternative for developing nursing knowledge. *Research in Nursing and Health*, 20(2): 169–177.

Thorne SE (2008). *Interpretive Description*. Walnut Creek: Left Coast Press.

Timmermans S and Tavory I (2012). Theory construction in qualitative research: from grounded theory to abductive analysis. *Sociological Theory*, 30(3): 167–186.

Tong A, Sainsbury P and Craig J (2007). Consolidated criteria for reporting qualitative research (COREQ): a 32-item checklist for interviews and focus groups. *International Journal for Quality in Health Care*, 19(6): 349–357.

Tricco AC et al. (2015). A scoping review of rapid review methods. *BMC Medicine*, 13(1): 1–15.

Tricco AC et al. (2018). PRISMA Extension for Scoping Reviews (PRISMA-ScR): checklist and explanation. *Annals of Internal Medicine*, 169(7): 467–473.

Tuffour I (2017). A critical overview of interpretative phenomenological analysis: a contemporary qualitative research approach. *Journal of Healthcare Communications*, 2(4): 52.

Uman LS (2011). Systematic reviews and meta-analyses. *Journal of the Canadian Academy of Child and Adolescent Psychiatry*, 20(1): 57.

University of Hertfordshire (2021). *About us*. Available at: www.herts.ac.uk/about-us/the-history-of-our-university

Varpio L et al. (2020). The distinctions between theory, theoretical framework, and conceptual framework. *Academic Medicine*, 95(7): 989–994.

Vassar M and Matthew H (2013). The retrospective chart review: important methodological considerations. *Journal of Educational Evaluation for Health Professions*, 10: 12.

von Koskull C (2020). Increasing rigor and relevance in service research through ethnography. *Journal of Services Marketing*, 34(1): 74–77.

von Kries R et al. (1999). Breast feeding and obesity: cross sectional study. *BMJ*, 319(7203): 147–150.

Wei Lam SS et al. (2013). Reducing ambulance response times using discrete event simulation. *Prehospital Emergency Care*, 18(2): 207–216.

West M and Farr JL (1990). *Innovation and Creativity at Work: Psychological and Organizational Strategies*. Hoboken: John Wiley and Sons.

West M, Eckert R, Collins B and Chowla R (2017). *Caring to Change: How Compassionate Leadership can Stimulate Innovation in Healthcare*. London: King's Fund.

References

White P (2017). *Developing Research Questions*, 2nd edn. Basingstoke: Palgrave.

Whitley GA (2020). Pre-hospital pain management in children: a mixed methods study. Unpublished PhD thesis, University of Lincoln. https://doi.org/10.24385/LINCOLN.24326401.V1

Whitley GA and Wilson C (2022). Paramedics... why do research? *British Paramedic Journal*, 7(1): 1–2.

Whitley GA et al. (2019). The complexity of pain management in children. *Journal of Paramedic Practice*, 11(11): 466–468.

Whitley GA et al. (2020a). Predictors of effective management of acute pain in children within a UK ambulance service: a cross-sectional study. *American Journal of Emergency Medicine*, 38(7): 1424–1430.

Whitley GA et al. (2020b). Mixed methods in prehospital research: understanding complex clinical problems. *British Paramedic Journal*, 5(3): 44–51.

Whitley GA et al. (2021a). The predictors, barriers and facilitators to effective management of acute pain in children by emergency medical services: a systematic mixed studies review. *Journal of Child Health Care*, 25(3): 481–503.

Whitley GA et al. (2021b). Ambulance clinician perspectives of disparity in prehospital child pain management: a mixed methods study. *Health Science Reports*, 4(2): e261.

Wilkinson-Stokes M (2021). Right ventricular myocardial infarction and adverse events from nitrates: a narrative review. *Australasian Journal of Paramedicine*, 18: 1–8.

Williams J (2012). Qualitative research in paramedic practice; an overview. In: Griffiths P and Mooney G (eds) *The Paramedic's Guide to Research: An Introduction*. New York: McGraw Hill, pp. 73–89.

Wilson C et al. (2022a). The role of feedback in emergency ambulance services: a qualitative interview study. *BMC Health Services Research*, 22(1): 296.

Wilson C, Janes G and Williams J (2022b). Identity, positionality and reflexivity – relevance and application to research paramedics. *British Paramedic Journal*, 7(2): 43–49.

Wilson P and Petticrew M (2008). Why promote the findings of single research studies? *BMJ*, 336(7646): 722.

Wiltshire G (2018). A case for critical realism in the pursuit of interdisciplinarity and impact. *Qualitative Research in Sport, Exercise and Health*, 10(5): 525–542.

Wood K (2012). Integrating clinical research into paramedic practice: current trends and influences. *Journal of Paramedic Practice*, 4(9): 502–508.

Woodall J et al. (2007). Impact of advanced cardiac life support-skilled paramedics on survival from out-of-hospital cardiac arrest in a statewide emergency medical service. *Emergency Medicine Journal*, 24(2): 134–138.

World Health Organization (2012). *Knowledge Translation Framework for Age and Health*. Geneva: World Health Organization.

World Health Organization (2021a). *Cardiovascular Diseases (CVDs) Fact Sheet*. Available at: https://www.who.int/news-room/fact-sheets/detail/cardiovascular-diseases-(cvds)

World Health Organization (2021b). *Knowledge translation mechanisms to translate evidence into public health policy in emergencies: Rapid response*. Available at: https://www.who.int/europe/publications/i/item/WHO-EURO--2021-2719-42477-58997

World Medical Association (2024). *Declaration of Helsinki*. Available at: www.wma.net/policies-post/wma-declaration-of-helsinki-ethical-principles-for-medical-research-involving-human-subjects/

Worster A and Haines T (2004). Advanced statistics: understanding medical record review (MRR) studies. *Academic Emergency Medicine*, 11(2): 187–192.

Xie F et al. (2021). Economic analysis of mobile integrated health care delivered by emergency medical services paramedic teams. *JAMA Network Open*, 4(2): 210055.

Yin RK (2014). *Case Study Research Design and Methods*. Thousand Oaks: Sage.

Index

A

Abductive approach, 175–176
Absolute risk, 128
Abstract screening, 62–63
Academic journals, 238–239
Action research, 147–148
AIRWAYS-2 trial, 133, 237
Alternative hypothesis, 131–132
Ambulance service research, 211, 259
Anonymity, 109, 114, 163
ANOVA, 133–134
Approval
    ethical, 209–211
    Health Research Authority (HRA), 210
Assessment, 217–218
Assumption-free tests. See Non-parametric tests
Attrition bias, 119
Autonomy, 120, 165, 204–205, 219
Axiology, 44, 199

B

Bayesian methods, 93
Beneficence, 120, 205
Bias, 118–119
    confirmation, 118
    researcher, 118
    selection, 119
    self-reporting, 118
Big data, 40
Boolean operators, 62
Budget, 12, 23–24, 35, 74, 211, 260–261

C

CAG. See Confidentiality Advisory Group
Capability assessment, 211
Capacity assessment, 211
CAQDAS. See Computer-aided qualitative data analysis software
Case–control studies, 103
Case series
    observational design, 84–85
Case study
    data collection, 153
    definition of, 151–152
    management of data, 153
    sampling strategy, 152–153
    strategies, 153
    type of, 154
    uses, 152
Chi-square, 134
Clinical audit
    definition of, 30
    history of, 31
Clinical trials of investigational medicinal products (CTIMP), 120, 212
Cluster randomised designs, 97–98
Cochrane Collaboration, 25, 58
Cochrane Library, 10, 20
Cohort studies, 90–91, 104–105
Computer-aided qualitative data analysis software (CAQDAS), 183–184
Conceptual frameworks, 52
Confidence interval (CI), 131
Confidentiality Advisory Group (CAG), 210, 214
Confounding, 119

Index

Consequentialist, 204
Content analysis, 177–178
Continuing professional development (CPD), 10
Continuous data, 124, 127
Control group, 84, 92–93, 117–118
Convergent design, 194–195
Conversation analysis, 182
Correlational analysis, 134–135
Cost-benefit analysis, 228
Cost-effectiveness analysis, 225–226
Cost-utility analysis, 226
Critical appraisal, 65–66
CTIMP. *See* Clinical trials of investigational medicinal products

D

Data analysis, 183–186
Data collection. *See* Experimental studies; Prospective data collection; Retrospective data collection
   ROSIER tool, 113
   sources of observational data, 105
   surveys
      closed questions, 108
      design of, 107–108
      electronic survey, 109
      open-ended questions, 108–109
      purposes of, 105–106
   tools of, 110–112
Data extraction, 64–65, 102–103, 104
Decision tree, 230
Declaration of Helsinki, 206
Deferred consent, 209
Deontology, 204
Dependent variable, 116–117
DES. *See* Discrete event simulation
Descriptive observational designs, 84–85
Descriptive statistics, 125–126
Discourse analysis, 183
Discrete event simulation (DES), 231
Dissemination, 26, 216, 234–244, 252
Documentary research, 167–169
Doxology, 44

E

EBP. *See* Evidence-based practice
Economic evaluation, 225–228
Embedded design, 197–198

Epidemiological studies, 127
Epistemology, 45–46
Ethical considerations, 109, 120, 251
Ethnography, 149–151
Evidence-based practice (EBP), 9–17
Externally-controlled experimental, 92–93
Experimental designs, 95–99, 116

F

Feasibility, 79, 256
Feedback-seeking behaviour (FSB), 176
Focus groups, 158–161
Framework analysis, 178–179
Funding applications, 23

G

Generic qualitative research, 142–144
Good Clinical Practice (GCP), 120, 206
Grant application, 256
Grounded theory, 180–181

H

Hawthorne effect, 165–166
Hazard ratio, 129–130
HCPC. *See* Health and Care Professions Council
Health and Care Professions Council (HCPC), 11
Health economics, 221–232
Healthcare systems, 223
Health research authority (HRA), 209–210
Hermeneutic, 145
HRA. *See* Health research authority
Hypothesis, research, 72–74
Hypothesis testing, 131–132

I

ICH. *See* International Conference on Harmonisation
Individually randomised designs, 96–97, 132–133
Innovation in healthcare, 36–38
Integrated Research Application System (IRAS), 209
International Conference on Harmonisation (ICH), 206
Interpretivism, 50
Interrupted time-series, 94–95
Interviews, 158–161

Index

IRAS. *See* Integrated Research Application System

J
JBI. *See* Joanna Briggs Institute
Joanna Briggs Institute (JBI), 66
Joint Royal Colleges Ambulance Liaison Committee (JRCALC), 13
    guidelines, 14–16
Journals, academic, 238–239
JRCALC. *See* Joint Royal Colleges Ambulance Liaison Committee

K
Knowledge translation
    definition of, 14
    Ottawa model, 15

L
Literature in research, 55–67
Literature review, 57–58
Literature search, 20, 60

M
Markov models, 230–231
Mean, 126
Measures of central tendency, 126
Median, 126
Medical Subject Headings (MeSH), 60
Medicines for Human Use (Clinical Trials) (Amendment) (EU Exit), 206
MeSH. *See* Medical Subject Headings
Methodology, 46
Mixed methods research, 189–200
Mode, 126
Modelling, 229–232
Multi-methods, 190
Multivariate regression analysis, 135–136

N
Narrative interview, 159
Narrative literature review, 57–58
NARSG. *See* National Ambulance Research Steering Group
National Ambulance Research Steering Group (NARSG), 15
National Institute for Health and Care Excellence (NICE), 31, 228, 232
National Institute for Health and Care Research (NIHR), 23, 255, 266
Negative predictive value, 138–139
Networking, 179, 268–269
NICE. *See* National Institute for Health and Care Excellence
NIHR. *See* National Institute for Health and Care Research
Non-normal distribution, 124–125
Non-parametric tests, 132, 134
Non-probability sampling, 87, 89
Non-randomised experimental, 91–92
Normal distribution, 124, 132
Null hypothesis, 131–132
Nuremberg Code, 206

O
Observational design, 84–91
Observational study, 164–166
Observer bias, 166
Ontology, 44–45

P
Paradigm, 199–200
PARAMEDIC2 trial, 102, 106–107, 132, 146
Paramedic Acute Stroke Treatment Assessment (PASTA), 197
Paramedic research
    definition of, 4–7
PASTA. *See* Paramedic Acute Stroke Treatment Assessment
Patient and public involvement and engagement (PPIE) research, 214–219
PDSA. *See* Plan, Do, Study, Act
Peer review, 10, 185–186
Plan, Do, Study, Act (PDSA), 31, 34
Population, Intervention, Comparator and Outcome (PICo), 59–62, 75–78
positive predictive value (PPV), 138–139
Preferred Reporting Items for Systematic reviews and Meta-Analyses (PRISMA), 56, 63–64, 67
Prehospital care research, 223–224
pre-test post-test, paired, 94–95
PRISMA. *See* Preferred Reporting Items for Systematic reviews and Meta-Analyses (PRISMA)

297

Index

Probability sampling, 86–87, 89
Prospective data collection, 104
PROSPERO, 20, 56, 67
PubMed, 55–56, 60–62
Purposive sampling, 87

Q
QALY. *See* Quality-adjusted life year
QI. *See* Quality improvement
Qualitative data collection, 157–171
Quality-adjusted life year (QALY), 227–228
Quality assessment, 65–66
Quality improvement (QI), 33–35
Quantitative data, 123–140
Quantitative research design, 83–99
Qualitative questionnaire, 162–164
Quasi-experimental designs, 91–95
Quasi-experimental research, 117–118

R
Randomised controlled trial, 95–97
Randomised stepped wedge designs, 98–99
Rapid review, 57–58
RCN. *See* Royal College of Nursing
Recognition of Stroke in the Emergency Room (ROSIER), 112–113
Relative risk, 128
Research aim, 72
Research careers for paramedics
   doctorate, 268
   getting started, 267–268
   longer-term research careers, 269–270
   tips for, 270–272
Research funding, 255–263
Research governance, 211
Research hypothesis, 72–74
Research objectives, 72
Research paramedic, 12
Research problem, 69–74
Research process
   aims, questions, hypotheses and objectives, 21
   analysis, 25
   apply for funding, 23
   choice of study design, 21–22
   dissemination activities, 26
   ethics and governance approvals, 23–24
   identify stakeholders, 21
   practice and policy, 20
   primary data, 24
   research protocol, 22–23
   review of, 20
   secondary data, 24–25
   write-up, 25–26
Research proposal, 245–254
Research question, 21, 69–70, 74–78
Research Support Service (RSS), 257
Retrospective data collection
   approaches, 102–103
   case–control studies, 103
   definition of, 101–102
   overview of, 102
   role of, 103–104
Retrospective record review, 85–86
Rigour, 146, 148, 151, 153, 156
ROSIER. *See* Recognition of Stroke in the Emergency Room
Royal College of Nursing (RCN), 36
RSS. *See* Research Support Service

S
Sample size calculations, 139
Sampling
   convenience, 84, 87, 89
   non-probability, 87, 89
   probability, 86–87, 89
   purposive, 87
Scoping review, 57–58
Search strategy, 60
Selection bias, 119
Sensitivity analysis, 231–232
Sequential design, 191–192
Service evaluation, 35–36
Service users. *See* Patient and public involvement and engagement (PPIE) research
Share research findings
   fundamentals of dissemination
      aim of, 237–238
      engaging in, 234–235
      formal method, 237
      key messages, 235
      target audience, 235–236
      target of, 235
   platforms for dissemination
      academic journals, 238–239

Index

oral presentation, 239–240
podcasts, 243
poster preparation, 241–242
social media, 242–243
Social media, 242–243
SPIDER (Sample, Phenomenon of Interest, Design, Evaluation, Research type), 59, 77
Subjectivism. *See* Interpretivism
Surveys
    closed questions, 108
    design of, 107–108
    electronic survey, 109
    open-ended questions, 108–109
    purposes of, 105–106
Systematic review, 57

T

Tagging, 176–177
Team approach, 185
Thematic analysis, 179–180
Transferability, 46, 121
Transparency, 209

Trial Steering Committee, 24
Triangulation, 151, 191, 194

U

Uncertainty, 222, 231–232

V

Validity
    external, 89, 92, 121–122, 139
    internal, 65, 93, 119, 122
    scientific, 208
Variable
    dependent, 116–118, 134–135
    independent, 88, 116–117, 135

W

WHO. *See* World Health Organization
World Health Organization (WHO), 14
Writing for publication, 268

Y

Young Persons Advisory Group (YPAG), 215
YPAG. *See* Young Persons Advisory Group